A SYSTEMATIC APPROACH
TO THE NURSING CARE PLAN

Second Edition

A SYSTEMATIC APPROACH TO THE NURSING CARE PLAN

MARLENE G. MAYERS, R.N., M.S., F.A.A.N.
Director, Nursing Services
El Camino Hospital
Mountain View, California

Consultant
Health Care Services

 APPLETON-CENTURY-CROFTS/New York

TO MY THREE SONS

78   79   80   81   82 / 10   9   8   7   6   5   4   3   2

Prentice-Hall International, Inc., London
Prentice-Hall of Australia, Pty. Ltd., Sydney
Prentice-Hall of India Private Limited, New Delhi
Prentice-Hall of Japan, Inc., Tokyo
Prentice-Hall of Southeast Asia (Pte.) Ltd., Singapore
Whitehall Books Ltd., Wellington, New Zealand

Library of Congress Cataloging in Publication Data
Mayers, Marlene Glover
  A systematic approach to the nursing care plan

  Bibliography:
  1. Nursing—Planning.   I. Title.   [DNLM: 1. Nursing care.
2. Patient care planning.   WY100.3 M468s]
RT42.M247   1978   610.73   78-4496
ISBN 0-8385-8790-9

Text design: Kristin Herzog

PRINTED IN THE UNITED STATES OF AMERICA

Contents

Preface

During the five years since the first edition of this book was written, nursing has taken tremendous strides toward formalizing and actualizing the nursing process. Care planning, in a variety of forms, has become an expected part of a professional nurse's practice. There is clear recognition of the crucial role that nursing plays in generating, processing, and transmitting tremendous amounts of patient care information among nurses, between disciplines, and with patients.

The care-planning component of the nursing process has become the foundation for other quality assurance processes: retrospective audit, concurrent audit, and multidisciplinary care planning. Care planning has also evoked and been affected by a trend toward formulating theoretical frameworks for nursing practice and has influenced beginning efforts toward developing a taxonomy of nursing diagnoses. This edition of *A Systematic Approach to the Nursing Care Plan* describes and incorporates these concepts.

Chapter 1 provides an overview of contemporary professional nursing practice. It defines the nursing process and its relationship to care planning in nursing service and in nursing education. This chapter also introduces the subject of conceptual frameworks for nursing practice.

Chapters 2 through 6 explain and illustrate the care-planning process. Numerous new examples have been added and outcome criteria have been revised and clarified throughout. Patient outcome charting is explained and illustrated in detail.

Chapter 7 explains how standard care plans provide not only functional day-to-day care-planning information but also shows how these standard protocols are, in fact, the clinical standards that are required by accrediting bodies and that are necessary for formulating the criteria for quality evaluation processes.

Chapters 8 and 9 carefully illustrate how standard and individualized plans can be adapted to meet patient needs in a variety of service settings. And Chapter 10 illustrates the differences necessary to the learner in educational settings. Included also is a suggested teaching/learning sequence for a nursing education curriculum. Specific guides are illustrated and explained. Audiovisual, graphic, autotutorial, modular, and other teaching methods are discussed and sources for teaching aids are included.

Chapter 11 enlarges upon the entire issue of the data base. It explains and illustrates data gathering in relation to conceptual frameworks and empirical practice. Numerous examples of nursing histories and assessment guides are provided.

Chapter 12 describes well-tested strategies for teaching and implementing the nursing process in the service setting. This chapter also shows how care-planning adaptations can be made in forms, terminology, and computer applications.

Chapter 13 ties care planning into the quality assurance cycle by showing the relationships between care plans, retrospective audit criteria (process and outcome), concurrent care criteria, and the remedial action/reevaluation components of quality assurance. This chapter also develops the "accountability" element of quality assurance and describes accountability in its many dimensions and processes.

It is with pleasure and great pride in the nursing profession that I have written this edition of *A Systematic Approach to the Nursing Care Plan*, for it reflects substantive changes in the state of the art of nursing practice—changes that were only amorphous concepts five years ago. I look forward with excitement and confidence to the patient care innovations that nurses will create during the next five years.

Acknowledgments

Thousands of nurses in the United States and Canada have provided suggestions and refinements and have greatly influenced my thinking. I wish I could mention them all by name. I wish especially to acknowledge the assistance, criticism, and support of Annita Watson, Sandra Hall, Jessie Mantle, Margo Cook, Geni Hushower, Joan Bsharah, Debbie Bietz, Barbara Sherer, Diane Gamberg, Nancy Smith, Helen Scott, and Ann Huntsman.

Special appreciation is extended to the nursing staff of El Camino Hospital who have patiently and creatively pioneered new ways to make care planning a real benefit to patients and to make the nursing process an integral part of professional nursing practice.

Marlene Glover Mayers

1

Care Planning: An Integral Part of Professional Nursing Practice

PROFESSIONAL NURSING PRACTICE

Patient care planning involves systematically assessing and identifying a patient's problems, setting objectives, establishing interventions, and evaluating results. Planning is universally employed to assure that, in complex situations, future events and results will be those that are intended. Planning is designed to prevent unpleasant surprises. Whether one plans a trip, a budget, a social event, or a patient's care, a sequence of decisions and actions is followed to make sure that all will be well. Making sure means controlling. Control requires responsibility, and responsibility for purposeful, planned patient care is one requirement of professional nursing practice. Today's health care world is replete with changing variables, both adding to and detracting from the fulfillment of nursing's responsibility for the coordination of purposeful, effective nursing care.

Definitions of nursing practice are continually reviewed by nurses themselves. Should nurses officially expand their roles to assume many functions previously the prerogative of physicians? Should nurses relinquish certain traditional nursing prerogatives to other health workers? Should nursing operate from a generally agreed-upon theory of illness-wellness? If so, which one? Should nurses legitimately be caregivers as well as care managers? Is nursing an independent discipline? Should nursing allow itself many definitions of practice depending upon the needs of clients or patients?

Consumers are scrutinizing nursing. National legislative groups see nursing as a huge health care resource that is virtually untapped in terms of its potential for lower cost and higher quality care. Other groups are looking to nursing for leadership in planning for more valid licensure and accreditation methods, for enhanced quality monitoring systems, and for more precise information about health care needs. Individual patients look to their nurses for support, comfort, safety, information, and sophisticated technical care.

Colleagues in the health professions see nursing as either a strong ally or a formidable foe when efforts for change must be set in motion. The large numbers of nurses and their powerful formal and informal positions in the health care industry place nursing in a position of great responsibility. This responsibility requires strong leadership to mold and guide the giant health care industry toward relevant, humanized, technically sophisticated, cost-effective services. Whether a nurse is concerned with one patient, a caseload of patients, a hospital full of patients, or a community of consumers, the leadership responsibility for patient centeredness and for purposeful, defensible decisions is inherent in the role of the professional nurse.

Within the contexts of scrutiny, change, and high expectations, the professional nurse utilizes the principles of the scientific method in the form of systematic problem solving and planning in order to assure herself and her patients that future events and results will be according to plan.

WELLNESS-ILLNESS THEORIES

There are many definitions of wellness. Most theoretical frameworks for nursing include statements of philosophy incorporating definitions of wellness. Most theories and definitions reflect either a developmental or a systems model as a framework for understanding wellness or illness. Maslow's well-known hierarchy of needs is one example of a developmental theory.[1] Erickson's stages of life is another.[2]

Rogers' assumptions,[3] basic to her theory of nursing, imply that wellness is a feeling of wholeness and uniqueness: a state of homeodynamic balance of energy requirements and energy demands, a continually evolving direction of growth, a sense of predictability, pattern, and organization of life, as well as a sense of satisfaction with one's ability to conceptualize, think, imagine, communicate, and experience sensations and feelings.

A total person definition of wellness can be derived from the Newman model.[4] The assumptions of this model lead one to see wellness as a dynamic composite of physical, psychologic, sociocultural, and developmental balance that is flexible yet retains an unbroken ability to resist disequilibrium.

Sister Callista Roy's adaptation model implies that wellness is positive, nonexhausting responses to stimuli that affect physiologic needs, self-concept, role function, and interdependence.

Another definition of wellness is derived from Loma Linda University's wholeness model.[5] Wellness, in this context, is seen to be a sense of harmony and balance between an individual and several concentric layers of his internal and external environment. A well person feels a high degree of physical, mental, social, and spiritual integrity. He is one who uses existing potentials and abilities to the fullest and prepares for the future.

Within the context of patient care planning, the functional use of a theory, model, or definition of wellness is crucial. Problems are identified when there are substantial variances from states of wellness. Thus, problem definition relies upon either a formal or an intuitive definition of wellness. Formal, generally accepted definitions are helpful. They provide mutually understood analytic and evaluative reference points for many professionals who may be supporting or critiquing a plan of care.

Very broadly stated, nursing's purpose is to deliberately intervene where there is variance from wellness. Nursing's interventions are purposive and are designed to produce positive change. The changes or results should be explained or measured according to an accepted model, theory, or definition of wellness.

To accomplish nursing's purposes of facilitating change or movement toward the positive end of the wellness–illness continuum, a nurse needs:

A philosophy   A set of beliefs about human beings: their needs, motivations, interactions, defense mechanisms, adaptation methods, stages of growth and development.

An operational model   A set of theories about and definitions of wellness, of illness, and of definable stages in between: criteria for data gathering and for making decisions about variances (nursing diagnosis), the goals (corrected variances), the types of interactions required, and valid evaluation methods.

An example of a theoretical framework and its associated operational model is illustrated and explained in Chapter 11.

THE NURSING PROCESS

The technical, behavioral, and intellectual skills of nursing practice are based upon theories and principles from the physical and social sciences. All of these elements are utilized in the nursing process and thus in planning patient care.

Technical Skills

The technical skills of nursing are perhaps the best known. These skills, which range from simple to complex and from supportive to restorative, are critical and basic to the care of many patients. They must be used with intelligence and a high degree of skill and discrimination.

Behavioral Skills

Behavioral skills in nursing refer to skills needed for communication and interpersonal relationships and to coordination and facilitative leadership roles. To intervene effectively in the wellness-illness milieu, a nurse must base her communication and interpersonal methods not upon intuition but upon a sound theoretical base. In her appraisal of a situation, the nurse consciously utilizes an approach that is most likely to be helpful to the patient at that time. In order to be an effective leader, facilitating patient care, she plans her activities and responds to her staff and patients in ways that reflect an understanding of people and how they relate to and work with one another.

Intellectual Skills

The intellectual components of the nursing process may be considered in terms of lateral, vertical, and discriminative thinking.

Lateral Thinking.   Lateral thinking[6] refers to those thought processes that are uniquely concerned with the creation of new ideas. It concerns itself with gathering information and looking at it in new ways or in new configurations. It is thinking that considers new connections, new applications, or possible variations. Lateral thinking is used when a nurse gathers information about a patient and a situation. Once a body of facts is collected, a nurse uses lateral thinking to scan the information and to start developing ideas about the meaning of it. Lateral thinking is most effective when one is willing to consider several possibilities of meaning before finally concluding that a certan one is, in all probability, the actual meaning. Once a series of possible meanings has been abstracted from a collection of facts, the time then comes for problem solving.

Vertical Thinking.   Vertical thinking, or problem solving, is the kind of thought process that is used to define problems based upon the meanings of interpretations made in the lateral thinking phase. Defining and stating a problem, determining the intended solution, developing methods for achieving the solution, and evaluating the effectiveness of those methods is the problem solving, or scientific, process. This is the process that is most commonly taught and utilized in nursing education and nursing service. Both lateral and vertical levels of thinking are essential when a nurse is responsible for assessing and deriving relevant meaning in an unstructured setting.

Discriminative Thinking.   The third major type of thought process is discriminative thinking. In nursing, when problems have been defined, it is necessary to make judgments regarding their relative importance. Some problems must be given higher priority for immediate care or for long-range care. Discrimination must be used to place more emphasis upon some strategies and less upon others.

These three intellectual processes can be developed to function simultaneously. When a nurse has a broad base of understanding relative to her client and his wellness–illness milieu, these thought processes are more likely to result in sound decisions and methodologies for patient care.

In order to make the best use of the technical, behavioral, and intellectual skills, and to combine these with lateral, vertical, and discriminative thinking, certain decision processes are used. In nursing, these sequential, interrelated steps are referred to as the "nursing process." This process is not unique to nursing. It is used by every professional discipline, occupational group, or human being. It is problem solving, and it is made up of several components: data gathering, problem identification, goal setting, method implementation, and evaluation.

The analagous terms in nursing are, as quoted from Little and

Carnevali,[7] assessment, diagnosis, presciption, implementation, and evaluation. Other terms of similar meaning are used by others. Bailey and Claus[8] define the process as a series of steps:

Step 1. Defining overall needs, purposes, and goals
Step 2. Defining the problem
Step 3. Weighing the constraints versus the capabilities and resources
Step 4. Specifying an approach to solving the problem
Step 5. Stating decision objectives and performance criteria
Step 6. Generating alternative solutions
Step 7. Analyzing options
Step 8. Choosing best options
Step 9. Controlling and implementing decision
Step 10. Evaluating effectiveness of decision

For the purpose of patient care planning in a service setting, this author suggests the following steps:

Gathering data
Identifying problems (variances from expected states of wellness)
Defining expected outcomes (ongoing evaluation criteria)
Prescribing best solutions (after considering options, constraints, and resources)
Evaluating at periodic and endpoint intervals

Whatever the author, whatever the nursing specialty, whatever the problem situation, the nursing process is well summarized by Yura and Walsh[9] as "an orderly, systematic manner of determining the client's problems, making plans to solve them, initiating the plan or assigning others to implement it, and evaluating the extent to which the plan was effective in resolving the problem identified."

CARE PLANNING IN SERVICE SETTINGS

Since the beginnings of organized nursing practice, patient care planning has been an integral, if not explicit, part of the delivery of care. As nursing has developed, there has been increasing concern for planning intervention strategies that will move a patient from one level of wellness to a higher one. This concern and planning have generally been an informal but basic part of nursing practice.

Nursing service professionals are formalizing and making more explicit the planning elements of nursing practice. Nursing care plans are a required part of the health team's information about patients—what needs to be done and why. Nurses are setting up policies, protocols, forms, performance evaluation tools, and audit procedures to enhance and to monitor the care planning system. Standards of care for specific patient populations are being formulated. Nurses are assessing and formulating statements of patient problems which are known as "nursing diagnoses." A large number of nurses are collaborating to formulate a framework for an official nursing nomenclature and lists of nursing diagnoses. All of this effort is designed to make explicit the functions and responsibilities of nursing so that patients will continuously receive well-considered, high-quality care.

In nursing service, implementation of the concept of nursing care planning varies from agency to agency and from nursing unit to nursing unit. As in nursing education, the principle of problem solving as the basis for nursing care planning is implicit, if not explicit. Various reminder systems are used to maximize the possibility that comprehensive patient care planning will occur.

Although many nursing service agencies are making significant progress toward the implementation of a workable and useful system for nursing care planning, many agencies find care planning implementation to be a major problem. Some of the reasons cited as causes for the difficulty relate to the pressures of short staffing with insufficient time to devote to writing care plans, to nursing staffs who are unclear about what nursing care plans are and how to use them, and to recent graduates who are frustrated in their attempts to implement the educational concept of nursing care planning in the service setting.

There are four additional basic underlying reasons for the difficulty:

1. A lack of general understanding among nursing educators and nursing services that there is and should be a significant difference between a detailed, time-consuming educational tool for learning and a functional, efficient service tool for nursing care delivery
2. Unclear definitions in the service setting regarding the meaning and purpose of a nursing care plan and ambiguity regarding the agency's definition of patient problems and needs or objectives and approaches
3. A lack of clear delegation of responsibility to certain nursing personnel who are to be responsible for initiating and updating care plans
4. An absence of a clear, well-defined rationale for ruling in and

ruling out the problems and items that should appear on a nursing care plan.

When all these basic problems are operative in a given nursing service setting it is not surprising that the concept of patient care planning causes great difficulty and frustration for both nursing service staff and administration.

Nursing care planning has been seen by federal and state governing and review agencies, as well as by nursing itself, to be a most basic requirement for the subsequent evaluation of nursing success or failure. Care planning is so important that it has become a universal requirement for licensing and accreditation of nursing service agencies.

Because of these factors and the intrinsic professional pressures occurring during the past few years, nearly all nursing service agencies have incorporated some system referred to as "nursing care planning." Upon closer examination, however, one finds much disparity and lack of consensus about implementing nursing care planning at the operational level. Much has been said and written about the need to establish objectives and to design nursing interventions. Yet, on the operational level, these concepts seem difficult to implement. Most care plan formats are designed to summarize or to abstract certain patient data. But a collection of data cannot be called a plan. Many nursing services that attempt to plan for care find that in reality they are only scheduling physicians' orders.

Many agencies have become more sophisticated. They have developed a care plan format that guides nurses to state patients' problems or needs and to follow that statement with nursing approaches. In actual practice, however, nurses are left with the forms but without specific instructions about using them. Each nurse has her own perception of needs or problems, and many questions arise: Which needs should she write? All persons have many needs. Must all of these be written on each patient's care plan? If not, on what basis does she decide which ones to include and which ones to omit? Are needs and problems the same? How does she write an objective? How is a nursing approach different from a doctor's order? Must the nurse copy all the doctor's orders under the "nursing approach" column? Does anyone really read and systematically act upon anything written on the care plan? Is the care plan just a suggestion box? Must every patient have at least one problem or need identified? Is the time spent writing a care plan really worthwhile, or is it just an exercise for the record? These questions are relevant and they deserve to be answered.

CARE PLANNING IN EDUCATIONAL SETTINGS

In nursing education, nursing care plans are among the basic tools by which students learn to identify patient problems and to plan in a scientific and systematic way for individualized patient care. Although specific formats vary from instructor to instructor and from student to student, the principle underlying the intellectual process in the educational setting is that of problem solving. Students generally make comprehensive theoretical and actual patient assessments, and they specify and define a complete range of physical, emotional, and sociologic problems for each assigned patient. The identification of problems or needs usually is followed by a statement of the cause, or etiology, of each problem identified and a statement of the objectives or nursing actions required for solving the problem. Inherent also in the educational concept of nursing care planning is a statement of the rationale for the nursing action taken. This statement reinforces for the student the basic principles of care as those principles relate to the identified problems or needs. Very frequently there is also included an evaluative statement. The evaluative statement clarifies how successful or unsuccessful the nursing actions are and the reasons for success or failure, with recommendations for necessary changes in nursing actions. Each nursing care plan developed in the present educational setting is a comprehensive and detailed analysis of the patient as well as a plan for his care.

This concept of nursing care planning is an integral part of the educational experience of almost every student of nursing today, regardless of the type of program. Diploma, Associate of Arts degree, and Baccalaureate degree programs all utilize some variation of the problem-solving approach in the teaching–learning process. As a result, most students graduate and become practitioners with the educational model of nursing care planning as their frame of reference for service and care delivery. Although in nursing service and nursing education the basic intellectual process, that is, problem solving, is the same, the objectives sought are different. With different objectives, different strategies or techniques must be employed.

Care planning as an educational tool is valid and useful, but it is not immediately transferable to a care delivery or service setting. The primary purpose of an educational tool is to provide a medium for learning about patients' health problems and the rationales for solving them. The primary purpose of a care delivery tool is to communicate relevant data rapidly and efficiently to other team members regarding the required strategies for care which contribute to overall patient objectives. The differences must be recognized.

SUMMARY

Patient care planning has long been an implicit, if not explicit, part of nursing practice. Whether a plan is written or not, nurses have always had one in mind as they cared for patients. However, with increasing sophistication among all health care disciplines regarding the evaluation of the effectiveness of care plans and with increasing pressures from government agencies, fiscal intermediaries, and consumers, it has become essential to become explicit. It is now mandatory for the health professions to assume leadership in developing viable strategies for care evaluation as it relates to consumer benefits, cost accounting, program planning, service, and role responsibilities.

Nursing as a profession is feeling these external pressures. It is also reacting to internal pressures—pressures relating to burgeoning client populations, rapidly changing roles and responsibilities, new classifications of nursing practitioners, and so forth. Nursing also feels the need to define its own purposes and objectives and to account for its successes and failures in the delivery of nursing care. The concept of care planning is one way to meet this responsibility.

One current element of confusion concerning nursing care planning is caused by the significant differences of purpose between educational and service care plans without a clear recognition that these differences exist. The primary purpose of an educational tool is to provide a medium for learning about a patient's health problems and to discover the rationale for solving them. The primary purpose of a care delivery tool is to communicate relevant data rapidly and efficiently to other team members. The differences are important and must be recognized if the confusion is to be resolved.

Nursing service agencies have met many obstacles in their attempts to implement nursing care planning—obstacles related to (1) lack of general understanding of the differences between an educational care plan and a delivery of service care plan; (2) unclear definitions regarding what is meant by a care plan and its purposes—ambiguity regarding the agency's definitions of problems, objectives, and approaches; (3) a lack of clear delegation of responsibility for care planning; (4) an absence of a clear, well-defined rationale for deciding which problems to enter on a care plan.

These and other problems must be solved. The system of care planning described in this volume is one possible solution. It deals specifically and in a systematic way with overall goals, patients' problems, interim goals (and deadlines), and nursing actions.

Within this system's frame of reference, a nursing care plan is an abstract of data regarding a specific patient. The data are organized in a concise and systematic manner. They facilitate overall medical and nursing goals, and they clearly communicate the nature of the patient's problems and the nature of the related medical and nursing orders.

REFERENCES

1. Maslow A: Toward a Psychology of Being. Princeton, Nostrand, 1962
2. Erikson E: Childhood and Society, New York, Norton, 1950, pp 86-320
3. Rogers M: An Introduction to the Theoretical Basis of Nursing. Philadelphia, Davis, 1970, p 3
4. Neuman B, Young RJ: A model for teaching total person approach to patient problems. Nurs Res 21:3, May-June 1972
5. Riehl J: Interaction models. In Riehl J and Roy C (eds): Conceptual Models for Nursing Practice. New York, Appleton-Century-Crofts, 1974, pp 272-273
6. De Bono E: Po: A Device for Successful Thinking. New York, Simon and Schuster, 1972
7. Little D, Carnevali D: Nursing Care Planning. Philadelphia, Lippincott, 1976, p 14
8. Bailey J, Claus K: Decision Making in Nursing. St. Louis, Mosby, 1975
9. Yura H, Walsh M: The Nursing Process. New York. Appleton-Century-Crofts, 1973, p 23

BIBLIOGRAPHY

Bower F: The Process of Planning Nursing Care—A Theoretical Model. St. Louis, Mosby, 1972
Eckelberry G: Comprehensive Nursing Care. New York, Appleton-Century-Crofts, 1971
Johnson M, Davis M, and Bilitch M: Problem-solving in Nursing Practice. Dubuque Iowa, Wm C Brown, 1970
King I: Toward A Theory for Nursing, New York, Wiley, 1971
Kron T: The Management of Patient Care. Philadelphia, Saunders, 1971
Lewis L: Planning Patient Care. Dubuque Iowa, Wm C Brown, 1970
Ryan B: Nursing care plans: A systems approach to developing criteria for planning and evaluation. In J Nurs Admin Editorial Staff (eds): Planning and Evaluating Nursing Care, 2nd ed. Wakefield Mass, Contemporary Publishing, 1976
Saxton D, Hyland P: Planning and Implementing Nursing Intervention. St. Louis, Mosby, 1975
Stevens B: First-line Patient Care Management. Wakefield Mass, Contemporary Publishing, 1975
Watson A, Mayers M: How to Write Nursing Care Plans, Stockton Cal, KP Co Medical Systems, 1976
Yura H, Walsh M: The Nursing Process. New York, Appleton-Century-Crofts, 1973

2

The Patient Care Plan:
Nursing Process in Action

DEFINITION OF A CARE PLAN

A patient care plan is an abstract of data concerning a specific patient organized in a concise and systematic manner. The plan facilitates achievement of the patient's goals. It clearly communicates the nature of the patient's problems and specifies what nursing and medical interventions are planned.

More specifically, a patient care plan contains all the information normally found in flip charts or other systems utilized in most patient care settings. It includes medication, treatment, laboratory, and other orders. It includes the patient's preferences. It also has a section that identifies certain specific unusual patient problems, expected outcomes, and prescribed nursing actions. And, of course, it includes a statement of the physician's purposes and expectations for progress as well as nursing's overall objectives for care.

According to Watson and Mayers[1] a care plan is a written guideline for patient care that is organized in such a way that "anyone can quickly visualize what care is needed and why." Care plan forms can be structured in various ways: Kardex or Rand cards, 8½ by 11 inch clipboard forms, or computer printouts. Size and form are important only insofar as they assist in organizing and writing (1) the patient's problems, (2) what should be done about the problems, and (3) what criteria should be used to evaluate progress toward positive outcomes.

The basic nursing care plan form that is used in this book has three major columns: PROBLEMS, EXPECTED OUTCOMES, and NURSING ORDERS. This three-column form can be adapted in many ways to meet the needs of a specific agency.

Other elements of a total care plan format are discussed and illustrated. They are physician's expectations of course of treatment, nursing criteria for discharge or maintenance, and physician's orders.

An example of the nursing care plan format that is used in this book as the tool for learning is shown in Figure 2-1. Figure 2-2 illustrates a form for summarizing physician's orders and checklist items.

Physician's expectations regarding treatment regimen or course of convalescence: ( ) typical or routine
                                        ( ) atypical or complicated
If atypical or complicated, in what way?

Identifying Information: _____

Diagnosis: _____

Criteria for discharge: _____

Home Care Coordination activities: _____

Other relevant data: _____

Date	Unusual Problems	Expected Outcomes	Dead-lines	Nursing Orders

FIGURE 2-1. Kardex care plan.

Date	Medications	Date	Treatments	Date	Diagnosis Tests

CHECKLIST OF STANDARD AND FREQUENTLY ORDERED CARE—
SURGICAL UNIT

Standard Care Plans

☐ Preoperative
☐ Early postoperative
☐ Late postoperative
☐ Chest approach surgery
☐ Abdominoperineal resection
☐ Amputation, leg
☐ Mastectomy, radical
☐ Tracheostomy
☐ Laryngectomy
☐ Laminectomy
☐ Skin care
☐ Indwelling catheter care
☐ Mouth care
Activity

Hygiene

☐ Bed bath
☐ Tub bath
☐ Shower
☐ With assistance
☐ Self, total
Intake
☐ Intake-output
Diet

Frequently Ordered Items

☐ Oral temperature
☐ Rectal temperature
☐ Pulse, respiration
☐ Blood pressure
☐ Neuro signs
☐ CVP
☐ Sp gr (urine)

☐
☐
☐
☐

Patient Preferences. Miscellaneous Information

FIGURE 2-2. Physician's orders and checklist, a Kardex or Rand form.

ELEMENTS OF A PATIENT CARE PLAN

Effective care planning is facilitated by common definitions and terminology. The following terms and definitions are basic to the care planning method that is described in this book.

Physician's expectations   The physician's statement of his general purpose or his expectations for the patient's current hospitalization or treatment regimen and, in particular, his concerns for any potentials for complications.

Nursing criteria for discharge or maintenance   The nurses' statements of the expected or desired patient outcomes as a result of the current hospitalization or treatment regimen. These criteria (or outcomes) are analogous to long-term objectives.

Physician's orders	Those specific activities delegated to nursing by the physician, including medication, treatment, and the coordination of other patient care services, such as laboratory, radiology, dietetics, and so forth.
Usual problems	The typically expected problems that most patients with a specific diagnosis experience. Usual problems are predictable difficulties or concerns.
Unusual problems	An unexpected or atypical difficulty or concern with which a patient is not coping satisfactorily.
Expected outcomes	A statement of the desired patient behavior or clinical manifestation which will indicate that the problem is resolved, resolving, or prevented. An expected outcome is also a criterion for evaluating the patient's progress.
Nursing orders	Nursing orders are those specific, itemized nursing activities which are designed to solve a problem by a projected point in time. They are nurse-initiated prescriptions for care.
Patient responses	A statement of the patient's actual behavior or clinical situation as compared with the expected outcomes. This type of statement appears only on the patient's progress notes or on nursing notes.
Standard care plan	A protocol (or plan) that is developed and prewritten for patients who are experiencing usual problems. A standard care plan represents nursing's standard of care.

OVERVIEW OF THE PLANNING PROCESS

In this section, each definition is explained and illustrated in greater depth.

Physician's Expectations

The physician usually has goals, purposes, or concerns about his patient, which, when made known, assist nurses to anticipate and to collaborate effectively. This information has been found to be as important to nursing care planning as is the medical diagnosis. When a new patient comes to a nursing service for care, his record already contains certain basic identifying and socioeconomic data as well as the medical diagnosis. Knowledge of these factors is, of course, essential, but it does not answer other questions the nurse is concerned with, such as: "Is this likely to be a typical case, or can we expect complications?" "If complications are likely, what is the doctor's perception of their nature?" "Approximately how long does the physician expect the patient to be under care?" "Does the physician believe the patient will be able to return to his usual way of life, or will it be altered—and if so, in what way?" It is easy to see that answers to these kinds of questions will provide a frame of reference for the nursing diagnosis and can save much time and effort in setting priorities for care.

Underlining the importance of having more information from the physician than just the diagnosis is an example that relates to a relatively common occurrence. Suppose that two patients are admitted to a hospital medical unit, both with a diagnosis of cancer of a certain part of the body. Both patients have had a long series of chemotherapy and radiation. One, however, has not responded well and is rapidly deteriorating. The other is responding, and the metastatic process seems to be allayed. Although both patients may have the same admitting diagnosis, the rationale for nursing care for the two patients will be very different. The patient who has responded well to treatment will generally be cared for in such a way that facilitates his return to the activities of daily life. The other patient, who is deteriorating rapidly and who is very unlikely to ever return to his home, will be cared for in a way that facilitates his comfort and enables him to live his last days in a way most meaningful to him. Unfortunately, too many patients come and go through a nursing service experience without nurses knowing until very late that the patient is dying or that his life style is being significantly altered. Early knowledge of this kind of information can assist a nurse significantly in planning effective and relevant care.

For effective care planning it is recommended, then, that part of the admission information requested from the physician be a statement regarding his expectations of the course of the illness or treatment regimen and whether he believes it will be a typical case or one with certain complications. The responsible nurse needs this information before she can effectively formulate a plan for care.

Nursing Criteria for Discharge or Maintenance

Nursing's statement of the outcomes that are expected as a result of the current hospitalization or treatment regimen should address itself to the overall, or long-range, patient objectives. The term "criteria" refers to statements of measurable patient-centered objectives or expected outcomes. The phrase "discharge or maintenance" refers to the time limit by which the outcomes should be achieved. "Discharge" refers to the time when nursing, or a given nursing service, need no longer bear responsibility for care. In the hospital setting, this normally is the time a patient is discharged. Therefore, the overall expected outcomes consist of statements of expected or intended patient behavior or of expected clinical status at the time of discharge. In other settings, such as in the home or in an extended care facility, nursing will want to maintain a given patient at a given level, although that patient is not likely to be discharged. In these cases, criteria for maintenance are written.

In the case of either discharge or maintenance, it is crucial to state the criteria because they provide the overall or long-range frame of reference against which to measure the success or failure of the total care regimen.

For instance, consider a patient who has been newly diagnosed as a diabetic and is hospitalized. All other factors being within reasonable norms, the care plan might indicate nursing criteria for discharge (expected patient behavior at time of discharge) as follows:

1. Verbalize appropriate understanding of dietary regimen
2. Demonstrate correct urine testing technique and verbalize understanding of meaning of test
3. Demonstrate correct insulin injection and dosage technique
4. Give correct verbal responses to questions regarding insulin shock and diabetic coma
5. Verbalize understanding of physician's plan for follow-up supervision and indicate an ability and willingness to comply

The preceding example itemizes those criteria for discharge that nursing would expect to document as having been accomplished by the patient before relinquishing responsibility for his care. Just as a physician will not discharge a patient from his responsibility if an important laboratory value is still significantly outside normal ranges, so too nursing, as a responsible professional discipline, must know and state criteria for an assessment of normalcy or satisfactory status under the circumstances. Nursing must document the patient's level of compliance before relinquishing responsibility. To do less is to function irresponsibly.

If a hospitalized patient has not met the specified criteria for discharge, one of several actions might be taken. A serious variance from predetermined criteria for discharge should be discussed with the physician to determine whether or not an extension of hospitalization should be made to allow time for meeting the criteria. Another alternative would be for nursing to document a definite referral to a service agency which will undertake to help the patient meet the established criteria. Only when a referral designed to fulfill unattained criteria that have been documented as such on the patient's record is made will the standards for care have been met.

Criteria for discharge serve another purpose. They provide the basis for formulating audit criteria for retrospective chart review. Chapter 15 discusses this concept in detail.

Physicians' Orders

Physicians' orders or plans are those specific activities which nurses or others are willing to have delegated to them. These activities usually include medications, treatments, and coordination of other patient care services. Physician's orders are so well known to nurses that it is unnecessary to elaborate further. The point to be made is that a total system of care planning considers the physician's plans to be a part of the patient's plan for care. It must be remembered, however, that the physician's orders DO NOT constitute the total plan for care. Nursing exercises its responsibility for diagnosing, prescribing, evaluating, and coordinating the patient's total plan of care, which includes the input of physicians and of other disciplines.

Usual Problems

Usual problems are predictable or frequently occurring among most patients with a given diagnosis. The identification and validation of predictable problems within certain diagnoses or situations is the work (empirical and research) that must be done to explicate nursing's body of knowledge. Usual problems have associated expected outcomes and standard nursing orders. This sequence of usual problem, usual expected outcome, and usual nursing orders forms the basis for standard care plans. Standard care plans are the operational versions of standards of clinical nursing care.

Unusual Problems

The unusual problem is one of the critical elements of systematic care planning. An unusual problem is a difficulty or concern that is atypical or not usually expected, or it is one with which a patient is not coping satisfactorily.

When assessing and analyzing the available information about a patient, certain problems emerge as items for special consideration. When reviewing the list of a patient's problems, the nurse will find that certain of the problems are expected and predictable and that the usual or standard medical and nursing care is likely to offer a satisfactory resolution. These expected and predictable difficulties are not considered to be unusual problems.

By this definition, an unusual problem is a difficulty that is not typical and not usually predictable. It is not compatible with satisfactory attainment of overall criteria for discharge. Unusual problems must be specifically handwritten and must be followed by written expected outcomes and nursing orders.

Expected Outcomes

An expected outcome is a statement of the desired patient behavior or clinical status. The expected outcome is another way of saying "objective." It is a short-term criterion that must be met before the criteria for discharge can be achieved. Just as the overall criteria for discharge are statements of intended patient responses or behavior at the time of discharge, the expected outcomes are statements of intended interim patient responses or behavior.

The expected outcome statement follows the statement of the problem. It specifies what behavior or clinical status will represent a correction of the problem. In addition, the expected outcome includes a deadline, since without projected time limits there is no effective way to evaluate the attainment of an objective. If the nurse does not state whether a problem should be corrected in five days, five weeks, or five years, the statement has no real value. The care planning format designed for use in this book includes a space for deadlines.

Nursing Orders

Prescribed nursing actions are those specifically itemized nursing activities that are designed to solve a problem by a projected point in time. The term "prescribed" is used to refer to an activity that is ordered by nurses for nurses. It does not refer to activities ordered or prescribed by a physician. When a nurse orders certain nursing actions, she should write with great specificity, leaving as little as possible to varying interpretations. Nursing orders, just as a physician's orders, must specify all major variables so that there is no question regarding what the physician intends.

The nursing order should say (1) what is to be done (2) under what circumstances, and (3) when. If a nursing order requires special skin care at frequent intervals, it should state what is meant by "special skin care": what areas of the body to include and at what hours of the day or night care it is to be done. Only when nursing orders are explicit are they likely to result in the intended care and the desired outcomes.

Patient Responses

The patient response is his reaction to the prescribed nursing actions. The patient response statement—or patient's status—does not appear on the care plan. It should be recorded in the patient's record either in the nurses' notes or on the progress notes.

The patient's response, when compared with the expected outcomes at the required intervals, provides a basis for measuring progress toward the intended correction of the problem. This comparison provides for an evaluation of an individual patient's situation. It also provides the basic documentation for retrospective audit procedures. Chapter 15 describes retrospective auditing.

Standard Care Plan

A standard care plan is a specific protocol for care that is appropriate for patients who are experiencing the usual or predictable problems associated with a given diagnosis or disease process. It is a prewritten plan of care that can be ordered by a nurse to assist a patient in solving usual, expected problems. Because the standard care plan is predetermined, it need not be written in detail each time it is ordered. It is referred to by title. It directs that all the predetermined nursing actions related to it be used. A standard care plan can also be duplicated and placed in the Kardex or Rand for reference when it is ordered for a patient.

BEING SYSTEMATIC

The elements of care planning just described are accomplished by following a systematic step-by-step process.

1. Observe and interview the patient, and others as necessary, to gather all relevant facts and information
2. Analyze the data and identify all the patient's apparent problems at this time
3. Separate the problems into categories of usual and unusual
4. Prescribe appropriate standard care for the usual problems
5. Write the unusual problems on a specified section of the care plan
6. For each unusual problem write an expected outcome statement, then design the relevant nursing actions
7. Sign or initial all nursing orders
8. See that the nursing orders are implemented into the system of care just as systematically as are physician's orders
9. Reevaluate the patient at appropriate intervals and update the plan of care as needed

Once a nurse has become familiar with the mechanics of this system, it can be used rapidly and effectively. Each patient will have been assessed and a plan of care instituted.

One reason this system is efficient is that it assumes that many patients at a given time are, for all practical purposes, coping satisfactorily with their problems. For these patients, specifically prescribed standard nursing care is appropriate and significant. It is necessary to handwrite only those problems that are unusual or beyond the normal range. Utilizing this unusual-problems concept, the nurse has a way of deciding what specifically to identify and write on a nursing care plan, and she has a rational and valid guide for decision making. It obliges her to write only those items of information specifically relevant to unique or unusual patient problems. This rationale for deciding what to write on a nursing care plan form keeps unnecessary writing to a minimum.

Subsequent chapters deal specifically with the various components of this system of care planning. Specific case examples are provided for demonstrating and illustrating the various aspects of the planning of nursing care. Applications are made for all major areas of nursing services, from acute care settings (operating room, emergency room, acute medical or surgical units), to convalescent and extended care, to home care services.

FORMAT FOR THE CARE PLAN

As a result of testing this system of care planning in various agencies and settings, a format for recording patient care data was designed. The basic design, with minor internal modifications, works well in any service setting.

The format has four major components. They can be placed in any sequence that is the most manageable or logical for a given care unit. The four parts of the total patient care plan are:

1. Physician's expectations of course of treatment and nursing's criteria for discharge (overall planning information)
2. Medications, treatments, and diagnostic tests
3. Checklist of standard and frequently ordered care
4. Unusual problems

Each of the four components of the total patient care plan is briefly described and illustrated below.

Overall Planning Information

This part of the care plan devotes itself primarily to a statement of the physician's expectations regarding the course of the treatment regimen and nursing's criteria for discharge. It sets the background or frame of reference for the remainder of the plan. Thus, it is most valuable if placed first in the flip chart or at the top of a series of pages in a notebook, depending upon the type of medium used in the agency.

In addition to the physician's and nurse's statements, this section of the care plan contains basic identifying information, such as name, room number or address, age, sex, religion, and so forth. This information can be spaced and varied to meet the needs of the agency or unit.

Included also is the diagnosis, both primary and secondary diagnoses if at all possible. This must be updated if the diagnosis changes, if surgery is done, or if anything happens to alter the first diagnostic impressions.

A further item in this section of the care plan is a space for noting home care coordination activities. If the home care coordinator has been called into the case, or if a referral is made to another home care agency, it is noted in this space.

A final portion of this section is devoted to space for writing any other relevant data, such as important socioeconomic or cultural information, visitor's schedules that are different from the ordinary, overnight or evening leave schedules, and so forth. This part of the care plan is shown below. Figure 2.1 also illustrates this part of the care plan form.

Overall Planning Information

Physician's expectations regarding treatment regimen or course of convalescence: ( ) typical or routine
( ) atypical or complicated
If atypical or complicated, in what way?
_____
_____

Identifying Information: _____
_____
_____
Diagnosis: _____
_____
_____
_____

Nursing's criteria for discharge or maintenance (overall expected outcomes): _____
_____
_____
_____

Home Care Coordination activities: _____

Other relevant data: _____
_____
_____

Medications, Treatments, and Diagnostic Tests

This part of the total patient care plan is familiar to most nurses. On it are copied the current physician's orders for medications, for special treatments and procedures, and for laboratory work. This form is constantly updated to provide a current abstract of the physician's orders. It is part of the total plan for care shown below. Figure 2-2 illustrates a Kardex or Rand card format for this information.

Medications, Treatments, Diagnostic Tests

Date—Medications	Date—Treatments	Date—Diagnostic Tests

Checklist of Standard and Frequently Ordered Care

This part is a variation of a form in quite common use throughout many acute care agencies. In addition to listing many of the commonly ordered medical and nursing procedures, such as vital signs, bed rest, catheter irrigation, diet, and the like, it also lists the titles of the unit's standard card plans, such as bowel care, skin care, colostomy care, and so forth. The checklist of all of these frequently ordered items makes it possible to indicate quickly and efficiently that certain items of care are ordered or are in effect.

Also included in this section is a space for writing a patient's preferences as well as other miscellaneous data. Patient preferences include such items as: likes tea at bedtime, likes to nap in afternoon, wants to sleep until 8:30 AM, likes bath in evening, and so on. This is an important part of the total care plan. A surgical unit's version of the checklist is shown below. Figure 2.2 illustrates another version of this part of the Kardex or Rand form.

Checklist of Standard and Frequently Ordered Care—Surgical Unit

Standard Care Plan	Hygiene	Frequently Ordered Items
_Preoperative	_Bed bath	_Oral temperature
_Early postoperative	_Tub bath	_Rectal temperature
_Late postoperative	_Shower	_Pulse, respiration
_Chest approach surgery	_With assistance	_Blood pressure
_Abdominoperineal resection	_Self, total	_Neuro signs
_Amputation, leg	Intake	_CVP
_Mastectomy, radical	_Intake-output	_Sp gr (urine)
_Tracheostomy	Diet	
_Laryngectomy	————————	
_Laminectomy	————————	
_Skin care	————————	
_Indwelling catheter care		
_Mouth care		
Activity ————————	Patient preferences, Miscellaneous information
————————	—————————————————
————————	—————————————————
————————	—————————————————

Unusual Problems

The unusual problems section is the portion of the care plan devoted to unusual problems, expected outcomes, deadlines, and nursing orders. The correct use of this section is explained in detail in the remainder of this volume.

The headings for the unusual problems section of the patient care plan are shown below. Figure 2-1 illustrates how an actual Kardex care plan form might look. Figure 2-3 shows a care plan with written entries.

CARE PLAN MADE OPERATIONAL

To put the care-planning process into operation, keep in mind the working definitions and examples below. Figure 2-3 shows a typical care plan.

| Physician's expectations regarding treatment regimen or course of convalescence: ( ) typical or routine ( ) atypical or complicated
If atypical or complicated, in what way? | Identifying Information: *Age 82*
Adm. 3/28
Catholic—male
Diagnosis: *Perineal excision of rectal*
stump and presacral abscess
(Ca) 3/14
Metastasis—old colostomy |

Criteria for Discharge: *By 6/30*
1. *Demonstrate ability to manage own colostomy.*
2. *Verbalize understanding of health problem and reveal sense of confidence in own ability to follow-up on MD's orders at home.*
3. *Verbalization by next-of-kin that he is willing and able to help at home.*

Home Care Coordination activities:_____

Other relevant data: *Retired fireman*

Date	Unusual Problems	Expected Outcomes	Dead-lines	Nursing Orders
4/5	*(1) Anxiety and depression due to recurrence of problem (Ca)*	*(1) Ability to verbalize fears and concerns* *Reflects a sense of satisfaction with each day of life*	√*qd*	*(1) Establish a trust relationship—listen, problem solve, and assist with working out a good way of life. (Delegated to S. Holman, RN)*
4/5	*(2) Potential general weakness and immobility due to pain when ambulating*	*(2) Verbalize that rectal area is comfortable when walking* *Demonstrate willingness to walk about much of day* *In bed during day no more than 2° at a time*	*(4/8)* √*AM & PM*	*(2)a. Ambulate with walker to day room tid—spray rectal area with local anesthetic before ambulating. Provide comfortable chair in day room and beside bed* *b. Reinforce idea that strength is maintained with reasonable activity* *Ruth Harmon, RN*

FIGURE 2-3. A care plan form with written entries. (From Mayers and Watson: *A Workbook for Patient Care Planning*, 1973, p 5. A. Watson, Sacramento Calif., used with permission)

Working Definitions

Unusual problems	Special difficulties or concerns experienced by a patient at a given point in time. For example:

A. Reddened area, ½ inch diameter, coccyx, due to immobility.
B. Anxiety and depression due to terminal prognosis.

Problems may be classified as "actual" or "potential."

Expected outcomes   Projected patient behavior or clinical manifestations which represent resolution, progress toward resolution, or prevention of the unusual problem. These are the same as short-term objectives. For example:

A. Decrease size of area.
B. Openly verbalize fears and concerns to staff.

Deadlines   Projected point in time by which the expected outcome(s) should be reached—and/or interim evaluation and documentation points. For example:

A. Decrease in size—within 24 hours. Interim deadlines, q 8h.
B. Openly verbalize fears and concerns—within one week. Interim deadlines, q d.

Nursing orders   Those nursing actions that are designed to produce the expected outcome(s) by the deadline. For example:

A. Turn side to side and abdomen (not back) even hours day and night. Massage bony areas each time turned. (M. Mayers, RN)
B. Spend time daily, listening and clarifying. Delegated to J. Jones. (M. Mayers, RN)

SUMMARY

Patient care planning is a method of organizing the nursing process into a functional written form. It is a plan of care that is derived from initial data gathering and that is continually updated through ongoing evaluative assessments. The patient care plan contains certain classifications of information: physician's expectations, nursing's criteria for discharge, unusual and usual problems, expected outcomes, nursing orders, physician's orders, and checklist of standard and frequently ordered care.

The nursing process component of the care plan is specifically directed to:

Problem identification (nursing diagnosis)
Expected outcome determination (patient-centered goals)
Deadline determination (evaluation points)
Nursing orders (nurse-initiated prescriptions)
Patient response documentation (charting that describes the patient's status in relation to the expected outcomes)

Patient care planning helps evaluate the effects of the nursing process through ongoing assessment at periodic intervals. Because of the distinction between usual and unusual problems, the nurse makes sophisticated nursing diagnostic judgments. Standard care plans help to strengthen and streamline care planning. Systematic care planning and charting help to ensure comprehensive assessment, planning, and documentation.

REFERENCES

1. Watson A, Mayers M: How to Write Nursing Care Plans. Stockton Cal, KP Co Medical Systems, 1976, p 9
2. Mayers M, Watson A: Workbook for Patient Care. Sacramento Cal, 1973, p 4

BIBLIOGRAPHY

Little ·D, Carnevali D: Nursing Care Planning, 2nd ed. Philadelphia, Lippincott, 1976.
Nursing Care Systems: Patient Care Planning—A Syllabus. Chicago, Medicus Systems Corp, 1974
Saxton D, Hyland P: Planning and Implementing Nursing Intervention. Louis, Mosby, 1975.
Yura H, Walsh M: The Nursing Process, 2nd ed. New York, Appleton-Century-Crofts, 1973

3

The Problem: Basis for Planning

FORMULATION OF PROBLEM STATEMENTS

Phrasing for Clarity

Whenever the scientific method is used, it is essential to explicitly define the presenting problem in order for the subsequent steps of the problem-solving process to become clear. The steps should follow in logical sequence. When the statement of the problem is ambiguous, vague, or rambling, the remaining steps of the problem-solving process will also be unclear and indefinite. An unclear problem statement cannot provide the basis for a relevant and effective plan.

Problem solving in the planning of patient care is no exception. Efficient and time-saving nursing care plans cannot be developed unless clear and specific problem identification is accomplished in early steps. To omit this step or to assume that it is understood violates a basic premise of problem solving. Staff personnel who are actually working with patient care planning information cannot be expected to know and understand, or to follow through with appropriate nursing action, unless a clear and specific statement of the patient's problem has been set forth.

Many conceptual frameworks in nursing refer to human needs. Maslow's hierarchy of needs is a good example. If a person's need for security is unmet or threatened in significant ways, a discrepancy or problem exists. If the need for security is satisfied, a problem (relative to that need) does not exist. This example is used to illustrate one source of confusion when formulating a problem statement. In terms of simple semantics, the words *needs* may lead to confusion when communicating about a patient's problem. The term *needs* almost automatically leads one to think in terms of a helping phrase, such as "needs encouragement and positive support." This kind of phrasing sidetracks one from making a clear statement of the discrepancy or problem and goes on instead to a solution to the as yet unstated problem. For the purpose of clarity in communicating a patient's problem, it is advisable to avoid the word "needs" in the problem statement.

Basic to care planning, then, is the requirement that a clear statement of the patient's problem or problems be made. This means that the problems will not only be mentally noted but that they will also be written on the care plan form. The *problem* in the context of nursing is analogous to the *diagnosis* in the context of medicine. A diagnosis gives everyone a clear idea about the patient's medical problem and provides a basic rationale for care. If a physician writes orders without stating the patient's medical problem, all of the disciplines involved have difficulty in focusing and in making their interventions relevant. Similarly, nurses list their perceptions of the patient's problems (nursing diagnoses) to provide a basic frame of reference for any care they, the nurses, subsequently order.

In nursing, a problem statement usually refers to a discrepancy between what is desirable and what actually is the case. To identify a discrepancy in a patient's situation it is necessary (1) to know what is expected at a given point in time, (2) to make a valid assessment of the actual situation, and (3) to come to a conclusion as to the consequence of any differences between desired and actual status.

Linkage to Conceptual Models

When a nurse has a working conceptual framework in mind, an appropriate data-gathering guide in hand, and interviewing, listening, observational, and clinical inspection skills in her repertory, she can identify the consequential discrepancies in a patient's situation. These discrepancies are the concepts that, in written form, become problem statements on the care plan.

One client-centered conceptual framework has been set forth by Carl Rogers,[1,2] who eloquently shows how listening, caring, and trusting help the client to identify and express his problems as he experiences them. The client also is aided in finding the most workable solution to his problems.

Another client-centered model is one referred to as *ethnography*.[3] Ethnocentric methods are based on a belief that a client (or person) represents his own group's theories, values, learned knowledge, and coping strategies. Thus, ethnographers listen for a client's (person) or family's (group) clues to their own values, classification system, taxonomy, and definitions. This is in contradistinction to that of a practitioner who brings a model (with its definitions, taxonomies, and functional components) to the client situation and proceeds to force or select the data so as to fit the model.

It may be that further study, by persons supplying health care, of client-centered methods of practice can ultimately yield new bodies of knowledge that can substantially assist caregivers to become care coaches. Because client-centered methods, such as Rogers', have become quite familiar to most nurses, more rigorous application of that philosophy, those values, and those processes could be employed and formulated in a model that other nursing practitioners could learn and utilize in their plans of care. Or further investigation of ethnocentric beliefs and processes, such as the study by Ragucci,[4] could yield a human-centered model for nursing practice. Many of the models well known in nursing today tend to be client centered in their basic essence and may only be limited by the addition of professionals' biases about people, how to classify them, and how to intervene for them.

This brief discussion provides the reader with some background for the operational definitions that are set forth in this text. The operational definitions lend themselves to a variety of client-centered models for nursing practice. The definitions can be modified to provide for a clear operational linkage to almost any specific conceptual framework.

For the purposes of illustrating the principles of care planning, the definitions and examples in this book are consistent with a client-centered basis for nursing. What the patient states, implies, or makes indirectly apparent as a difficulty or concern becomes the basis for identifying a problem. Thus, the definition of a problem is "... a difficulty or concern experienced by a patient at a given point of time."[5]

The key to writing a good care plan is to perceive the problem from the patient's or family's perspective. To achieve a client-centered perspective, keep the following kinds of questions in mind. Their answers lead one to formulate a problem in terms of the patient's perspective.[6]

What is happening to the patient physiologically?
What clinical signs and symptoms are causing him difficulties?
What is happening to him emotionally? socially? spiritually?
What feelings are the patient or his family experiencing?
How is the patient or his family adapting to what is happening?

Some examples of patient perspectives problems are:

1. Extreme thirst and lethargy (physiologic difficulty or concern)
2. Unrelieved pain (clinical symptom)
3. Fear (emotional). Loneliness (social). Doubtful of previously held values (spiritual)
4. Extreme concern (feelings about what's happening)
5. Denial (adapting)

Usual, predictable problems are those difficulties that the science of nursing has identified as common to large numbers of patients. Usual problems can be classified in various ways: by physicians' diagnoses, by nurses' diagnoses,[6] by age groups, by stages of growth and development, or by organizing themes within a conceptual framework. The most common classification for usual problems is by diagnosis, medical or nursing. Examples of medical diagnoses are diabetes mellitus, cholecystectomy, or acute renal failure. Nursing diagnoses might be immobility, acute grief, noncompliance, or alterations in trust. Usual problems and their classifications are discussed and illustrated in Chapters 7 and 8.

Unusual or special problems are those that are unique to an individual. Unusual problems are not predictable, nor are they necessarily common to most patients within certain diagnoses or classifications. They are unique to him because of his values, his experiences, his self-concept, his physiologic state, or his life style.

DEFINITION OF USUAL VERSUS UNUSUAL PROBLEM

For the purposes of the method described in this volume, a problem is described as usual or unusual. This distinction is basic to an understanding of the system.

Usual problem	A predictable difficulty or concern experienced by many patients with the same diagnosis.
Unusual problem	A special difficulty or concern experienced by a patient at a given point in time.

Thus, identifying problems (making a nursing diagnosis) is extremely helpful if the nurse attempts to preceive the problem from the patient's perspective. The closer one comes to understanding how the patient feels—how HE sees his difficulties or concerns—the closer the plan of care will come to solving HIS problems.

The patient is very much aware of some of his problems and can express them quite eloquently either verbally or nonverbally. Other problems may be outside his fields of awareness and knowledge. Certain emotional problems and complicated physiologic problems fall into these categories. However, whether or not the patient is knowledgeable or aware, the nurse can make defensible deductions about his difficulties or concerns. When the problem is phrased in such a way that it communicates the patient's difficulties and concerns, it eloquently and effectively sets the stage for patient-centered nursing interventions.

Causes of Problems

In addition to making a clear statement of the patient's difficulty, the nurse sets forth a brief statement of her understanding of the cause of the problem. For the patient who has a decubitus ulcer of the coccyx, the nurse might write an unusual problem statement such as "Decubitus ulcer, 3 inches in diameter, 1/4 inch deep, coccyx area, *due to lack of turning and poor nutrition.*" Or for a patient with a low fluid intake there might be an unusual problem statement such as "Low fluid intake (900 ml daily) *due to weakness, fatigue, and inability to handle water glass.*" Another patient with a low fluid intake might have this kind of statement: "Low fluid intake (900 ml daily) *due to lifetime habit of inadequate fluid intake.*" Obviously, the nursing action prescribed for the first patient with a low fluid intake will be quite different from the nursing actions prescribed for the second patient with the same apparent problem. These examples clarify why the cause of the problem should also be stated. Careful assessment, interviewing, and consultation with the physician, the clinical nurse specialist, the patient, or the family should in most cases provide the information necessary not only for defining the problem but also for understanding and stating its cause.

Notice that throughout this text every problem statement contains an etiologic phrase, which is the nurse's perception of the cause of the patient's problem. The mental process and attitude required of the nurse in developing this portion of the statement will inevitably make the individual patient a more real person to her and will enable her to plan the most effective care for that person.

DIFFERENTIATION OF ACTUAL, POTENTIAL, AND POSSIBLE PROBLEMS

A further guide to writing problem statements is to deal with them in terms of the three major categories into which all types of patients' problems may fall, whether the problems be physiologic, psychologic, sociologic, or economic. The three categories are actual, potential, and possible.

Actual Problems

Actual problems are those patient concerns and difficulties which, in the nurse's judgment, are present at the time the assessment is made. They are problems that, in fact, exist. They are actually present. For instance, the patient with a decubitus ulcer of the coccyx has an actual problem. So do the patients previously mentioned with the actual low daily fluid intake.

Actual Problem Statement Examples

1. Depression and embarrassment due to facial disfigurement from lacerations
2. Impaired circulation over coccyx, sacrum, and thoracic spine due to emaciation, malnutrition, and immobility
3. Acute grief due to death of husband in same accident (husband died March 16)
4. Multiple decubiti: Rt trochanter, 3 inch diameter, 1½ inch deep, Lt trochanter, 4 inch diameter, 1 inch deep, Sacrum and coccyx, 5 inch diameter, ¼–½ inch deep, due to immobility, pressure, and poor nutrition
5. Anxiety and restlessness due to dyspnea

Actual problems are not prefaced by the word *actual* when written on the care plan. They are assumed to be actual if they are not otherwise indicated.

Potential Problems

A potential problem is a difficulty or concern that a patient has an unusually high risk of developing or experiencing. For instance, an elderly, emaciated patient with a fractured hip is at unusually high risk of developing skin breakdown over pressure areas. At the time of the nurse's assessment, the skin breakdown has not actually occurred, but the nurse knows that it is likely to occur unless certain nursing measures are instituted immediately. Another example is a patient who is experiencing nonacceptance of the diagnosis of diabetes mellitus. He is at unusually high risk of uncontrolled diabetes after leaving the hospital environment. Just as with actual problems, potential problems must also include a statement of the cause or reason for their being at high risk in that particular case.

Potential Problem Statement Examples

1. Potential postoperative bleeding due to hemophilia
2. Potential pressure areas of back and hips due to casting and traction of both legs
3. Potential uncontrolled diabetes due to language and cultural differences and subsequent lack of understanding of instructions
4. Potential postpartum vaginal hemorrhage due to atonic uterus
5. Potential injury from falling due to poor coordination and weakness

Any potential problem, when written on a care plan, is prefaced by the word "potential."

Possible Problems

A possible problem is a situation requiring more information before it can be ruled in or ruled out as a problem. Until more data are gathered, a statement of the possible problem should be made so that it will not be forgotten and so that more information can be obtained and evaluated.

There are innumerable instances when, for various reasons, it is impossible or inappropriate to gather all necessary data at a given time—data which would make it possible to clearly identify and define an actual problem. It, therefore, becomes necessary that a patient care planning system provide for writing statements of possible problems. Unless possible problems are written, they are likely to be lost to follow-up at an appropriate future time. The nurse is in a particularly strategic position to identify possible problems. By noting them in the care plan she makes them known to those who will be assessing and providing care in the future.

For example, a young mother is being admitted on an emergency basis. She has a tentative diagnosis of congestive heart failure and is experiencing significant dyspnea, pain, and apprehension. She mentions some concern about her three preschoolers at home, although she also says that she made babysitting arrangements for them. Because her physiologic problems are of primary importance for the first few hours after admission, it may not be appropriate for the nurse immediately to interview her further regarding her concern about her children. When the patient's breathing is easier, her pain subsided, and her apprehension relieved, her concern for her children can be pursued and can be ruled in or ruled out as an unusual problem. If a change of shift should occur before the patient has become reasonably stabilized, it would be necessary to write, in the unusual problems column of the patient's care plan, that there is "Possible concern regarding babysitting arrangements." Prescribed nursing actions would be to "Gather more information regarding this as soon as the patient is reasonably well stabilized." After gathering more data, the nurse may find that the babysitting arrangement is satisfactory to the mother, and, therefore, the problem may be ruled out. Or she may find that this is a real concern to the patient and that certain assistance is needed in making better arrangements.

Frequently patients will give certain clues to emotional or social problems. But because of lack of time, lack of the necessary rapport with the nursing staff, or for other reasons, they may not provide enough information for a clear identification of the problem. In these cases the nurse should write, in the unusual problems category, a phrase or two which generally describes the clues the patient has revealed. The nursing actions will then be to "gather more data" in whatever way and at whatever time the nurse believes is appropriate. The inclusion of the possible problems category, in addition to the actual and potential problems categories, increases the likelihood that important clues to further data for problem identification will not be lost.

Possible Problem Statement Examples.   Following are listed several examples of how possible problem statements can be written on a nursing care plan:

1. Possible financial problems due to long convalescence
2. Possible worry over teenage children at home
3. Possible concern regarding meaning of diagnosis
4. Possible lack of understanding of physician's treatment regimen
5. Possible worry over job and family adjustments to illness

A possible problem should be preceded by the word "possible" when entered on a care plan.

COMPOSITION OF A PLAN

Handwrite Unusual Problems Only

The major principle that makes patient care planning efficient and effective is that there is a basic rationale for deciding which problems need be handwritten on a care plan and which need not be. Only unusual problems are handwritten.

Some people recommend that a nurse use her judgment about which problems should be entered on a care plan. Others recommend a priority system based on basic human needs, while others recommend, explicitly or implicitly, that a comprehensive list of problems and needs be written. A common system (or nonsystem) for deciding what to write on a nursing care plan appears to be based on the theory that every patient has at least one problem.

Many nurses feel uncomfortable when they see a blank nursing care plan. Their concern is understandable, particularly if there is no other way to determine whether or not a patient has been assessed. This is where the every-patient-has-at-least-one-problem syndrome comes into being. It takes a nurse of great fortitude to resist the urge to write something, no matter what, in that demanding blank space.

The principle that this system recommends as basic to a decision about what to write on a care plan is: Every patient has physiologic or other problems, but he may be coping with them satisfactorily. Illness or surgical intervention may not make him unable to cope with or manage his own problems.

Since nurses believe that persons receiving care have a right to appropriate independence, interdependence, and dependence, it is important that nursing not intervene when a patient is already managing satisfactorily. To safeguard a patient's independence, a nurse makes as complete an assessment as possible and then decides which problems the patient is not coping with or managing adequately. These are the problems that must be written on the care plan and for which expected outcomes and individualized nursing actions must be formulated. These are the unusual problems. Unusual problems must be handwritten.

Usual Problems

Basic to efficient, effective care planning is the assumption that a patient may be progressing satisfactorily and may, therefore, have no unusual problems to be written on the nursing care plan. Probably a majority of patients on a typical surgical unit may fall into this category. Everyone has problems, patients and nurses alike. However, "What are the problems?" is not the only question to ask. Rather, having identified the problems, one asks, "Is the person responding or progressing satisfactorily with respect to his situation and to his medical and nursing objectives?" Distinguishing between usual and unusual problems also upgrades the decision-making process because, with every assessment, the nurse considers the patient's actual status in relation to expected or desired outcomes, and upon that basis she makes decisions. When the nurse constantly asks "Is this problem within expected parameters?" or "Is this patient coping satisfactorily with his problems?" her analysis and decision making are significantly refined.

Examples of Patients Who Do Not Have Unusual Problems

Following are five cases which portray situations where each patient is managing or is coping satisfactorily. Each one has no apparent unusual problems.

CASE 1

Harry J, age 17, is admitted on 2/17 for an emergency appendectomy after several hours of abdominal pain.

On 2/18, postoperative day[1], the registered nurse asseses his status. After completing a nursing history, following through on two or three possible concerns, and explaining to him the care he will be receiving, the nurse concludes that Harry has no unusual problems and that he is coping satisfactorily with the usual problems of postoperative pain, ambulation, intake, and so forth. He apparently has a supportive family, and his hospitalization costs are covered by his family's health insurance plan. Harry verbalizes realistic plans for keeping up with his schoolwork.

As a result of her assessment and analysis, the nurse makes the following notation on his patient care plan form:

Date	Unusual Problems
2/18	No apparent unusual problems at this time

CASE 2

Mrs. Carol J, age 25, is being admitted to a medical unit with a diagnosis of acute cystitis. The physician's purpose for hospitalization is to control the infection and to do further diagnostic work in order to determine the cause of the pattern of recurrent bladder infections. He foresees no significant complications for her recovery. The registered nurse responsible for Mrs. J's care interviews her and completes an assessment of her status. The nurse finds that Mrs. J has had previous bladder infections and that she is familiar with the symptoms and the treatment. Her family doctor has treated her previously and is managing her medical care again. Upon admission Mrs. J is feeling general malaise and burning upon urination, and she has an elevated temperature. The physician's orders for pain, fever, the infection, and sleep seem likely to keep Mrs. J. comfortable and rested. The estimated length of hospitalization is two or three days. Mrs. J states that she has no children and that her hospitalization is covered by her health insurance. She expresses no apparent signs of emotional distress or evidence of being unable to cope with the expected course of convalescence.

As a result of this assessment the nurse concludes that Mrs. J has no unusual problems and that she appears to be coping satisfactorily with the symptoms of her illness. The nurse's notation on Mrs. J's patient care plan is as follows:

Date	Unusual Problems
2/19	Apparently coping satisfactorily at this time

CASE 3

Mr. James R, age 48, is recovering from a lumbar laminectomy. When the nurse assesses his progress she finds that Mr. R is getting satisfactory relief from his pain medication, that he demonstrates that he is able to "log roll," and that he verbalizes satisfactory understanding of his condition and his medical and nursing care. He is having slight distress from flatulence, but the physician's orders provide satisfactory relief. His morale seems good. Since his is a planned hospitalization, he has made appropriate prehospitalization plans for his work, family, and finances.

As a result of these findings the nurse enters on Mr. R's patient care plan the following notation:

Date	Unusual Problems
2/17	No apparent unusual problems at this time

CASE 4

Mrs. Alice M, age 37, is being admitted for an A and P repair. The registered nurse responsible for her care interviews her upon admission and does a total assessment.

In summary, the nurse finds that Mrs. M has been seeing her physician for some time regarding her stress incontinence and the associated symptoms of a relaxed pelvic floor. Mrs. M verbalizes appropriate understanding of her physical problem and of the surgical procedure that is planned, as well as an understanding of the expected postoperative course. The nurse explains the nursing care that she can expect during her hospitalization.

Since this is a planned hospitalization, Mrs. M has made arrangements for the care of her three children, who are preteenager and early teenagers. Her husband also indicates satisfaction with the arrangements and has accepted the added home responsibilities that will be his during his wife's hospitalization. He states that his health insurance will cover his wife's medical care costs.

As a result of this admission interview and assessment, the nurse makes the following notation on Mrs. M's patient care plan:

Date	Unusual Problems
2/12	No apparent unusual problems at this time

CASE 5

Mrs. Joyce H, age 52, has had an abdominal hysterectomy due to fibroids. It is her third postoperative day.

The registered nurse who assesses her status on the third postoperative day finds that Mrs. H is ambulating well and is taking oral foods and fluids in amounts consistent with satisfactory postoperative progress. Pain in the surgical area seems to be decreasing, consistent with the usual abdominal hysterectomy postoperative pattern. When needed, her pain medication orders provide satisfactory relief.

Mrs. H has the usual questions and concerns that a woman experiencing a hysterectomy so frequently has. The nurse's responses and clarification appear to be understood and accepted by Mrs. H. She gives every indication by her questions, responses, and verbalization of feelings that she is coping satisfactorily with the effects of surgery. Since her surgery has been planned in advance, Mrs. H has made arrangements for her husband, her home, and for the financial aspects of her care.

As a result of her findings, the nurse makes the following entry under the unusual problems section of the patient care plan:

Date	Unusual Problems
4/20	Apparently coping and progressing well

Unusual Problems

As previously indicated, many patients are coping well with their problems. It is thus superfluous for nurses to write down these usual problems. Rather, the nurse should determine, by use of a nursing history or other assessment method, whether or not the patient has unusual problems at this time. Valuable nursing time should be spent in defining unusual problems and in designing meaningful nursing care. Priorities of this nature must be set if nurses are to meet their responsibilities to all patients and, in particular, to patients who have overwhelming problems.

How to Write Unusual Problem Statements

For purposes of clarity and efficiency, an unusual problem statement must meet the following criteria:

1. It must be a statement of an unexpected, unusual, or atypical difficulty or concern being experienced by a patient.
2. It must be a difficulty or concern with which the patient is not coping in ways consistent with expected or desired outcomes or objectives.
3. It must be defined as the result of a systematic assessment by the responsible registered nurse.
4. It must be categorized as either an actual, potential, or possible problem.

5. It must contain a brief statement of the nurse's perception of the cause of the problem.
6. It must have implications for care which are not already covered by physician's orders or by standard nursing care orders.

Examples of Unusual Problem Statements. The following list of selected statements illustrates the brevity, clarity, and specificity required of unusual problem statements.

1. Low fluid intake (800 ml on 3/24) due to lifelong habit of not drinking much
2. Decubitus ulcer (2 inch diameter and ¼ inch deep) over coccyx due to immobility and poor nutrition
3. Extreme anxiety due to unknown diagnosis
4. Reluctant to take IPPB because of embarrassment from urinary incontinence caused by coughing when using IPPB
5. Low caloric intake (1,000 calories on 3/24) due to confusion and distraction of hospital environment
6. Worried and upset due to complex family problems
7. Anxiety and fear due to dyspnea
8. Feelings of panic caused by memory loss due to cerebrovascular accident

The statements in the previous examples are brief and specific, yet they give a precise indication of the nature of the problems that must be solved. When unusual problem statements are written this clearly, the subsequent steps of the problem-solving process are greatly facilitated. The prescribed care is most likely to be directly relevant and to result in an effective solution of the problem.

In brief, a nurse makes a complete assessment of the patient's status and problems. She then makes a decision regarding whether or not the patient is coping satisfactorily with each of the problems. After making that appraisal she writes the unusual problems on the nursing care plan. In reality, the nurse also finds that the amount of writing necessary for most patients is significantly decreased when she limits herself only to entries of unusual problems. It is true that many patients have many unusual problems. For those patients there will of necessity be a significant number of entries concerning their problems and nursing interventions. However, many other patients do not have unusual problems and, for them, little or no comment is required. This frees the nurse to devote her time and energy more profitably to the priority problems and to the patients who do require her valuable decision-making and intervention skills. When nurses recognize this principle and act upon it, they use their time and energy effectively.

Decision Making for Unusual Problem Identification. Decisions about what to write on a nursing care plan take into consideration whether or not a patient is functioning satisfactorily. When unusual or exceptional patient problems have been identified, they must be entered as unusual problems on the care plan. In order for the problem statements to provide a sound basis for effective problem solving, four requirements should be met. Each problem must be listed separately. Each problem statement must be specific, concise, and to the point. Each problem statement must include a short statement, in the nurse's judgment, of the cause of the problem. And, finally, each problem must be categorized and termed as actual, potential, or possible.

Case Study Applications

The following five case histories clarify problem identification and the associated decision-making process about which items to hand-write on a nursing care plan.

CASE 1. RICHARD M, MULTIPLE TRAUMATIC INJURY

Richard M, a 16-year-old boy, normally lives with his parents and an older sister. Several days ago he was in a motorcycle accident and sustained multiple injuries.

The following paragraphs outline the basic background information for his nursing care planning.

Medical Impression: Multiple trauma
    Fractured zygoma, mandible, clavicle
    Probably basilar skull fracture
    Intracranial clot
    Multiple facial lacerations
Surgical Intervention:
    Tracheostomy
    Open reduction, debridement, and repair of facial and neck
        lacerations
Physician's Orders (Current orders, six days postaccident and post-

operative, when patient was transferred from intensive care to a regular medical-surgical unit):

    Osterized diet

    Intake and output

    Ambulate

    Vital signs q shift

    Do not turn on right side—patient has fractured clavicle

    Tight clavicle brace q AM

    Clean inner cannula q shift

    Remove inner cannula and change q day

    Suction prn

    Tracheostomy tube can be changed prn every few days

    Liquid ferrous sulfate po, 300 mg tid

    Valium, 5 mg prn

    Darvon, prn

Analyzing the Problems.   Mrs. Fullington, the registered nurse who evaluates the patient's status at the time of admission to the medical-surgical unit, identifies several problems. Each problem she identifies is followed in this text by a sample of the nurse's analysis of the problem. After thinking through the total range of concerns, the nurse would enter on the patient care plan only those problems that are unusual, those outside the expected range of problems, or those the patient seems unable to manage satisfactorily.

Following is a complete list of the problems that Mrs. Fullington identifies at the time of Richard's admission to the medical-surgical unit on 4/20.

1. There is some mucus in tracheostomy cannula.
   Analysis: There is a minimal amount of mucus. It poses no real threat to respiration or to potential aspiration even with infrequent suctioning of the tracheostomy. Suctioning has been ordered by the physician. This situation seems to be under control.
2. He apparently is very much afraid of being suctioned.
   Analysis: He guards the tracheostomy when the nurse wishes to suction. His facial expression reveals fear when it is suctioned. He tries to push the nurse away. This is an unusual response and represents real fears and concerns on the part of the patient.
3. He is at high risk for choking on fluids because of his wired jaws.
   Analysis: This is an expected problem when a jaw wiring is

done. The suction machine is at the bedside. There should be no unusual, unanticipated problems in this area.

4. He communicates that he has soreness and tenderness of his head and face.
   Analysis: This is expected in his case. The pain order appears to keep him comfortable, so significant discomfort is not likely as long as he is appropriately medicated.

5. He cannot express his needs because of his inability to speak due to the tracheostomy and his unwillingness to plug it, even temporarily.
   Analysis: Because he appears fearful and because the nursing staff does not often care for teenages, he may have many unmet, unanticipated problems that he is not able to express. This is an unusual problem.

6. Because of the tracheostomy he has a potential for pulmonary infection.
   Analysis: This is always a potential when there is a tracheostomy. The routine tracheostomy care which requires sterile technique is appropriate. The physician checks the patient's chest sounds daily. For these reasons, the patient probably is not at unusually high risk for pulmonary infection.

7. His facial expressions and manner reveal that he has fear and anxiety, possibly due to a lack of knowledge and understanding of the meaning of the tracheostomy as well as many of the other medical and nursing procedures.
   Analysis: Because of his guarding and his pushing away of the nurses, and because of his facial expressions of fear, one can safely conclude that he probably is not coping well. This is a real problem.

8. He must feel lonely and alienated because of the infrequent visits of his family.
   Analysis: His family lives 40 miles away and can't visit often. In addition, he is surrounded by adult patients and staff. This could be an exceptional difficulty for a teenager.

9. He is very likely to become bored with the osterized diet.
   Analysis: To a teenager, dietary likes and dislikes are important. Osterized foods can be quite unpalatable as they are so different from one's usual diet. A call to the dietition can solve this.

10. He could be at risk for some of the side effects of immobility.
    Analysis: He ambulates well. He walks about the room and down the hall for bathing. Probably immobility is not a real problem area for him.

11. His parents may feel real concern and a sense of lack of know-

ledge regarding his progress and the physician's treatment plans.

Analysis: There's not enough information to evaluate this as yet, but it is a real possibility that his parents are quite uninformed. This should be checked out.

12. The patient and his family may be concerned about his loss of school time.

Analysis: There is not enough information available to evaluate as yet, but this should be explored with the parents.

After analyzing the problems Mrs. Fullington, the nurse, would make certain entries on Richard's care plan under the unusual problems section. Examples of expected outcomes and nursing orders for this case are found in the following chapters.

Richard M's Patient Care Plan

Physician's expectations regarding course of treatment and convalescence:
( ) typical or routine
(√) atypical or complicated
If atypical or complicated, in what way?
Some possible unknown injuries, delayed reduction of mandible. Keep tracheostomy open for anesthesia for mandible reduction.

Identifying Information: _____
_____
_____
Diagnosis: Multiple trauma, _____
Fr zygoma, mandible, clavicle, _____
basilar skull _____
Intracranial clot _____
Facial lacerations _____
Tracheostomy _____
_____

Nursing's criteria for discharge or maintenance (overall expected outcomes):
(a) Patient and family will verbalize appropriate understanding of course of
   convalescence and indicate ability to follow through.
(b) They will demonstrate ability to manage any necessary care.
                                        M. Fullington, RN

Home Care Coordination activities: _____

Other relevant information (socioeconomic, etc): _____

Date	Unusual Problems
4/20	(1) Extreme fear and anxiety, probably due to lack of understanding of tracheostomy and possibly due to lack of trust in staff—guards, pushes away staff from trachestomy—has facial expressions of fear
4/20	(2) Potential frustration and depression due to inability to communicate needs well. (Can't speak because of tracheostomy)
4/20	(3) Potential feelings of isolation and loneliness—due to parents and friends who live out of town and can't visit often
4/20	(4) Possible concern and lack of knowledge by parents re treatment progress and plans
4/20	(5) Possible concern of patient and family re loss of school time

Summary. Although on 4/20 Mrs. Fullington identifies a total of 12 actual, potential, and possible problems, only five problems qualify as unusual. The five problems entered on the patient care plan require for their solution other than the standard nursing care or the currently ordered medical care. The dietary problem can be solved by a call to the food service department requesting that a dietition assess Richard's nutritional problems and set up a good selection of liquefied foods for his diet. The new diet order can then be entered in the appropriate space on the care plan. The diet problem would not be entered as an unusual problem because it is solved on the spot.

The two possible problems are written to remind the staff to obtain further information so that these clues can ultimately be ruled in or ruled out as actual or potential problems.

CASE 2. MARY R, COLOSTOMY

Mrs. R. is 72 years of age, a widow, and is being evaluated by the registered nurse on 4/14, postoperative day 5. Current information and orders are outlined in the subsequent paragraphs.

History: Peptic ulcer 1½ years duration. Appendectomy and hysterectomy performed 20 years ago. Acute myocardial infarction three years ago

Present Illness: Patient's chief complaint: Abdominal cramps accompanied by increasing distention. No bowel movement for two days. March 22, seen in ER c̄ distended abdomen. X-ray showed massive free air in abdominal cavity. Admitted for diagnostic celiotomy

Preop. Diagnosis: Perforated ulcer

Postop. Diagnosis: Perforated ascending colon, 2° volvulus

Operation: Celiotomy, cecostomy, double-barreled colostomy

Physician's Orders:
    CBC
    Ambulate 10 minutes tid
    Rectal temperature q 4°
    VS qid
    Tub bath q d
    Stool GUIAC x 3-2-1
    Reg diet, hi-pro, lo residue
    Irrigate wound c̄ H_2O_2 and NS. Pack c̄ wet fine mesh gauze
        and 4 by 4s covering. Change qid
    Teach patient colostomy care

Medications:
  FeSo₄ 300 mg 9-1-5
  Librium 10 mg po 9-1-5
  Multivits tid 9-1-5
  Colace 100 mg po 9-1-5
  Darvon 65 mg po q 4° prn pain
  Chlortrimeton 4 mg po q 4° prn

Analyzing the Problems.   Mrs. Walker, the nurse who evaluates Mrs. R's status on postoperative day 5, identifies several problems. Each problem is followed in this text by some of the nurse's thinking which results in decisions regarding the magnitude of the problems:

1. The patient is upset and embarrassed by the continuous smell and mess of the colostomy, due to leakage around the bag. *Analysis:* Her facial expressions and her tone of voice reinforce that the smell and mess are intolerable. She cannot cope with it.
2. She seems very emotionally upset over the feuding of her four adult sons and daughters over who will be "stuck with" caring for her. *Analysis:* She weeps when she tells of the feelings of anger and resentment among her sons and daughters. She's sorry she's a burden but knows she can't help it right now. It's a very difficult situation for her.
3. Mrs. R is worried about the elevated temperature which has occurred during the past several hours. *Analysis:* She verbalized real concern over a possible setback due to the fever. The doctor explained to her that he is running some laboratory work to determine what antibiotic to use and that it should soon be under control; she now seems appropriately reassured.
4. She states that she has pain in the surgical area but that it is "not too bad" when she gets pain medication periodically. *Analysis:* The pain medication which is given every six to eight hours seems to provide satisfactory comfort. This is not an unusual pain problem.
5. She expresses concern over how she will manage her own colostomy after she goes to one of her children's homes. *Analysis:* Mrs. R seems willing and eager to learn about her own care. She is strong enough now to get up to the bathroom to manage her own irrigation.
6. There is potential for surgical wound infection because of the leakage around the colostomy bag. *Analysis:* The incision still is not completely healed. There are

no signs of wound infection yet. It is still a potential problem, however, because of the leaking colostomy. This definitely is a potential problem.

7. There is potential for skin excoriation around the stoma due to the drainage.

   Analysis: No excoriation at present. Routine skin care apparently is adequate. This is not an unusual situation now.

8. There is potential for fluid, electrolyte, and nutritional imbalance due to the constant fluid drainage from the colostomy. *Analysis:* At present, blood chemistries reveal the electrolytes to be within normal limits. The doctor is monitoring this daily. Her special diet order and the supplementary vitamins and iron help reduce this possibility. This situation seems to be under control.

After analyzing the problems, Mrs. Walker, RN, would make the entries in the unusual problems column of Mrs. R's care plan as illustrated in the following section. Examples of expected outcomes and nursing orders for this patient are portrayed in subsequent chapters.

Mary R's Patient Care Plan.

Physician's expectations regarding course of treatment and convalescence:

( ) typical or routine

(√) atypical or complicated

If atypical or complicated, in what way?

Obese—abdominal wound will heal slowly.

Identifying Information: _____

Diagnosis: Celiotomy, cecostomy, double-barreled colostomy, 4/8

Nursing's criteria for discharge or maintenance (overall expected outcomes):

(a) Will verbalize appropriate understanding of medical regimen and follow-up.

(b) Will demonstrate satisfactory ability to irrigate own colostomy.

(c) Will verbalize feelings about colostomy and state realistic plans for home care.   Mrs. Walker, RN

Home Care Coordination activities: HCC notified on 4/14

Other relevant information (socioeconomic, etc.): _____

Date	Unusual Problems
4/14	(1) Very upset and embarrassed by smell and mess of colostomy due to leakage
4/14	(2) Emotionally upset by feuding of adult children over who will have to care for her
4/14	(3) Potential surgical wound infection due to colostomy leakage

Summary. Although on 4/14 the nurse identifies a total of eight actual and potential problems, only three problems are considered by her to be unusual. These three would be written on the patient care plan because they require other than the standard postoperative colostomy care.

Mrs. R's anxiety about learning her own colostomy care is evaluated by the nurse to be a normal concern because Mrs. R expresses a desire and a willingness to learn.

Under "criteria for discharge" the nurse indicates that the patient should be able to demonstrate an ability to manage her own colostomy care, including the dietary management aspect. Since from all available data it seems that the patient will not have unusual difficulty learning to do her own colostomy care, this would not be entered under the unusual problems section.

CASE 3.   RALPH L, FRACTURED HIP AND ACTIVE PULMONARY TUBERCULOSIS

Mr. L, age 66, is evaluated by L. Pratt, registered nurse, a few hours after his transfer to a medical-surgical unit from intensive care. Current information and orders as reviewed by Mrs. Pratt, RN, are outlined in the following paragraphs:

Present History and Illness: The patient is a 66-year-old man, whose last admission to the hospital six years previously was for a stasis ulcer of the left lower leg. He was brought to the hospital by ambulance on 3/14 from the downtown skid row area. He had nonobtainable blood pressure and a weak and thready pulse. He was incoherent and confused.

Past Medical and Social History: A skin graft to the left leg was done 10 years previously. He had stasis ulcers of the left leg with atrophic dermatitis 7 years ago. He is a transient worker who is said to have been smoking one pack of cigarettes per day. One uncle died of diabetes mellitus.

Impression: Dehydration and malnutrition
  R/O chronic renal disease vs prerenal azotemia
  Pulmonary tuberculosis, active
  Left hip fracture (hip pinning done on 3/20)

Doctor's Orders:
  Do not get patient out of bed
  Weigh daily with bed scale
  Foot cradle
  VS q shift

C/A 6:30, 11:30, 4:30, hs
IPPB c̄ NS q 4°
Cough qid
Clamp Foley catheter 9-1-5-9-1-5
Unclamp Foley 8:30, 12:30, 4:30, etc
Irrigate Foley c̄ ¼% acetic acid 9-1-6
I & O
Sputum culture Tuesdays and Fridays
Rainbow insulin coverage
Clean decubitus with pHisoHex. Leave uncovered
Gavage feedings
D/10/W, 300 ml by drip NG q 4°
Skim milk, 100 ml 9-5 with INH
Bouillon, 200 ml 9 AM daily

Medications:
NPH insulin, 15 U of U 40 8:30 daily
Thexforte, 1 ml 9 AM daily
Ethambutal, 400 mg 9 AM daily
Phridoxine, 100 mg 9 AM daily
INH, 100 mg c̄ 100 ml skim mile/NG bid
KCL, 20% tsp ÿ 9 AM daily
Elase and neosporin to decubitus
Tolwin prn
Thorazine, prm for hiccoughs
ASA, ÿ po q 4° for temp 101.8

Analyzing the Problems. Mrs. Pratt, RN, identifies several problems. As in the previous case examples, each problem is followed here by some of the nurse's thinking that results in decisions regarding the magnitude of the various problems.

Following is a total list of the patient's problems as identified on 4/5, the sixteenth postoperative day:

1. Patient has a potential for pulmonary hemorrhage or spontaneous pneumothorax because of his active tuberculosis. *Analysis:* He has been having some streaking. His pulmonary cavitation is large. He is at unusually high risk for this problem to occur.
2. There is a potential for constipation because of his immobility and his liquid diet. *Analysis:* He apparently has been having bowel movements. The record is not precise regarding amounts and consistency. This needs careful watching.

3. He is a potential source of infection (tbc) to others.
   Analysis: Isolation procedures for airborne infections have been instituted. This should be adequate.
4. He has very severe pain upon moving and turning due to his fractured left hip and the decubitus ulcer.
   Analysis: He moans as though he is in severe pain when he is turned. His rigid posture and facial expressions reinforce that he is having real difficulty coping with his pain.
5. He has a decubitus ulcer, 2 inch diameter, ¼ inch deep, over the sacrum due to immobility and poor tissue nutrition.
   Analysis: There is no necrotic tissue noticeable. There is no sign of granulation tissue around the edges, however. The ulcer probably is increasing in size at the present time. This is a real problem.
6. He has dry, scaly, itchy skin due to dehydration and due to the frequent bathing schedule of the hospital.
   Analysis: He says his skin is uncomfortably dry and itchy. It looks dry and scaly. This is a real problem.
7. He has a potential for hypostatic pneumonia because of his immobility.
   Analysis: He is on an IPPB and coughing regimen. The doctor listens to his chest daily. The "turning" routine will help. Because of his chest infection and his significant immobility, he is at very high risk for stasis pneumonia.
8. There is a potential for contractures of his joints due to his immobility.
   Analysis: Passive range of motion of his legs reveals that he is experiencing beginning joint stiffness. Foot drop is a real possibility unless aggressive action is immediately instituted.
9. He has a painful right arm due to a wound secondary to a previous intracath procedure.
   Analysis: Mr. L says it's much better, though still painful. The pain medications and warm pad seem to maintain reasonable comfort.
10. He has a dry, uncomfortable mouth and nose due to the nasogastric tube.
    Analysis: His mouth seems very dry. He needs more aggressive action than the routine mouth care provides.
11. There is potential for urinary infection due to the indwelling catheter.
    Analysis: The doctor's orders include fluid intake, a closed bladder irrigation system, and a urinary antiseptic. Urinalyses are done frequently. Urine appears clear now.

12. He must have feelings of loneliness and depression, since he has no family or home. This is compounded by his hospital isolation.

    Analysis: He says he has no family left anymore. He lived in a hotel room before hospital admission. He has no idea where he will go when he is discharged. This is a real problem.

13. He may have financial problems.

    Analysis: He is unclear in stating his source of income. His hospitalization is being covered by Medicare funds. He may be eligible for a categorical welfare grant upon discharge. The social worker must be informed about him.

14. It is reasonable to assume that he may feel fear and anxiety because of the many unfamiliar procedures and because of the staff who wear masks, caps, gowns, and gloves when caring for him.

    Analysis: He seems lonely. He responds to questions with facial expressions and tones of voice that convey feelings of low self-esteem—"Nobody should bother with me." He has a tense, rigid posture in bed. This seems to be a significant problem.

After analyzing all of the problems, Mrs. Pratt would write the following unusual problems on Mr. L's care plan. Examples of expected outcomes and nursing orders for him are illustrated in subsequent chapters.

Ralph L's Patient Care Plan

Physician's expectations regarding course of treatment and convalescence:

( ) typical or routine

(√) atypical or complicated

If atypical or complicated, in what way?
Malnourished, expect slow healing and slow progress regarding ambulation.

Identifying Information: _____

Diagnosis: Dehydration, malnutrition, active pulmonary tbc, left hip fracture—pinned, 3/20

Nursing's criteria for discharge or maintenance (overall expected outcomes):
(a) Will verbalize approval of convalescent facility or home care.
(b) Will demonstrate safe and efficient transfer and ambulation techniques.
(c) Will verbalize understanding of and demonstrate safe isolation technique for tbc.
(d) Will verbalize appropriate understanding of medical care regimen and ability to follow up.   L. Pratt, RN

Home Care Coordination activities: HCC notified on 4/5.

Other relevant information (socioeconomic, etc): On Medicare hospital insurance. Social worker notified on 4/5.

Date	Unusual Problems
4/5	(1) Potential pulmonary hemorrhage or spontaneous pneumothorax due to active pulmonary tbc
4/5	(2) Potential constipation due to immobility and liquid diet
4/5	(3) Severe pain upon moving and turning due to fr left hip and decubitus of sacrum
4/5	(4) Decubitus ulcer (sacrum) 2 inch diameter, ¼ inch deep due to immobility and poor tissue nutrition
4/5	(5) Dry, itchy skin due to dehydration and frequent bathing
4/5	(6) Potential joint contractures due to immobility in bed
4/5	(7) Dry, uncomfortable mouth and nose due to nasogastric tube and dehydration
4/5	(8) Feelings of loneliness, fear, and depression due to no family, hospital isolation, and many unfamiliar procedures

Summary. Although the nurse identifies a total of 14 actual, potential, and possible problems, only eight of them meet the criteria for unusual problems.

The possible financial problem would not be written on the care plan because Mrs. Pratt immediately informs the home care coordinator and the social worker, as noted under the home care and other information section.[5]

CASE 4. STEPHEN F, CHOLECYSTECTOMY

Mr. Stephen F, age 58, is interviewed by J. Roth, RN, upon his admission to a medical-surgical unit. He is scheduled for a cholecystectomy the following morning. Mrs. Roth reviewed his record and notes the following background information.

History: Mr. F is an outgoing, friendly person, is married, and has two adult daughters with families of their own. Twenty years previously he had a laminectomy with no subsequent problems. He experienced a mild CVA about five months prior to this admission and still has some left-sided weakness requiring the use of a cane for walking. Several months of recurring bouts of cholecystitis have resulted in the decision by his physician to perform a cholecystectomy. He is experiencing no acute symptoms at the time of admission.

Medical Orders: His preoperative orders are routine for a cholecystectomy.

Analyzing the Problems. J. Roth, RN, identifies several problems as a result of her admission interview. As in the previous case examples, each problem she identifies is followed in the text by some of the thinking that results in a decision regarding the magnitude of each of the problems.

Following is a list of the problems identified on 3/29, the day of admission.

1. Patient has a potential for postoperative hypostatic pneumonia due to the high incision of a cholecystectomy.
   Analysis: Routine preoperative teaching of deep breathing and coughing and vigorous postoperative follow-up as well as the anticipated orders for IPPB and ambulation postoperatively should be adequate. This should not be an unusually difficult problem.
2. He has some fear and anxiety regarding the impending major surgery.
   Analysis: His questions reveal an appropriate level of fear and a desire to know more about what to expect. He seems to be coping well with his fears.
3. He may have financial problems related to the expense of surgery and hospitalization.
   Analysis: He states that his hospitalization is covered by health insurance and that his sick leave will be used. He doesn't anticipate an overwhelming financial burden.

After analyzing the problems, Mrs. Roth would write the following notation under the unusual problems of Mr. F's care plan. Examples of expected outcomes and nursing orders for this patient are shown in subsequent chapters.

Stephen F's Patient Care Plan

Physician's expectations regarding course of treatment and convalescence:
(√) typical or routine
( ) atypical or complicated
If atypical or complicated, in what way?

Identifying Information: _____
_____
_____
Diagnosis: Cholecystectomy, 3/29 _____
_____
_____

Nursing's criteria for discharge or maintenance (overall expected outcomes):
See standard postoperative expected outcomes.   J. Roth, RN

Home Care Coordination activities: _____

Other relevant information (socioeconomic, etc.): _____

Date	Unusual Problems
3/29	Appears to be coping satisfactorily, both physiologically and psychologically

Summary. For the three problems identified, it would be decided by Mrs. Roth that the standard cholecystectomy care will be appropriate. The patient's fear of surgery is normal. He appears to be coping satisfactorily with his fears, so that this is not considered to be an unusual problem. The routine preoperative support and teaching provided by the nursing staff should be adequate in his case. Standard postoperative criteria for discharge are appropriate. His is an example of a situation that can be managed quickly, yet appropriately, without long detailed entries on the patient care plan.

CASE 5. HELEN H, RADICAL MASTECTOMY

Mrs. Helen H has had a radical mastectomy. She is 38 years of age, married, and the mother of two children in their early teens. She is experiencing her first postoperative day. The team leader, Miss Hiskin, is seeing her for the first time and intends to start a nursing care plan. As she reviews the record, she sees that Mrs. H had first noticed a small, hard lump in the upper outer quadrant of the right breast. She waited two weeks before seeing a physician, hoping that the lump would disappear. Upon examination, her doctor recommended that the lump be biopsied as soon as possible. She was admitted to the hospital, and in surgery the tissue was found, by rapid frozen section, to be malignant. A later pathology report confirmed adenocarcinoma of the breast with metastasis to regional lymph nodes. A right radical mastectomy was done, removing the pectoralis major and minor, axillary fat, and the entire breast. A drain was inserted and a pressure dressing applied.

The recovery room notes and nurse's notes over the past 24 hours reveal that she is apparently well stabilized physiologically. Her vital signs are within normal range for her. She is voiding, turning, and deep breathing with help and is taking surgical liquids.

Current medical orders:
   Demerol, 100 mg prn q 4° for pain
   Connect drain to suction machine
   Liquids postnausea as tolerated, then diet as tolerated
   Catheterize q 8° if necessary
   Seconal 100 mg prn at hs
   Out of bed

Miss Hiskin, the nurse, enters the room and finds Mrs. H lying on her back, her body posture rigid, and her face drawn and tense. As the two begin speaking with one another, Miss Hiskin sits down to enable her to listen and to respond with less sense of distraction.

After talking for some time and after inspecting Mrs. H's dressing and drain, Miss Hiskin would review the information she has gathered in order to make decisions about her patient's problems.

Analyzing the Problems. The nurse identifies several problems as listed in the succeeding paragraphs. Each is followed by a description of some of Miss Hiskin's thinking that would result in decisions regarding the significance (usual or unusual) of the problems.

1. Serosanguineous drainage through drain, moderate amount for the first postoperative day. No seepage through dressing.
   Analysis: The drainage through the tube is of the expected color and amount for the first postoperative day. Since there is no seepage of blood through the dressing and since her vital signs are stable, it is reasonable to assume that there is no excessive incisional bleeding. The problem seems to be within the normal range.
2. Severe pain in operative site and aching of arm.
   Analysis: Mrs. H states that the Demerol does effectively relieve the pain, but that the aching returns about two hours after the last dosage and that she feels quite uncomfortable until it is again time for the medication. There is moderate edema of the right hand and arm. The episodes of severe aching that the patient experiences are a problem that nursing should attempt to resolve.
3. She is at high risk for hypostatic pneumonia because of the surgical immobilization of the chest.
   Analysis: Because she is deep breathing well and demonstrates this satisfactorily for Miss Hiskin and because she is physiologically stable, she is likely to ambulate and move about as necessary. Potential hypostatic pneumonia is probably not an unusual problem at this time.
4. The patient expresses anger, bitterness, and a sense of desperation about the loss of her breast and the cancer. She wonders whether they "really got it all." She says, "I can't bear this mutilation"; "I know my husband will say it makes no difference, but I'm afraid it will"; "I don't know that I want to go on living facing this, yet I'm afraid to die of cancer"; "This is terrible, I can't bear it"; "My whole life is changed, what can I do?"
   Analysis: Mrs. H is experiencing grief which is normal and expected. However, she seems unable at this time to cope with all of the ramifications of the problem. She needs special help.
5. Her husband is likely to be experiencing a great deal of stress

and worry over his wife's diagnosis. He may not know and understand the meaning of it nor feel adequate to support his wife through the crisis.

Analysis: This is definitely a possibility that should be checked out. Mr. H may be the critical element in Mrs. H's psychologic recovery.

6. There may be financial difficulties involved in this unexpected, long-term illness. Mrs. H has been working as a secretary prior to surgery.

Analysis: This is a problem that should be explored. It may become a significant problem for the family.

After reviewing and analyzing the problems, Miss Hiskin would write the following unusual problems on the care plan. Examples of the expected outcomes and nursing actions for Mrs. H are illustrated in subsequent chapters.

Helen H's Patient Care Plan

Physician's expectations regarding course of treatment convalescence:

(√) typical or routine

( ) atypical or complicated

If atypical or complicated, in what way?

Identifying information: _____

_____

_____

Diagnosis: Adenocarcinoma, rt _____

breast c̄ metastasis to regional _____

lymph nodes _____

Radical mastectomy, 6/3 _____

Nursing's criteria for discharge or maintenance (overall expected outcomes):

(a) Will demonstrate ability to do arm exercises correctly and to manage any necessary self-care.

(b) Will verbalize correct understanding of what to do in case of swelling, fatigue, or other complications.

(c) Ongoing verbalization (c̄ associated congruent feelings) of ability to cope c̄ the changes in her life.

   —active plans for getting and using prosthesis.

   —active plans for getting back into normal life style.

(d) Ongoing verbalization (c̄ associated congruent feelings) by husband re: ability to give his wife the necessary support.   S. Hiskin, RN

Home Care Coordination activities: _____

Other relevant information (socioeconomic, etc.): _____

Date	Unusual Problems
6/4	(1) Severe incisional pain and aching of right arm 3 hr after each pain medication, due to surgical trauma and pressure (edema) of rt arm
6/4	(2) Acute grief response and feelings of desperation due to loss of breast and associated changes in life style

Date	Unusual Problems
6/4	(3) Possible worry and concern by husband due to impact of diagnosis
6/5	(4) Possible financial problems associated with unexpected surgery and long convalescence

Summary. Although Miss Hiskin has identified a total of six problems, only four of them, in her judgment, would be considered unusual or possible problems. These are the only four that she writes in the unusual problems section of the care plan. She has set priorities based upon her judgment of whether the problems are usual or unusual.

SUMMARY

A clear statement of the patient's problem or problems is the obvious first step in the problem-solving process. The listing by a nurse of a patient's difficulties or concerns associated with a health problem is analogous to the physician's writing of his diagnosis. The listing of a patient's difficulties can be said to be the nursing diagnosis.

Since most patients have a wide range of problems, it is necessary for nurses to distinguish between the usual and unusual problems. It is time consuming and not necessarily productive to list on a patient's care plan all of the problems he may have. This system of care planning utilizes as its rationale for setting priorities the assigning of problems to the categories of "usual" and "unusual." Usual problems are not specifically handwritten in detail on the care plan but are managed through prewritten standard care plans. Only those problems considered to be unusual are entered in brief detail on the care plan and become the basis for subsequent setting of objectives (expected outcomes) and the writing of nursing orders.

For ease in thinking about and organizing unusual problems once they are identified, they are divided into three categories: actual, potential, and possible. Actual problems are those that do, in fact, exist at a given time, the time of the nurse's appraisal. Potential problems are those at unusually high risk for occurring in a given patient's situation. Possible problems are those that may or may not be actual or potential problems; further information must be obtained before a decision can be made.

Success in stating a problem requires brevity, clarity, and specificity. Since the problem statement is the first step in the problem-solving process, it must be on target. And it must be the patient's problems, not the nurse's, that are being described.

The process of gathering relevant data, mentally scanning them, developing hypotheses about problems, and then ruling them in or out as usual or unusual can be done quickly and easily once a nurse understands the basic guidelines and rationale for problem identification. The plan of care that emerges as a result of this systematic method of thinking and managing data yields relevant and highly useful information. At the same time it conserves and directs a nurse's time and energy for the priority problems constantly facing her.

REFERENCES

1. Rogers C: Client-centered Therapy. New York, Houghton-Mifflin, 1951
2. Rogers C: On Becoming a Person. New York, Houghton-Mifflin, 1961
3. Gebbit K, Lavin M (eds): Classification of Nursing Diagnoses. St. Louis, Mosby, 1976
4. Ragucci A: The ethnographic approach and nursing research. Nurs Res 21:6, Nov-Dec 1972
5. Spradley J, McCurdy D: The Cultural Experience: Ethnography in Complex Society. Chicago, Science Research Associates, 1972
6. Watson A, Mayers M: How to Write Nursing Care Plans. Stockton Cal, KP Co Medical Systems, 1976, p 17

BIBLIOGRAPHY

Bailey J, Claus K: Decision Making in Nursing. St. Louis, Mosby, 1975

Bower F: The Process of Planning Nursing Care. St. Louis, Mosby, 1972

Doona M: the judgment process in nursing. Image 8:27, June 1976, pp. 27—29

Johnson M, Davis M, Bilitch M: Problem-solving in Nursing Practice. Dubuque Iowa, Wm C Brown, 1970

Kelly M, Roessler L: Development of interdisciplinary problem-oriented recording in a public health nursing agency. J Nurs Admin 6:24, Dec 1976

Little D, Carnevali D: Nursing Care Planning, 2nd ed. Philadelphia, Lippincott, 1976

Lofland J: Analyzing Social Settings. Belmont Cal, Wadsworth Publishing Co, 1971

Schulman E: Intervention in Human Services. St. Louis, Mosby, 1974

Speir M: How to Observe Face-to-Face Communication: A Sociological Introduction. Pacific Palisades Cal, Goodyear Publishing Co, 1975

Sudnow D: Passing On: The Social Organization of Dying. Englewood Cliffs NJ, Prentice-Hall, 1967

Woolley F, Warnick M, Kane R, Dyer E: Problem-oriented Nursing. New York, Springer, 1974

4

The Expected Outcome: Criterion for Evaluation

FORMULATION OF EXPECTED OUTCOMES

A deficiency in some methods of care planning is the failure to recognize the need for stating criteria, or expected outcomes and deadlines, against which to measure nursing success or failure. A further failing is that the term *objectives* has generally been used by nursing to summarize the goals sought in individualized patient care planning. However, when the term *objectives* is used, the nurse's goals rather than the patient's goals tend to be the focus of the written plan and thus of the actual treatment. The use of the word *objectives* tends to distract the nurse from thinking in terms of the patient's goals. The utilization of the phrase *expected outcome* facilitates the use of a patient-centered problem-solving process. Therefore, instead of the word *objective*, the phrase *expected outcome* is consistently used in the working vocabulary of care planning in this text.

How to Write the Expected Outcome

After a nurse has specifically identified and stated an unusual patient problem, her next step is to follow it with a similarly concise statement of the intended or expected outcome. An expected outcome is a statement of the desired, or realistically expected, correction of the patient's problem by a certain point in time. Expected outcomes are those desired patient behaviors or clinical manifestations that will indicate that the problem is being resolved, is resolved, or has been prevented. [1,2]

For every unusual problem written on a care plan, a statement of the expected outcome must follow. In addition there must also be a projection of the point in time at which a correction, or partial correction, is expected to occur. For example, a patient mentioned in a previous chapter who had a low fluid intake (900 ml daily) might have an expected outcome statement such as: "2,500 ml fluid intake" by a date two days from the time of identification of the problem.

Like problem statements, expected outcome statements are brief and concise. An expected outcome statement should specify as clearly as possible what patient behavioral clinical manifestations will represent correction of the problem. When written definitively, the expected outcome becomes the standard, or criterion, for measuring the success or failure of nursing intervention. When the time for correction is reached, the expected outcome should be reached. This is the time to evaluate the situation. If the expected outcome has not been achieved on time, the obvious question is, "Why not?" Thus, the expected outcome statement and its deadline provide the basis for ongoing patient care evaluation.

Deadlines. Every expected outcome statement should have a projected deadline. Without deadlines or checking intervals, expected outcome statements are open-ended. There is no built-in safeguard for periodically evaluating the effectiveness or noneffectivensss of nursing actions. As the responsible registered nurse checks through the patient care plan, the deadline column should be reviewed to see which patients must be checked on this date or during this shift for progress toward expected outcome standards. Each patient with a deadline or checking interval for that day must be assessed regarding the specific problem and the expected outcome. A notation must then be made relevant to that item on the patient's progress notes or nursing care notes. If at this time it is seen that the patient is responding satisfactorily to the nursing care regimen, the prescribed nursing action will remain in effect. If, however, it is seen that the patient is not responding so as to meet the projected deadline, or if he is not meeting the standards for maintenance or for prevention of potential problems, it is then the nurse's responsibility to revise the prescribed nursing actions in such a way that the expected outcomes are most likely to be met. A reassessment of the problem may reveal that the problem itself was inaccurately stated, in which case a revised problem and plan are set up.

When it is not reasonably possible to set a date for the ultimate correction of a problem, intervals for checking progress should be indicated under the deadline column. In most cases, it is necessary to state checking intervals in addition to the ultimate deadline. Intervals for checking guarantee that a patient will receive interim evaluations of progress by the nurse.

Phrasing Expected Outcomes.   It takes practice to phrase expected outcomes so that they are clear enough to be measured or observed. Mager,[3] in his book on writing objectives, states that ". . . it is one thing to know what . . . represents the essence of your goal(s)," but it is something else to describe the nature or amount of behavior or performance that would cause you or a colleague to agree that the outcome is achieved. The task is to write brief phrases that describe the performance, behavior, level of knowledge, skill or ability in self-care, or the clinical manifestation(s) that can be observed or measured from shift to shift or day to day.

A practical guide for selecting the words and phrases that become the expected outcome statement is to ask, "What do I see or hear that makes me believe that the patient has a problem?" Is it what he says, how he looks, how he behaves, how his family behaves, or what? Whatever makes the nurse recognize a problem also provides her with the clues for determining the expected outcome. For instance, if a patient is thrashing about, groaning constantly, has tense and anxious facial expressions, and is bitterly complaining of severe pain in his right side, this behavior is the key to the criteria that should be listed as part of the expected outcome statement. In this case, the expected outcome statement can be set forth:

Date	Unusual Problems	Expected Outcomes	Deadlines
3/10	Severe pain, RLQ	Quiet and relaxed in bed Relaxed, peaceful facial expressions Statements by pt that pain is decreasing or absent	(3/11)

The criteria listed as expected outcomes in this example are taken directly from the patient's behavior, which indicates that he is in acute pain. They are stated so as to serve as specific guides for evaluating the resolution of the patient's pain. The more specifically expected outcome statements are written and the more clearly they refer to clues for evaluating the patient's progress, the more effective a nursing staff will be in measuring the success of their interventions.

The Expected Outcome as a Criterion for Evaluation

The expected outcome statement is the standard against which the success or failure of the nursing regimen is evaluated. This statement is essential to the evaluation of care. Without it, nursing cannot responsibly assess its own usefulness; it cannot ascertain the relative progress of a patient.

Common Categories of Expected Outcomes

As nurses increasingly use the concept of expected outcomes they find that most clues to patients' problems, and thus to expected outcome criteria, fall within four major categories.

1. *Patients' Verbalizations Regarding What They Know or Understand or How They Feel about a Situation or Circumstance.* This includes such factors as what a patient says about his illness, about its treatment, or about the physician's plans and expectations. It refers to his statements about his feelings or attitudes about his illness, his situation, events in his past, expected events, and so forth. Most of these factors can be appraised only by listening to a patient's verbalizations about them. Therefore, many criteria that are listed under expected outcomes are prefaced with "Verbalizations relating to . . . ," because that is the only way certain information becomes accessible to someone else, such as a nurse.

2. *Patients' Behavior Patterns Relating to Specific Situations.* This category refers to behavior or activities the nurse can observe, such as observations regarding a patient's socialization patterns, his dietary patterns, his employment patterns, and others. It specifically refers to competencies in any given area. For instance, a patient may demonstrate a minimal level of competence in managing his diabetic regimen. Several weeks later he may demonstrate significantly improved competence. Criteria for expected outcome statements that fall into this general category usually begin with the phrase "Demonstrates a satisfactory ability to. . . ." What a patient demonstrates to a nurse, either formally or informally, is the only way that certain information about his progress can be obtained.

3. *Patients' Traits, Behaviors, and Symptoms Relating to Illness, Disease Process, or Emotional Disability.* This category of behaviors is well known to most clinicians because it embodies the concept of the signs and symptoms of health or illness. Identification and measurement of these traits is accomplished in many ways—through laboratory and diagnostic tests, checking of vital signs, and observing behavior. By various means the signs and symptoms of a patient's health or illness status become known to a nurse. Checking one set of observations against another at a different point in time provides clues for the measurement of progress.

4. *Patients' Environment.* This fourth category refers to those circumstances in the patient's environment which have significance. How he keeps up his home, his clothing, or how his family functions around him are elements of this category. Expected outcome criteria referring to environmental conditions are stated descriptively, depending upon what is to be observed as significant.

These four categories provide a general framework for thinking about how to write expected outcome statements. *An expected outcome is a statement of what the nurse expects to observe, hear, or see demonstrated at a given point in time.* With practice and repetition, this process of setting standards, or defining expected outcomes, becomes easier, and it results in the acquisition of new intellectual skills that facilitate all aspects of patient care.

CRITERIA FOR DISCHARGE

An important ingredient of any patient care plan is a statement of the overall or long-range expected outcomes. In the system of care planning presented here, space for these statements is included in Chapter 1, p. 31.

As soon as enough information is available, the nurse should briefly but comprehensively state the criteria for discharge or maintenance, since these are the overall expected outcomes. The rules for writing statements of that sort are exactly the same as those previously elucidated except that these statements should indicate the expected behaviors, attitudes, competence, or signs and symptoms that represent a patient's satisfactory status at the time he is discharged from nursing's responsibility.

When patients are under long-term care, as in some extended care or home nursing settings, the overall expected outcomes refer to those conditions that are expected to be achieved and maintained.

With these overall criteria for discharge or maintenance as general guides for the ultimate expected status, more effective interim decisions can be made regarding the relative magnitude of problems that occur. If a problem occurs which, if left unresolved, will significantly interfere with reaching any of the overall expected outcomes by the time of discharge, it is apparent that that problem must be resolved.

At regular intervals, each patient's stated overall expected outcomes should be reviewed and evaluated to ascertain their current relevance. Significant unexpected changes in a patient's condition or diagnosis may well require a concomitant change in overall expected outcomes.

At the time of discharge, each patient's record should contain a brief documentation of the nurse's perception of the patient's status relative to each of the stated overall expected outcomes.

EXPECTED OUTCOMES FOR USUAL PROBLEMS

Patients who are listed as "having no unusual problems" require no handwritten expected outcome statements. The rationale for writing care plans for usual problems is detailed in Chapter 7.

For the usual problem patients analyzed in Chapter 3, the following plans illustrate how no unusual expected outcomes are handwritten on the form.

Case 1. Harry J, Emergency Appendectomy

Date	Unusual Problems	Expected Outcomes	Deadlines
2/18	No apparent unusual problems at this time		

Case 2. Carol J, Acute Cystitis

Date	Unusual Problems	Expected Outcomes	Deadlines
2/19	Apparently coping satisfactorily at this time		

Case 3. James R, Lumbar Laminectomy

Date	Unusual Problems	Expected Outcomes	Deadlines
2/17	No apparent unusual problems at this time		

Case 4. Alice M, A and P Repair

Date	Unusual Problems	Expected Outcomes	Deadlines
2/12	No apparent unusual problems at this time		

Case 5. Joyce H, Abdominal Hysterectomy

Date	Unusual Problems	Expected Outcomes	Deadlines
4/20	Apparently coping and progressing well		

EXPECTED OUTCOMES FOR UNUSUAL PROBLEMS

Further examples of expected outcome statements that might follow unusual problems are analyzed in the following paragraphs. The expected outcomes and deadlines are based on the 8 problems that are developed in Chapter 3.

Example 1

Date	Unusual Problems	Expected Outcomes	Deadlines
3/25	Low fluid intake (800 ml on 3/24) due to lifelong habit of "not drinking much"	Fluid intake: 1,200 ml by 3/25 1,800 ml by 3/26 2,500 ml by 3/27 and then daily	(3/27) √daily

Analysis. Because the problem statement clearly identifies the amount of low intake (800 ml), it is possible to write very specific expected outcome statements. The nurse would decide to make gradual increments so that, by the third day, the outcome of 2,500 ml will be reached and maintained. Each day the in-take-output sheet will confirm success or failure in reaching and maintaining the expected outcome.

Example 2

Date	Unusual Problems	Expected Outcomes	Deadlines
3/25	Decubitus ulcer (2 inch diameter, ¼ inch deep) over coccyx due to immobility and poor nutrition	↓ size and depth	√daily

Analysis.   Because the problem statement gives a clear baseline for measuring increase or decrease in the size and depth of the ulcer, daily documentation of its size and depth will indicate progress— or the lack of it. Because of the typically slow healing process of a decubitus ulcer, it may not be possible on a daily basis to measure decrease of size and depth. It would be possible, however, to note deterioration on a daily basis. It is for this reason that the checking interval is set for daily evaluation and documentation.

Example 3

Date	Unusual Problems	Expected Outcomes	Deadlines
3/25	Extreme anxiety due to unknown dx	Expressed fears Ask questions about dx	√daily

Analysis.   Since some anxiety regarding an unknown diagnosis is undoubtedly a normal response, the expected outcome is stated in terms of the behavioral clues that will indicate that the patient is coping more adequately. Daily (see deadlines column), a nurse will observe and interview the patient. She would document her findings regarding the expression of fears and asking of questions.

Example 4

Date	Unusual Problems	Expected Outcomes	Deadlines
3/24	Reluctant to take IPPB due to embarrassment from urinary incontinence due to to coughing when using IPPB	Actively participates in IPPB treatment	(3/26) √daily

Analysis.   Since the problem clearly states that the patient is "reluctant to take IPPB," his "active participation" will indicate progress. A nurse will observe or interview daily to ascertain whether the problem is resolving. Her findings will be documented on the patient's record. An ultimate deadline date of two days later has been entered because the nurse feels that the patient will be in jeopardy of hypostatic pneumonia if the problem is not totally corrected in a maximum of two days.

Example 5

Date	Unusual Problems	Expected Outcomes	Deadlines
3/24	Low caloric intake (1,000 calories on 3/24) due to confusion and distraction in hospital environment	Caloric intake: 1,500 calories by 3/25 2,000 calories by 3/26 2,500 calories by 3/27 and maintain	(3/27) √daily

Analysis.   Since the problem clearly defines the amount of low intake, it is possible to evaluate his progress toward the expected increments at daily intervals. The nurse would consult the physician and dietition in order to determine intelligently the ultimate desirable intake and the interim increments.

Example 6

Date	Unusual Problems	Expected Outcomes	Deadlines
3/26	Worried and upset due to complex family problems	Actively discuss how to deal with problems	√daily

Analysis.   At least daily, a nurse will document the patient's behavior relative to the criteria listed in the expected outcome statement. The nurse has not stated an ultimate deadline date because of the difficulty in predicting an individual's progress under these circumstances. She would, however, require daily evaluations (see deadlines column).

Example 7

Date	Unusual Problems	Expected Outcomes	Deadlines
3/15	Anxiety and fear due to dyspnea	Relaxed body posture Self-pacing of activities	√q8°

Analysis.   When checking every eight hours, the nurse will look for and document the patient's level of anxiety based upon the criteria listed under the expected outcome section. An ultimate deadline for the total resolution of the anxiety and fear is not listed because resolution will depend upon the correction of the dyspnea, which is a response to the physician's care. As a result, the time of the total relief of the dyspnea probably could not be predicted, and thus the associated relief of anxiety could not be predicted. Decreasing symptoms of anxiety, however, can be realistically expected.

Example 8

Date	Unusual Problems	Expected Outcomes	Deadlines
3/25	Feelings of panic due to memory loss due to CVA	Acknowledges memory lapses Relaxes when lapses occur Asks for memory joggers	√daily

Analysis.   This patient, who has feelings of panic and frustration due to memory loss associated with a cerebrovascular accident, will be evaluated daily regarding his ability to cope with his feelings. The nurse would interview or observe him to ascertain his progress. The results of the nurse's appraisal will be documented on the patient's record at daily intervals, as stated in the deadlines column.

EXPECTED OUTCOMES FOR ACTUAL, POTENTIAL, AND POSSIBLE PROBLEMS

For Actual Problems

When actual patient problems are identified and written on a care plan, the expected outcomes should be statements of the intended correction or solution of the problem. Included must be an ultimate deadline date for the total or partial correction of the problem. When deadlines for total or partial correction of a problem cannot realistically be predicted, it is necessary to determine the intervals at which documentation of progress (checking intervals) toward ultimate correction is to be made. In most cases, both an ultimate deadline for correction and periodic interim checking intervals should be written.

In order to illustrate how expected outcome statements should be written, the actual problem statements from Chapter 3 are rewritten below and are followed by an appropriate outcome statement. Deadlines and checking intervals are included. Ultimate deadlines are always placed within parentheses and checking intervals are written just below them.

Example 1

Date	Unusual Problems	Expected Outcomes	Deadlines
3/10	Depression and embarrassment (sad expression—speaks only when spoken to) due to facial disfigurement from lacerations	Smiles Initiates conversations	(3/20) √daily

Analysis. The patient's emotional status is assessed daily, as required by the deadline-checking interval. The nurse looks for evidence of decreasing depression (smiling and initiating conversation) in the patient's interactions. It has been predicted that by 3/20 there should be evidence of significant correction of the problem. If by 3/20 this does not occur, the problem will be reevaluated and rephrased, and new expected outcomes and deadlines would be written, or they might be left stated in the same way with new deadlines and checking intervals entered.

Example 2

Date	Unusual Problems	Expected Outcomes	Deadlines
3/12	Impaired circulation over coccyx, sacrum, and thoracic spine (3 inch diameter) due to emaciation, malnutrition, and immobility	↓ size of redness over areas	√daily

Analysis. The patient is evaluated daily as required by the deadline-checking interval. Since the sizes of the reddened areas are specified at the time the problem is identified, the nurse would observe and measure the size of the reddened areas to determine any relative decrease or increase in their size.

Example 3

Date	Unusual Problems	Expected Outcomes	Deadlines
3/20	Acute grief response due to death of husband in same accident (husband died 3/16)	Verbalizes loss Expresses emotions Increasing involvement c̄ personal needs and present problems	√q 8°

Analysis. Every eight hours a nurse will document that she has evaluated the patient's grief response. She will look for evidence of normal or abnormal emotional responses to loss. This would imply that the evaluating nurse has an adequate understanding of the process of loss so that the assessment will be meaningful and valid.

Example 4

Date	Unusual Problems	Expected Outcomes	Deadlines
3/8	Multiple decubiti: Rt trochanter, 3 inch diameter 1½ inch deep Lt trochanter, 4 inch diameter, 1 inch deep Sacrum and coccyx, 5 inch diameter, ¼-½ inch deep due to immobility, pressure, poor nutrition	↓ size and depth	√daily

Analysis.   At daily intervals a nurse will check the areas mentioned and will observe for an increase or decrease in the size and depth of the decubiti. Because the size and depth of each ulcer are described at the time the problem is identified, it would be possible at subsequent checking intervals to measure changes in their condition.

Example 5

Date	Unusual Problems	Expected Outcomes	Deadlines
3/10	Anxiety and restlessness due to dyspnea	Relaxed posture Self-pacing of effort and activity	√q 8°

Analysis.   At least every eight hours the nurse will document levels of relaxation and restfulness. Increasing or decreasing levels of these symptoms would indicate the failure or success of nursing intervention.

For Potential Problems

For potential problems, expected outcome statements must be somewhat different than for actual problems. For instance, most potential problem statements require that the expected outcomes be stated in terms of prevention or maintenance. They do not have an ultimate projected deadline for the correction or solution of the problem because the problem is only potential. It has not yet occurred. The difference, therefore, lies primarily in the fact that there is not an ultimate deadline date but, rather, specified checking intervals for documenting prevention, maintenance, or early detection. To illustrate, a patient in a previous chapter is described as elderly and emaciated, with a fractured hip. He has one potential problem, skin breakdown over the coccyx area. The expected outcome statement to follow such a potential problem might be "Prevention of skin breakdown over coccyx," or, better still, "No signs of redness over coccyx." Under the deadline column, a notation would require a nurse to check this every eight hours. For another instance, a surgical patient with a past history of recurrent chronic thrombophlebitis might have the problem, "Potential postoperative thrombophlebitis and pulmonary embolism." The expected outcome statement to follow might be, "Early detection of pain in calf of leg or pain in chest." Under the deadline column would be a notation requiring that a nurse check every eight hours.

In order to illustrate how expected outcome statements should be written, the potential problems from Chapter 3 are rewritten below and are followed by an appropriate outcome statement. Checking intervals are included in the deadline column.

Example 1

Date	Unusual Problems	Expected Outcomes	Deadlines
3/2	Potential postoperative bleeding due to hemophilia	Early detection of incisional bleeding	√q 8°

Analysis.   At least every eight hours a nurse will document that during the previous eight hours there has been no evidence of incisional bleeding. If there has been bleeding, the patient's record will reveal the time and magnitude of the bleeding as well as the follow-up measures that were instituted.

Example 2

Date	Unusual Problems	Expected Outcomes	Deadlines
3/10	Potential pressure areas of back and hips due to casting and traction of both legs	No redness over bony prominences of spine, sacrum, coccyx, and buttocks	√daily

Analysis.   In this case, at least daily a nurse will document that there are no reddened areas over the bony prominences indicated. In the event that reddened areas do develop, a new problem statement will need to be developed. The new statement would describe the size and location of redness.

Example 3

Date	Unusual Problems	Expected Outcomes	Deadlines
3/10	Potential uncontrolled diabetes due to language and culture difference, therefore lack of understanding of instructions	a. Db in control b. Verbal feedback indicating safe understanding of diabetes (diet, activity, insulin) c. Verbalizes ability to make applications to home setting	√qod

Analysis. At least every other day a nurse will document the level of the patient's understanding of diabetes and his plans for managing activity, diet, and insulin as it will apply in his own home. This is a problem that undoubtedly also would be referred to home care nursing supervision.

Example 4

Date	Unusual Problems	Expected Outcomes	Deadlines
3/8	Potential pp vaginal hemorrhage due to history of hemorrhage immediately postpartum	Early detection of bleeding	√q 8°

Analysis. The patient with potential postpartum hemorrhage will have entered into her record the status of her vaginal bleeding. Preferably it would be a pad count for the preceding eight hours. If hemorrhage has occurred during the preceding eight hours, the magnitude of the bleeding and any follow-up measures that have been instituted will have been documented at the time of occurrence.

Example 5

Date	Unusual Problems	Expected Outcomes	Deadlines
3/10	Potential injury from falling when ambulating due to poor coordination and weakness	No falls or near falls	√daily

Analysis.   At least daily, a nurse's statement on the patient's record would document the safety of ambulation during the prior 24 hours.

For Possible Problems

Items listed as possible problems do not have expected outcome statements written in the succeeding column. Since a specific problem has not been identified, it is impossible to make a statement of intended outcome. Only when further information has been gathered at an appropriate time and from appropriate sources can the possible problem be ruled out or found to be an actual or potential problem. It is then that a decision is made about whether it should appear on the nursing care plan format. If, when more information is obtained, the problem is found to be actual or potential—unusual—at that time an expected outcome statement will be written for it.

The possible problem statements listed in Chapter 3 will, when written on a care plan, have no entry under the expected outcome column. These are illustrated below.

Examples of Expected Outcome Statements for Possible Problems

Date	Unusual Problems	Expected Outcomes	Deadlines
3/8	Possible financial problems due to long convalescense		
3/10	Possibly worry over teenage children at home		
3/11	Possible concern regarding meaning of dx		
3/14	Possible lack of understanding of Dr's treatment regimen		
3/18	Possible worry over job and family adjustments to illness		

Analysis.   All of the possible problems, but none of the expected outcomes, should be entered on the care plan as shown in the preceding examples. Since an actual or potential problem has not yet been identified, it would not be possible to make an expected outcome statement about it.

The next chapter shows how the nursing actions column follows through from the statement of the possible problem.

CASE STUDY APPLICATIONS

Further examples of how to write expected outcomes for the five case studies cited in Chapter 3 are continued in the following paragraphs. Each case illustrates the next step of the problem-solving process—stating the expected outcome. Each care plan is followed by an analysis that explains how the expected outcomes are developed.

Case 1. Richard M, Multiple Traumatic Injury

Physician's expectations regarding course of treatment and convalescence:

( ) typical or routine

(√) atypical or complicated

If atypical or complicated, in what way?
Some possible unknown injuries, delayed reduction of mandible—Keep tracheostomy open for anesthesia for mandible reduction

Identifying Information: _____

_____

Diagnosis: Multiple trauma,

Fr zygoma, mandible, clavicle,

basilar skull

Intracranial clot

Facial lacerations

Tracheostomy

_____

Nursing's criteria for discharge or maintenance (overall expected outcomes):

(a) Patient and family will verbalize appropriate understanding of course of convalescence and indicate ability to follow through.

(b) They will demonstrate ability to manage any necessary care.

M. Fullington, RN

Home Care Coordination activities: _____

Other relevant information (socioeconomic, etc.): _____

Date	Unusual Problems	Expected Outcomes	Deadlines
4/20	(1) Extreme fear and anxiety, probably due to lack of understanding of tracheostomy and possibly due to lack of trust in staff—guards, pushes staff away from tracheostomy—has facial expressions of fear	(1) Facial expressions show trust No guarding	(1) (4/23) √daily
4/20	(2) Potential frustration and depression due to inability to communicate needs well. (Can't speak because of tracheostomy)	(2) Uses flash cards to communicate Expresses satisfaction (nonverbally) with staff's responses	(2) √daily
4/20	(3) Potential feelings of isolation and loneliness, because parents and friends live out of town and can't visit often	(3) Plays games with someone daily Makes friends with at least one person	(3) ∨daily

Date	Unusual Problems	Expected Outcomes	Deadlines
4/20	(4) Possible concern and lack of knowledge by parents re treatment progress and plans		
4/20	(5) Possible concern of patient and family re loss of school time		

Analysis. Problem (1), involving "extreme fear and anxiety," has an expected outcome statement: "Facial expressions show trust— No guarding." These items are the criteria for the nurse to look for when checking daily and for documenting progress on the patient's record. The nurse would chart the presence or absence of the behaviors that are listed.

Problem (2) lists "potential frustration and depression due to inability to communicate needs well." The expected outcome statement briefly indicates what behaviors are the criteria for assessing frustration and depression. At daily intervals the nurse would document the presence or absence of these behaviors.

Problem (3), "potential feelings of isolation and loneliness," has expected outcome statements indicating what behaviors will represent prevention of these feelings. At daily intervals the nurse would document on the patient's record the absence or presence of symptoms of isolation and loneliness.

Problem (4) and (5) are possible problems. As such, they are not followed by expected outcome statements. Once these possible problems are either ruled out or ruled in as actual or potential problems, they would be specifically restated and then be followed by appropriate expected outcome statements.

Case 2. Mary R, Postoperative Celiotomy, Cecostomy, Double-barreled Colostomy

Physician's expectations regarding course of treatment and convalescence:

( ) typical or routine

(√) atypical or complicated

If atypical or complicated, in what way?
Obese—abdominal wound will heal slowly.

Identifying Information: _____

_____

Diagnosis: Celiotomy, cecostomy, double-barreled colostomy, 4/8

_____

_____

Case 2. Mary R, Postoperative Celiotomy, Cecostomy, Double-barreled Colostomy (cont'd)

Nursing's criteria for discharge or maintenance (overall expected outcomes):
(a) Will verbalize appropriate understanding of medical regimen and follow-up.
(b) Will demonstrate satisfactory ability to irrigate own colostomy.
(c) Will verbalize feelings about colostomy, and state realistic plans for home
    care.   Mrs. Walker, RN
Home Care Coordination Activities: HCC notified on 4/14.

Other relevant information (socioeconomic, etc.):

Date	Unusual Problems	Expected Outcomes	Deadlines
4/14	(1) Very upset and embarrassed due to smell and mess of colostomy due to leakage	(1) No smell or mess Expresses approval of aesthetics	(1) (4/15) √a 8°
4/14	(2) Emotionally upset due to feuding of adult children over who will have to care for her	(2) Openly verbalize concerns Actively discusses "what to do"	(2) (4/17) √daily
4/14	(3) Potential surgical wound infection due to colostomy leakage	(3) No s/s of local redness or swelling No leakage to incision	(3) √q 8°

Analysis.   Problem (1), relating to "embarrassment over the smell and mess" of the colostomy, is followed by an expected outcome of "no smell and mess and approval of aesthetics" to be accomplished within one day.

On 4/15 a nurse will evaluate whether or not there is odor and leakage. If there is, more stringent nursing actions will be ordered. If successful, the originally prescribed orders will remain in effect. Every eight hours, and on 4/15, a nurse would enter a statement regarding the situation on the patient's record.

Problem (2) refers to the patient as being "emotionally upset." The expected outcome indicates two major criteria for ascertaining success or failure. The two criteria are (1) "openly verbalizes concerns" and (2) "actively discusses 'what to do.' " The final deadline is 4/17 (three days later), with interim daily checking intervals. By interview and observation the nurse will be able to assess whether the patient is making satisfactory or unsatisfactory progress toward the goal. Statements of progress would be entered in the patient's record at the required intervals.

Problem (3) states that there is "potential wound infection due to colostomy leakage." The major criterion, of course, is the absence of signs and symptoms of wound infection. However, once signs of wound infection develop, it is too late for prevention, so the nurse has added the second expected outcome criterion which is "no leakage to incision." The required intervals for documenting an evaluation of the patient against these criteria is every eight hours. At least every eight hours, the nurse will check the dressing to observe for incisional integrity and for the absence or presence of colostomy drainage to the incision. If, at the time of a sample inspection, the wound is free of leakage, she might make the assumption that this is consistently the case.

Case 3. Ralph L, Postoperative Right Hip Pinning and Active Pulmonary Tuberculosis

Physician's expectations regarding course of treatment and convalescence:

( ) typical or routine

($\sqrt{}$) atypical or complicated

If atypical or complicated, in what way? Malnourished, expect slow healing and slow progress regarding ambulation.

Identifying information: _____

_____

Diagnosis: Dehydration, malnutrition, active pulmonary tbc, left hip fracture pinned 3/20

_____

Nursing criteria for discharge or maintenance (overall expected outcomes):

(a) Will verbalize approval of convalescent facility or home care.

(b) Will demonstrate safe and efficient transfer and ambulation techniques.

(c) Will verbalize understanding of and demonstrate safe isolation technique for tbc.

(d) Will verbalize appropriate understanding of medical care regimen and ability to follow up.   L. Pratt, RN

Home Care Coordination activities: HCC notified on 4/5.

Other relevant information (socioeconomic, etc.): On Medicare hospital insurance. Social worker notified on 4/5.

Date	Unusual Problems	Expected Outcomes	Deadlines
4/5	(1) Potential pulmonary hemorrhage or spontaneous pneumothorax due to active pulmonary tbc	(1) Prevention and early detection—pt to verbalize understanding of s/s and his need to report	(1) $\sqrt{}$daily
4/5	(2) Potential constipation due to immobility and liquid diet	(2) Soft, formed stool, at least qod	(2) $\sqrt{}$even days
4/5	(3) Severe pain upon moving and turning due to fr left hip and decubitus of sacrum	(3) Reports that he is reasonably comfortable	(3) $\sqrt{}$q 8°

Case 3 Ralph L, Postoperative Right Hip Pinning and Active Pulmonary Tuberculosis (cont'd)

Date	Unusual Problems	Expected Outcomes	Deadlines
4/5	(4) Decubitus ulcer (sacrum) 2 inch diameter, ¼ inch deep due to immobility and poor tissue nutrition	(4) Continually ↓size and depth	(4) √daily
4/5	(5) Dry, itchy skin due to dehydration and frequent bathing	(5) Minimum or no dryness No itching	(5) (4/10) √daily
4/5	(6) Potential joint contractures due to immobility in bed	(6) Full range of motion, ankles	(6) √even days
4/5	(7) Dry, uncomfortable mouth and nose due to nasogastric tube and dehydration	(7) Moist, clean mucous membranes States that mouth and nose are comfortable	(7) (4/7) √q 8°
4/5	(8) Feelings of loneliness, fear, and depression due to no family, hospital isolation, and many unfamiliar procedures	(8) Participates in planning day's activities Asks questions and initiates conversations	(8) (4/10) √daily

Analysis.   Problem (1), "potential pulmonary hemorrhage" has an expected outcome of "prevention and early detection" as well as "patient verbalizes an understanding of the signs and symptoms" of spontaneous pneumothorax and understands that he should notify the nurse if any symptoms occur. The nurse will check daily and will record her appraisal of the presence or absence of signs and symptoms of pulmonary hemorrhage. She would also check the patient's knowledge about spontaneous pneumothorax.

Problem (2) refers to "potential constipation," and it is expected that the patient will have a "soft, formed stool at least every other day." The nurse will check every even day and would record what the bowel pattern is so as to ascertain success or failure in preventing constipation.

Problem (3) indicates "severe pain upon moving and turning." The expected outcome is that he will report that he is "reasonably comfortable." Every eight hours the nurse would document the patient's pain pattern to ascertain how effectively the problem of pain is being solved.

Problem (4) refers to the patient's "decubitus ulcer" and expects "continually decreasing size and depth." Because of the patient's poor general condition, the nurse would check the current size and depth of the ulcer frequently—every eight hours. Although a decrease in the size of an ulcer is difficult to detect as early as every eight hours, an increasing size and depth can be detected early. Therefore, it is imperative that it be checked that frequently.

Problem (5), "dry, itchy skin" is expected by 4/10 (five days later) to reveal "minimum or no dryness and no itching." A nurse would record her ongoing progress evaluations on a daily basis, as required by the deadlines column.

Problem (6), "potential joint contractures" is expected to be prevented. On even-numbered calender days, an RN would evaluate the patient's joint status and document her findings.

Problem (7), referring to "dry, uncomfortable mouth and nose," is expected to be resolved by 4/7 (two days later) with interim evaluation and documentation every eight hours.

Problem (8), "feelings of loneliness, fear, and depression," has expected outcomes that describe behaviors that would be consistent with decreasing depression and fear. This problem is projected to be resolved—so that the patient will be coping adequately—by 4/10, five days later, In the interim, an RN would interview, observe, and document his progress on a daily basis.

Case 4. Stephen F, Preoperative Cholecystectomy

Physician's expectations regarding course of treatment and convalescence:
   (√) typical or routine
   ( ) atypical or complicated
If atypical or complicated, in what way?

Identifying information: _____

Diagnosis: cholecystectomy 3/29

Nursing's criteria for discharge or maintenance (overall expected outcomes):
See standard postoperative expected outcomes.   J. Roth, RN

Home Care Coordination activities: _____

Other relevant information (socioeconomic, etc.): _____

Date	Unusual Problems	Expected Outcomes	Deadlines
3/29	Appears to be coping satisfactorily, both physiologically and psychologically.		√(3/31)

Analysis. Because on 3/29 the patient is "coping satisfactorily, both physiologically and psychologically," there is no need for an expected outcome statement. There is, however, a date of 3/31 listed under the deadlines column which means that, on that date, an RN will reevaluate him to determine his status. On 3/31 the patient will be experiencing his first postoperative day and will be at a point in his convalescence where new problems are likely to develop. It is for this reason that the patient would be scheduled to be rechecked on 3/31. Whenever a patient is listed as having no unusual problems, there still must be a date set for reevaluation. Judgments regarding the patient's health problem, his current general status, and his expected therapeutic episodes assist in setting a date for reevaluation.

Case 5. Mrs. Helen H, Radical Mastectomy

Physician's expectations regarding course of treatment and convalescence:
 (√) typical or routine
 ( ) atypical or complicated
If atypical or complicated, in what way?

Identifying information: _____
_____
Diagnosis: Adenocarcinoma, rt
breast c̄ metastasis to regional
lymph nodes.

Nursing's criteria for discharge or maintenance (overall expected outcomes):
(a) Will demonstrate ability to do arm exercises correctly and to manage
    any necessary self-care.
(b) Will verbalize correct understanding of what to do in case of swelling,
    fatigue, or other complications.
(c) Ongoing verbalization (c̄ associated congruent feelings) of ability to
    cope c̄ the changes in her life.
    —active plans for getting and using prosthesis.
    —active plans for getting back into normal life style.
(d) Ongoing verbalization (c̄ associated congruent feelings) by husband re:
    ability to give his wife the necessary support.   S. Hiskin, RN

Date	Unusual Problems	Expected Outcomes	Deadlines
6/4	(1) Severe incisional pain and aching of right arm 3 hr after each pain medication, due to surgical trauma and pressure (edema) of rt arm	(1) Statements by pt that arm is increasingly more comfortable	√q 8°
6/4	(2) Acute grief response and feelings of desperation due to loss of breast and associated changes in life style	(2) Verbalizes fears Looks at incision Asks questions and seeks information about recover Actively plans for prosthesis	√ daily

Date	Unusual Problems	Expected Outcomes	Deadlines
6/4	(3) Possible worry and concern by husband due to impact of diagnosis		
6/5	(4) Possible financial problems associated with unexpected surgery and long convalescence		

Analysis. Problem (1), "severe incisional pain and aching of right arm," is followed by an expected outcome statement which indicates that, if all progresses according to plan, the nurse expects Mrs. H when queried to state that the incision and her arm are increasingly more comfortable. Since pain is such a subjective phenomenon, statements by the patient regarding her own perceptions of the magnitude of the pain are, under the circumstances, the best criteria against which to measure progress. The deadlines column would require that a nurse check and document the patient's pain status every eight hours.

Problem (2) is "acute grief response and feelings of desperation." The expected outcome statement includes four criteria for evaluating the acute grief process. Miss Hiskin has indicated that a nurse should evaluate the patient's status against these criteria on a daily basis.

Problems (3) and (4) refer to possible problems. Since they have not yet been specifically identified nor ruled in or out, no expected outcomes are written.

SUMMARY

The expected outcome is a statement of the desired, or realistically expected, correction of the patient's problem. It logically follows the statement of the problem. It should specifically define the criteria a nurse must use when evaluating the patient's status. When written correctly, the expected outcome statement becomes an effective standard against which to compare the patient's actual response to care.

The expected outcome statement must also indicate the time or date by which the intended correction is expected to occur. When dates for ultimate correction of a problem cannot reasonably be stated, interim intervals for evaluating the patient's status must be indicated.

Expected outcomes are stated so as to provide definite clues to assessing, listening to, or observing the patient's status at specified deadlines. Most of the criteria and behaviors fall within four general categories: (1) Patients' verbalizations about what they know, understand, or feel, (2) patients' formal or informal demonstrations of competence, (3) patients' signs and symptoms related to their health or illness status, and (4) the significant elements in patients' environments.

The expected outcome statement is the standard against which the success or failure of the nursing regimen is evaluated. It is essential to the evaluation of care.

REFERENCES

1. Beitz D: Nursing Care Planning: A Teaching-Learning Module. Mountainview Cal, El Camino Hospital, 1976
2. Watson A, Mayers M: How to Write Nursing Care Plans. Stockton Cal, KP Co Medical Systems, 1976
3. Mager R: Goal Analysis. Belmont Cal, Fearon Publishers, 1972, pp 63–65

BIBLIOGRAPHY

Bailey J, Claus K: Decision Making in Nursing: Tools for Change. St. Louis, Mosby, 1975, p 131
Bower F: The Process of Planning Nursing Care. St. Louis, Mosby, 1972, p 117
Lewis L. Planning Patient Care. Dubuque Iowa, Wm C Brown, 1970 pp 57–64
Little D, Carnevali D: Nursing Care Planning. Philadelphia, Lippincott, 1976, pp 179–208

5

The Nursing Order: Process for Achieving Outcomes

DEFINITION OF NURSING ORDERS

With unusual or atypical patient problems identified and written, and with the expected outcomes and the deadline or checking intervals stated, it is then possible to decide upon and to write the nursing orders. A nursing order is a specifically recommended, individualized nursing activity designed to solve the patient's problem by a projected point in time. A nursing order is a nursing prescription.

In order to be useful to the staff, it is necessary that the nursing order be written concisely, clearly, and with specificity. Also it should be itemized if several nursing actions are necessary for the solution of one problem.

If prescribed nursing orders are to be effective and useful, it is important that they not repeat any other orders in the patient care system. For example, if a patient's problem is solved via a physician's order and requires no further specific nursing order to achieve an expected outcome, it should not be repeated under nursing orders. If only a medically prescribed action is necessary to achieve the expected outcome, it is not necessary for that specific problem to be identified or written in the unusual problems section. However, when certain nurse-prescribed orders are also necessary for solving the patient's problem, the requisite nursing order should be written in the appropriate section of the patient care plan. The medical orders regarding that particular problem and expected outcome will already be in the system via the physician's order section of the care plan; thus, they need not be repeated as a part of the nursing orders.

Before deciding upon one course of action, it is always wise to consider alternatives. What other methods might solve the problem? Little and Carnevali[1] discuss "branching logic" as a method of reconsidering alternatives, and Bailey and Claus[2] review a process for generating alternatives, for analyzing the alternatives, and for applying decision rules. Generating and considering various nursing interventions can be done in patient-care conferences, in consultation with a colleague, and, of course, in many circumstances with the patient himself or his family. Textbooks, past experiences, and assessment data also provide sources for ideas about alternatives. Each idea is carefully weighed in terms of its probability for success and its feasibility.

Lewis says:

> To develop creative and innovative approaches to any nursing problem requires . . . deliberative, critical thinking. . . . Each practitioner should have the time, energy and desire to develop creative and innovative approaches from time to time. Hopefully this will not be relegated only to the student, the researcher, or the clinical specialist. Rather, each nurse will come to know the joy and stimulation which can come from such an activity. It should be both a criterion for and a symbol of professional excellence.[3]

Whenever a nurse orders nursing actions for patient care, she should sign the order. As a professional person, she indicates by her signature that she is assuming responsibility for her decisions and judgments. The assumption of responsibility is a professional level of function. The signature has other beneficial side effects. Other staff members know with whom to discuss the orders for any necessary clarification. The signature also encourages colleagues to exchange ideas regarding care. A follow-up nurse may have a different perception of a patient's problems and care requirements from the ones that are written in the nursing orders. The signature lets her know with whom to share her perceptions. Nursing care can be significantly improved by a mutual sharing of ideas. Refinement of problem identification, goal setting, and care planning is the logical outcome of a mutual feedback process among staff persons.

NURSING ORDERS FOR USUAL PROBLEMS

Patients who are coping adequately with their problems may have standard nursing orders prescribed for them. For instance, an uncomplicated postoperative patient may very appropriately receive standard postoperative nursing care. However, for patients who do not have unusual problems, it is imperative that their care plans direct that continuing nursing assessments be made at appropriate intervals.

Examples

In previous chapters, case studies have been developed to show how to write care plan statements for patients with usual problems. Following are the same cases, with examples provided to show how to write nursing orders.

In these examples of "no unusual problems" the deadlines columns contain a date when the nurse must reevaluate the patient's progress.

In Table 5-1, the nurse has referred to the standard care section of the plan. She has ordered the postoperative standard care so that other nurses will know that certain specific care activities are required, including ambulation, deep breathing and coughing, vital signs at certain intervals, and so forth. The specific care that goes into a regular postoperative protocol is available for reference in many readily accessible places on the patient care unit. Orientation in the unit's standards of care should be part of every staff nurse's inservice education.

TABLE 5-1.   NURSING ORDERS FOR CASE 1, HARRY J, STANDARD CARE

Date	Unusual Problems	Expected Outcomes	Deadlines	Nursing Orders
2/18	No apparent unusual problems at this time		(2/20)	Standard care early postop J. Suchaki, RN

The nurse who sets up the postoperative routine for Harry J also uses the deadlines column, indicating that on 2/20 the patient must be reevaluated to determine whether or not he is still progressing satisfactorily. If at that time he is still progressing well, either another nursing care plan or the same one will be ordered. If, on or before 2/20, the patient is found to have an unusual problem, the problem will be written, followed by appropriate expected outcome and nursing order statements.

In any case, it is always necessary to set up deadlines for reevaluation of a patient.

Table 5-2 shows that because the nurse has assessed Mrs. J as coping satisfactorily with the symptoms and problems of her illness, the nurse orders a standard care plan. For this patient the nurse orders standard medical care, which includes such specific care items as vital signs at certain intervals, special observations, certain bathing and activity patterns, and so forth. Because these specific items are all outlined in the unit's care protocols, the nurse does not write all the items on the care plan. Rather, she indicates, "standard medical care," which automatically indicates that the specific items of that prewritten routine are ordered.

The nurse has indicated in the deadlines column that the patient should again be evaluated on 2/21, two days after the first assessment.

In the case of Mr. R (Table 5-3), who is assessed by the nurse on 2/17 and found to have no unusual problems, the standard care plan is referred to again. This time the nurse indicates "postoperative laminectomy." This plan includes certain turning, deep-breathing, active and passive exercises, vital signs, and other relevant items of care.

The nurse has indicated in the deadlines column that the patient should be reevaluated on 2/20.

Table 5-4 shows that the nurse evaluates Mrs. M preoperatively on admission and concludes that she has no apparent unusual problems at this time. The nurse refers to the standard care plans and indicates "standard preoperative care." This routine includes such specific care as vital signs at certain intervals, certain observations, teaching, and nursing support for the usual and appropriate apprehension prior to surgery, as well as other relevant care.

The nurse enters the date 2/22 in the deadline column. On 2/22, which will be the patients' first postoperative day, the patient will be reevaluated. If she is still found to have no unusual problems, she will have the appropriate "postoperative care" ordered.

Table 5-5 illustrates the care plan for Mrs. H. On her third postoperative day, Mrs. H is, in the nurse's judgment, coping well with the problems and concerns of a hysterectomy. As a result the nurse

TABLE 5-2.   NURSING ORDERS FOR CASE 2, CAROL J, STANDARD CARE

Date	Unusual Problems	Expected Outcomes	Deadlines	Nursing Orders
2/19	Apparently coping satisfactorily at this time		(2/21)	Standard medical care B. Garrison, RN

TABLE 5-3.   NURSING ORDERS FOR CASE 3, JAMES R, STANDARD CARE

Date	Unusual Problems	Expected Outcomes	Deadlines	Nursing Orders
2/17	No apparent unusual problems at this time		(2/20)	Postop laminectomy L. Christian, RN

TABLE 5-4.   NURSING ORDERS FOR CASE 4, ALICE M, STANDARD CARE

Date	Unusual Problems	Expected Outcomes	Deadlines	Nursing Orders
2/20	No apparent unusual problems at this time		(2/22)	Standard Pre op care J. Bennett, RN

TABLE 5-5.   NURSING ORDERS FOR CASE 5, JOYCE H, STANDARD CARE

Date	Unusual Problems	Expected Outcomes	Deadlines	Nursing Orders
4/20	Apparently coping and progressing well		(4/23)	Late postop care C. Deming, RN

orders the "late postoperative care." This includes certain observations, support, activity, and vital signs patterns which are different in nature and intensity from an "early postoperative care," which would normally be in effect for the first three days after surgery.

The nurse has indicated in the deadlines column that the patient should be reevaluated on 4/23, which is expected to be about the time of discharge from the hospital. In any case, if a patient is discharged before the anticipated date, a discharge evaluation is always necessary. A discharge evaluation is done to identify any previously undiscovered, relevant unusual problems and to make appropriate referrals to the physician or other community resources. The discharge evaluation also verifies that the patient understands his home care regimen and his doctor's appointment schedule and that he will be able to meet these requirements for his safe and satisfactory convalescence.

NURSING ORDERS FOR UNUSUAL PROBLEMS

Further examples of how to write nursing orders are illustrated on subsequent pages. The nursing actions that follow the unusual problems and their extension from Chapter 4 are portrayed.

Examples

In Table 5-6, the nursing order notifies the staff that the patient is involved in making and meeting his own intake schedule and that the staff's job is to give positive reinforcement.

TABLE 5-6. NURSING ORDERS FOR UNUSUAL PROBLEM, LOW FLUID INTAKE

Date	Unusual Problems	Expected Outcomes	Deadlines	Nursing Orders
3/25	Low fluid intake (800 ml, 3/24) due to lifelong habit of "not drinking much"	↑ fluid intake 1,200 ml, 3/25 2,000 ml, 3/26 2,500 ml, 3/27	(3/27) √daily	Give pt positive reinforcement in keeping track of intake and making and keeping an intake schedule (Pt knows and accepts need to drink more—will keep own records) I. Schulz, RN

In Table 5-7, the nursing orders clearly specify just how and when to provide care for the patient's decubitus ulcer. The nursing orders

TABLE 5-7. NURSING ORDERS FOR UNUSUAL PROBLEM,
DECUBITUS ULCER

Date	Unusual Problems	Expected Outcomes	Deadlines	Nursing Orders
3/25	Decubitus ulcer (2 inch diameter, ¼ inch deep) over coccyx due to immobility and poor nutrition	↓ size and depth	√daily	a. Turn alternately q 2 hr to rt and left sides and prone (no lying on back) b. At night, turn q 3 hr c. Digital circular mss to bony prominences of spine and hips when turned d. Clean sheepskin in direct contact c̄ skin at all times e. Take time necessary to assist c̄ total intake of special diet S. Haney, RN

statement could possibly be improved by giving specific hours for
turning rather than giving a general turning schedule.

Table 5-8 reveals, in the case of this patient who has extreme
anxiety due to unknown diagnosis, that the nursing action, which
requires developing a relationship and providing active support for
minimum amounts of time, has been delegated to two nurses, one

TABLE 5-8. NURSING ORDERS FOR UNUSUAL PROBLEM,
EXTREME ANXIETY

Date	Unusual Problems	Expected Outcomes	Deadlines	Nursing Orders
3/25	Extreme anxiety due to unknown dx	Express fears Asks quesstions about dx	√daily	a. Spend 30 min each AM and PM shift at bedside actively listening and responding to anxieties and concerns (Delegated to L. Swanson AM and M. Dains PM J. Canaris, RN

on each of the two daytime shifts. These two nurses need to communicate well with each other for both to be helpful to the patient.

In Table 5-9, the nursing actions designed to solve the patient's embarrassment are simply stated and outlined. The actions should certainly facilitate the expected outcome to be reached by 3/26.

TABLE 5-9.   NURSING ORDERS FOR UNUSUAL PROBLEM,
RELUCTANCE TO TAKE TREATMENT

Date	Unusual Problems	Expected Outcomes	Deadlines	Nursing Orders
3/24	Reluctant to take IPPB due to embarrassment from incontinence due to coughing when using IPPB	Actively participate in IPPB treatment	(3/26) √daily	a. Be matter-of-fact about problem b. Place pads under pt before each treatment c. Allow her to clean herself up after treatment d. Keep deodorant spray available B. Patterson, RN

Table 5-10 illustrates that, since the cause of the low intake is believed to be the distracting environment, the nursing actions are specifically designed to solve that basic problem.

TABLE 5-10.   NURSING ORDERS FOR UNUSUAL PROBLEM,
LOW CALORIC INTAKE

Date	Unusual Problems	Expected Outcomes	Deadlines	Nursing Orders
3/24	Low caloric intake (1,000 cal 3/24) due to confusion and distraction in hospital environment	↑ cal. intake 1,500 cal 3/25 2,000 cal 3/26 2,500 cal 3/27 and maintain	(3/27) √daily	a. Plan care to be completed 30 min in advance of each meal b. Stay c̄ pt at mealtime and encourage self-feeding Help to feed if necessary c. Keep conversation and mood calm and unhurried during meals G. Barnaby, RN

In Table 5-11, the emotional problem requires an ongoing trust relationship, so the task has been delegated to one nurse for follow-up. This nurse will be a resource to the remainder of the staff so that all of the patient's care will be within a consistent frame of reference.

TABLE 5-11. NURSING ORDERS FOR UNUSUAL PROBLEM, EMOTIONAL UPSET

Date	Unusual Problems	Expected Outcomes	Deadlines	Nursing Orders
3/26	Emotionally upset due to complex home and family problems	Actively discusses how to deal with problem	(3/30) √daily	Initiate conversations c̄ pt to clarify and explore concerns and ways of coping c̄ them (Delegated to R. Roberts, RN) J. Landers, RN

TABLE 5-12. NURSING ORDERS FOR UNUSUAL PROBLEM, ANXIETY AND FEAR

Date	Unusual Problems	Expected Outcomes	Deadlines	Nursing Orders
3/15	Anxiety and fear due to dyspnea	Relaxed body posture Self-pacing of activities	√q 8°	a. Keep bed elevated 30°-45° b. Space care to 10 min periods 45 min apart. Then allow 1 to 2° rest period, 4 times daily c. O to 8 l/min during periods of necessary exertion S. Sauer, RN

In Table 5-12, anxiety and fear are believed to be due to dyspnea. The nursing actions are designed to minimize the symptom. In this patient's case the nurse has found that frequent, short periods of care are the most effective. Such information, clearly written for all staff to implement, will certainly minimize trial and error and will conserve the patient's energy.

In Table 5-13, in order to help the patient cope with his panic over memory loss, two simple and clear nursing actions have been stated.

TABLE 5-13. NURSING ORDERS FOR UNUSUAL PROBLEMS,
FEELINGS OF PANIC

Date	Unusual Problems	Expected Outcomes	Deadlines	Nursing Orders
3/25	Feelings of panic due to memory loss due to CVA	Acknowledges memory lapses Relaxes when occur Asks for memory jogger	√daily	a. Respond postively and matter-of-factly to to pt's concerns b. Recall recent events with patient to reinforce feelings of ability to remember B. Wolfe, RN

NURSING ORDERS FOR ACTUAL, POTENTIAL, AND POSSIBLE PROBLEMS

When the unusual problem has been stated well and the expected outcome has been clearly indicated, along with deadlines or checking intervals, it then becomes possible to write nursing orders, or nursing action statements. To write nursing orders without having completed the first two steps is to run the risk of instituting care that does not have a specifically justified rationale.

Actual Problems

In order to illustrate how nursing orders should be written, the actual problems and expected outcome statements from Chapter 4 are rewritten on subsequent pages and are followed by an appropriate set of nursing orders.

Table 5-14 illustrates that nursing orders a, b, and c are specific actions which the nurse believes will result in achievement of the expected outcome by 3/20. Additionally, item d, "Discuss problem with family and physician and obtain their ideas and assistance for a positive coping process," is added. Notice that the particular order was delegated to an RN on the staff who the responsible nurse believes is able to follow through. Many orders requiring significant, well-coordinated follow-up are the best delegated to one nurse. That nurse then assumes responsibility for that phase of the care and becomes a resource person for the rest of the staff caring for the patient. If item d were not delegated to one RN, several nurses in succession might talk with the family and physician, each from a dif-

TABLE 5-14. NURSING ORDERS FOR UNUSUAL PROBLEM,
DEPRESSION AND WITHDRAWAL

Date	Unusual Problems	Expected Outcomes	Deadlines	Nursing Orders
3/10	Depression and withdrawal (sad expression, speaks only when spoken to) due to facial disfigurement from lacerations	Smiles Initiates conversation	(3/20) √daily	a. Use a positive, direct, matter-of-fact approach regarding face and lacerations b. Take time for patient to verbalize her feelings about her face c. Work aggressively with patient in devising ways to cope with problem Cosmetic surgery is a possibility d. Discuss problem c̄ family and physician and obtain their ideas and assistance for a positive coping process (To be done by B. Watters, RN P. Patterson, RN

ferent frame of reference, and ultimately only add confusion to the care process. Many nursing actions of this nature must be delegated to one particular nurse for follow-up. Delegation of specific patient care is done after consultation with the nurse and only with her positive acceptance of the responsibility.

Table 5-15 illustrates that the nursing orders for this problem are very specifically outlined, leaving no doubt as to the intended care regimen. The type of massage for the reddened areas is clearly stated, as well as the length of each massage treatment. Times for turning are also specifically stated, leaving no doubt or confusion about the schedule. Since the problem is partly caused by emaciation, the nursing orders include positive diet guides.

In Table 5-16, items a, b, and c give staff nurses direct guidance in responding to and working with the patient, to help her cope with her grief. Item d, "Discuss problem with physician and family to facilitate the 'grief work,'" is another order that has been delegated to one specific nurse. It is apparent that just one nurse following through can facilitate understanding among all members of the team, including the patient and family.

TABLE 5-15.   NURSING ORDERS FOR UNUSUAL PROBLEM,
PRESSURE AREAS

Date	Unusual Problems	Expected Outcomes	Deadlines	Nursing Orders
3/10	Reddened areas over coccyx and sacrum (3 inch diameter) due to emaciation, malnutrition, and immobility	↓ size of redness over areas	√daily	a. Clean, full-size sheepskin under patient at all times (No linen or pads between pt and sheepskin) b. Gentle digital circular massage to areas mentioned (3 min to each area) each time turned Same massage to all other bony prominences each time turned c. Turn q 2 hours during day—8-10-12-2-4-6-8 Turn q 3 to 4 hours at night—11-1-5 d. Assist with ordered meals and fluids so that total amount is taken Hi vit and pro diet (5 small feedings) 2,000 ml water or juice q 24° B. Valentine, RN

Table 5-17 illustrates nursing orders that outline specifically what should be done and when it should be done. Actions include giving attention to the special diet, which is certainly a relevant part of the solution of the problem..

Table 5-18 shows that, in order to achieve decreased symptoms of anxiety and diminishing restlessness, four nursing actions have been developed. Since the cause of the anxiety and restlessness is believed to be dyspnea, the nursing care is designed to minimize dyspnea. This, in turn, should result in decreased anxiety and restlessness. The nurse writing this care plan has found that the patient responds best to care performed in blocks of time between comparatively long periods of undisturbed rest. Stating this on the care plan will prevent each nurse having to find that fact out for herself and will result in less energy expenditure by all.

TABLE 5-16. NURSING ORDERS FOR UNUSUAL PROBLEM,
ACUTE GRIEF

Date	Unusual Problems	Expected Outcomes	Deadlines	Nursing Orders
3/17	Acute grief response due to death of husband in same accident (Husband died 3/16)	Verbalizes loss Expresses emotions Increasing involvement c̄ personal needs and present problems	√q 8 hr	a. Respond to patient's desire to be alone or to have company b. Be positive regarding at least minimal involvement c̄ meals and personal hygiene c. Make it ok for patient to express her emotions in presence of nurse d. Discuss problems c̄ physician and family to facilitate the "grief work" (Delegated to L. Swanson, RN) S. Forsman, RN

TABLE 5-17. NURSING ORDERS FOR UNUSUAL PROBLEM,
MULTIPLE DECUBITI

Date	Unusual Problems	Expected Outcomes	Deadlines	Nursing Orders
3/10	Multiple decubiti, rt trochanter, 3 inch diameter, ½ inch deep, lt trochanter 4 inch diameter, 1 inch deep, sacrum and coccyx 5 inch diameter, ¼-½ inch deep, due to immobility, pressure, poor nutrition	↓ size and depth	√daily	a. Circle bed: Prone position, 2° supine, and semisupine 1° Then repeat day and night b. Direct contact with sheepskin under total body—except for drsgs as ordered over ulcerated area c. Take time necessary to assist c̄ special hi vit, lo protein diet, and 2,500 ml water or juices q 24° L. Raminez, RN

TABLE 5-18. NURSING ORDERS FOR UNUSUAL PROBLEM,
ANXIETY AND RESTLESSNESS

Date	Unusual Problems	Expected Outcomes	Deadlines	Nursing Orders
3/10	Anxiety and restlessness due to dyspnea	Relaxed posture Self-pacing of effort and activity	$\sqrt{q}$ 8°	a. Keep bed elevated 20 to 45° b. Plan care to be done in blocks of time leaving long periods for undisturbed rest Turn up O_2 to 10 l/min during required exertional activities c. Use quick, smooth movements on the part of the patient and nurse to minimize energy output d. Explain what and why of care Give complete answers to questions J. Litizzette, RN

Potential Problems

For the category of problems that are potential, nursing orders are written just as for actual problems with the difference that these orders are geared toward preventing the onset of actual problems.

The examples below further develop the potential problem statements analyzed in Chapter 4.

Table 5-19 illustrates how, to guarantee early detection of incisional bleeding, very specific instructions are outlined for covering the first 24 hours after surgery when the danger of bleeding is greatest. The deadline date is 3/3, 24 hours later. At that time, depending upon the patient's progress, the orders should be discontinued or modified.

In Table 5-20, nursing care for preventing redness over bony prominences of back and hips is carefully and completely itemized so that all staff on all shifts will follow through in the same manner.

In Table 5-21, the nursing order that is designed to prevent potential uncontrolled diabetes in a patient with a language and cultural barrier has been delegated to one nurse for follow-through. Developing a relationship and communicating effectively for teaching–learning purposes are activities of such complex nature that

TABLE 5-19. NURSING ORDERS FOR UNUSUAL PROBLEM, POTENTIAL POSTOPERATIVE HEMORRHAGE

Date	Unusual Problems	Expected Outcomes	Deadlines	Nursing Orders
3/2	Potential bleeding due to hemophilia	Early detection of incisional bleeding No hematoma No bright red bleeding	(3/3) √q 8°	a. Note any bleeding through drsg (estimate size—dime, nickel, quarter, etc) √q 15 min 1st hr po √q 30 min 2nd and 3rd hr po √q 1 hr 4th to 12th hr po then q 2 hr remainder of 1st 24 hr b. √area around drsg for signs of subcutaneous hemorrhage B. Joynes, RN

TABLE 5-20. NURSING ORDERS FOR UNUSUAL PROBLEM, POTENTIAL PRESSURE AREAS

Date	Unusual Problems	Expected Outcomes	Deadlines	Nursing Orders
3/10	Potential pressure areas of back and hips due to casts and traction of both legs	No redness over bony prominences— spine, sacrum coccyx, and buttocks	√daily	a. Digital circular massage for 5 min over areas listed, q 2° during day, q 3° during night b. Lift pt straight up to do back care. Three persons needed—one on each side to support hips—third person to do back care c. Use hospital mss lotion for care—wipe off—apply cornstarch d. Keep all areas in direct contact c̄ clean sheepskin M. Reynolds, RN

TABLE 5-21.   NURSING ORDERS FOR UNUSUAL PROBLEM,
POTENTIAL UNCONTROLLED DIABETES

Date	Unusual Problems	Expected Outcomes	Deadlines	Nursing Orders
3/10	Potential uncontrolled diabetes due to language and cultural differences— lack of understanding of instructions	a. Db in control b. Verbal feedback indicating understanding c. Verbalizes ability to make applications to home setting	√qod	a. Ongoing teaching regimen (delegated to L. Swanson, RN— obtain skilled, Spanish interpreter, meal plans, and Spanish literature) of db, diet, activity, and insulin c̄ applications to home setting M. Ratekin, RN

one nurse performing them in a consistent manner is more likely to
be successful than several nurses each acting in her own manner.
That nurse can then become a resource person for other staff members so that their care will support, or at least not confuse, the major
teaching-learning activity.

TABLE 5-22.   NURSING ORDERS FOR UNUSUAL PROBLEM,
POTENTIAL INJURY

Date	Unusual Problems	Expected Outcomes	Deadlines	Nursing Orders
3/10	Potential injury from falling when ambulating due to poor coordination and weakness	No falls or near falls	√daily	a. Get pt out of bed from side of bed to his left b. With pt dangling, lower bed until feet are flat on floor. Face him—he will put hands on nurse's shoulders and stand up. Nurse assist c̄ her hands under axilla c. Pt will walk c̄ cane in rt hand Nurse walk on pts left d. Walk length of hall to lounge 2 times daily e. Back to bed—same way A. Finch, RN

Table 5-22 shows that, in order to accomplish the expected outcome of "no falls," a complete set of instructions for ambulating the patient has been outlined. Falls will be prevented not only because the instructions are specific and geared to the patient but also because all staff will function with the patient in the same way, minimizing confusion.

Table 5-23 illustrates that, to insure early detection of postpartum hemorrhage, a detailed pad-checking schedule for the first 24 hours is set up. On 3/9, 24 hours later, the care will be discontinued or modified, depending upon the patient's progress. For this patient, the doctor had ordered a safe schedule of vital signs evaluation. If that schedule had not been ordered by the doctor, the nurse herself would have added an appropriate schedule for vital signs checking. But when the doctor's order has covered certain care, the order is not repeated in the nursing orders. The doctor's orders already appear in another part of the total patient care plan.

TABLE 5-23. NURSING ORDERS FOR UNUSUAL PROBLEM,
POTENTIAL POSTPARTUM HEMORRHAGE

Date	Unusual Problems	Expected Outcomes	Deadlines	Nursing Orders
3/8	Potential pp vaginal hemorrhage due to history of hemorrhage in delivery room	Early detection of hemorrhage No more than one pad per hr	(3/9) √q 8°	a. √pads and mss fundus q 15 min 1st 2° pp, q 30 min next 4° pp, q 1° next 6° pp, then q 3° next 12° P. Toney, RN

Possible Problems

For problems listed as "possible," more information is needed before a decision can be made regarding whether they are problems at all. If they are, it must be decided whether they are unusual problems. Nursing orders are related to how, when, and from whom further information bearing on this point should be obtained. The deadlines column is used to indicate a time limit for obtaining further data and for ruling the possible problem in or out. To show that a date in the deadline column refers to a deadline for nursing action, not for patient progress, an arrow or line can be used.

The following pages illustrate how nursing orders might be written when they follow possible problems.

Table 5-24 shows that before 3/15 further information is expected that will clarify whether the possible financial problem should be ruled in or ruled out. Because of the personal nature of the family's finances and because a continuum of interviews may be needed to decide whether or not this is an unusual problem, the task has been delegated to one nurse for follow-through.

TABLE 5-24.   NURSING ORDERS FOR POSSIBLE FINANCIAL PROBLEM

Date	Unusual Problems	Expected Outcomes	Deadlines	Nursing Orders
3/8	Possible financial problems due to long convalescence		(3/15)	Discuss c̄ wife and make any appropriate referrals (Delegated to M. Dains, RN) P. McHugh, RN

On or before 3/15, M. Dains, RN, will either discontinue the possible problem or will write the actual financial problem she has found. She will then develop any appropriate new nursing orders. If the financial problem is delegated to a social worker or other resource person a notation to that effect should be made on the chart and the problem crossed off the unusual problems section of the care plan.

In Table 5-25, the "possible worry over teenage children at home" and the need to obtain more information by 3/15 has again been delegated to one nurse as the most effective way of following through.

TABLE 5-25.   NURSING ORDERS FOR POSSIBLE PROBLEM, WORRY

Date	Unusual Problems	Expected Outcomes	Deadlines	Nursing Orders
3/10	Possible worry over teenage children at home		(3/15)	Initiate conversations c̄ pt to ascertain (Delegated to M. Dains, RN) P. McHugh, RN

Tables 5-26, 5-27, and 5-28 show that the stated possible problems require further information and clarification to be obtained about the patient's concerns. In order to accomplish this effectively, the task in each case has been delegated to one nurse.

TABLE 5-26. NURSING ORDERS FOR POSSIBLE PROBLEM, IGNORANCE OF DIAGNOSIS

Date	Unusual Problems	Expected Outcomes	Deadlines	Nursing Orders
3/11	Possible concern regarding meaning of dx		(3/13)	Initiate conversations c̄ pt to clarify and ascertain her understanding and fears (Delegated to H. Moore, RN) R. Rote, RN

TABLE 5-27. NURSING ORDERS FOR POSSIBLE PROBLEM, MISUNDERSTANDING REGIMEN

Date	Unusual Problems	Expected Outcomes	Deadlines	Nursing Orders
3/14	Possible lack of understanding of Dr's treatment regimen		(3/15)	Initiate conversation c̄ pt to clarify and ascertain (Delegated to S. Hoffman, RN) R. Campos, RN

TABLE 5-28. NURSING ORDERS FOR POSSIBLE PROBLEM, ADJUSTMENT

Date	Unusual Problems	Expected Outcomes	Deadlines	Nursing Orders
3/18	Possible worry over job and family adjustment to illness		(3/21)	Initiate conversation c̄ pt to ascertain and clarify (Delegated to S. Hoffman, RN) L. Hurley, RN

CASE STUDY APPLICATIONS

The five example cases developed in the previous two chapters are continued here. In this section the nursing orders column is completed. Each nursing order is followed by an analysis.

Case 1. Richard M, Multiple Traumatic Injury

Physician's expectations regarding course of treatment and convalescence:

( ) typical or routine

(√) atypical or complicated

If atypical or complicated, in what way? Some possible unknown injuries, delayed reduction of mandible—Keep tracheostomy open for anesthesia for mandible reduction.

Identifying Information: _____

_____

_____

Diagnosis: Multiple trauma,

Fr zygoma, mandible, clavicle,

basilar skull,

Intracranial clot

Facial lacerations

Tracheostomy

Nursing criteria for discharge or maintenance (overall expected outcomes):

(a) Patient and family will verbalize appropriate understanding of course of convalescence and indicate ability to follow through.

(b) They will demonstrate ability to manage any necessary care.

M. Fullington, RN

Home Care Coordination activities: _____

Other relevant information (socioeconomic, etc): _____

Date	Unusual Problems	Expected Outcomes	Deadlines	Nursing Orders
4/20	(1) Extreme fear and anxiety, probably due to lack of understanding of tracheostomy and possibly due to lack of trust of staff— guards, pushes staff away from tracheostomy— has facial expressions of fear	(1) Facial expressions show trust No guarding	(1) (4/23) √daily	(1) a. On each shift *one* nurse to do tracheostomy care. AM nurse L. Swanson delegated to assume initial responsibility for setting up specific and consistent way of doing tracheostomy care and to write on care plan and explain to other shift nurses b. Take time to clarify and explain procedure Gradually teach him how to plug trach and to speak so he can express himself

Date	Unusual Problems	Expected Outcomes	Deadlines	Nursing Orders
				c. Include family in plan Allow them to express their concerns regarding tracheostomy Enlist their support and participation as appropriate M. Fullington, RN
4/20	(2) Potential frustration and depression due to inability to communicate needs well. (Can't speak because of tracheostomy)	(2) Uses flash cards to communicate Expresses satisfaction (nonverbally) with staff's responses	(2) √daily	(2) a. Gradually teach pt to plug tracheostomy so that he can communicate c̄ his voice (see bedside instructions) b. Develop a flash card system for the usual needs—bedpan, water, pain, etc (see bedside instructions) Keep a writing pad and pencil available c. Spend extra time c̄ pt to learn his needs and to anticipate them better and to facilitate a trust relationship M. Fullington, RN
4/20	(3) Potential feelings of isolation and loneliness, because parents and friends live out of town and can't visit often	(3) Plays games with someone daily Makes friends with at least one person	(3) √daily	(3) a. Enlist parents' support in getting friends to set up a rotating visiting schedule b. Introduce pt to other teenage pts on unit c. Continue to ascertain needs for books, hobby supplies, records, etc Enlist parents' active leadership d. On days when visitors can't come, spend more time c̄ pt— play games, etc M. Fullington, RN
4/20	(4) Possible concern and lack of knowledge by parents re treatment		4/23	(4) Initiate discussions c̄ parents to ascertain the accuracy of their understanding Clarify and enlist help as needed

Date	Unusual Problems	Expected Outcomes	Deadlines	Nursing Orders
	progress and plans			(Delegated to M. Brown, RN) M. Fullington, RN
4/20	(5) Possible concern of patient and family re loss of school time		4/23	(5) Initiate discussions c̄ family and patient to clarify plans (Delegated to M. Brown, RN M. Fullington, RN

Analysis of Nursing Orders, Mr. Richard M. Nursing order (1), a through c, specifically delegates to certain nurses the responsibility for various aspects of care. Items b and c provide a general frame of reference for the care. As soon as a specific tracheostomy care regimen for this patient has been developed, it will be clearly written in easy to understand steps, will be posted at the bedside, and will be referred to on the patient care plan. By delegating duties to certain nurses and by providing a general guide for care, the responsible nurse has minimized the possibility of further confusion and its consequent anxiety and lack of trust.

Nursing order (2), a through c, includes specific guides for preventing frustration due to the patient's inability to communicate well. All staff will utilize and implement these guides. The bedside instructions referred to would be developed and posted by the nurse delegated to do so in nursing action (1).

Nursing order (3), a through d, provides specific guidelines to staff for minimizing the patient's feelings of isolation. The staff is reminded to enlist his parents in assuming leadership in this project. Item d makes clear that part of his nursing care is for the staff to play games and spend time with him on days when other visitors are at a minimum.

Nursing orders (4) and (5) delegate to M. Brown, RN, the responsibility for gathering more information regarding the parents' possible lack of knowledge of treatment progress and their possible concern over his loss of school time. M. Brown has set a deadline of 4/23 for ruling in or ruling out these possible problems. On or before 4/23 she will gather the appropriate data and will report to the responsible nurse. Together they will either state the unusual problem as identified and will develop expected outcomes and nursing actions, or they will make a note on the patient's chart regarding the resolution of the problem. Or they will state that it is not a problem. They will then discontinue the specific items under the unusual problems section of the care plan.

Case 2. Mary R, Postoperative Celiotomy, Cecostomy, Double-barreled Colostomy

Physician's expectations regarding course of treatment and convalescence:

( ) typical or routine

(√) atypical or complicated

If atypical or complicated, in what way? Obese—abdominal wound will heal slowly.

Identifying Information: _____

_____

Diagnosis: Celiotomy, cecostomy, _____
double-barreled colostomy, 4/8. _____

_____

Nurisng's criteria for discharge or maintenance (overall expected outcomes):
(a) Will verbalize appropriate understanding of medical regimen and follow-up. _____
(b) Will demonstrate satisfactory ability to irrigate own colostomy. _____
(c) Will verbalize feelings about colostomy, and state realistic plans for _____
   home care.   Mrs. Walker, RN _____

Home Care Coordination activities: HCC notified on 4/14. _____

Other relevant information (socioeconomic, etc.): _____

Date	Unusual Problems	Expected Outcomes	Deadlines	Nursing Orders
4/14	(1) Very upset and embarrassed due to smell and mess of colostomy due to leakage	(1) No smell or mess Expresses approval of aesthetics	(1) (4/15) √q 8°	(1) a. Use largest diameter colostomy bag available Reinforce seal c̄ generous amount Karaya Jel Reinforce c̄ surgical pads because some leakage will occur Fasten entire drsg c̄ Montgomery straps b. Chg drsg and Montgomery straps frequently (q 2°) to prevent leakage onto gown and bedclothing c. Spray room c̄ deod before, during, and after drsg chg to minimize odor d. Prepare drsg and waste receptacle in advance so that

Date	Unusual Problems	Expected Outcomes	Deadlines	Nursing Orders
				change can be completed rapidly e. Clean around stoma c̄ clear water and clean washcloth M. Walker, RN
4/14	(2) Emotionally upset due to feuding of adult children over who will have to care for her	(2) Openly verbalizes concerns Actively discusses "what to do"	(2) (4/17) √daily	(2) Initiate discussion c̄ pt re problem Clarify concerns and assist c̄ problem solving (Delegated to L. Krusche, RN) M. Walker, RN
4/14	(3) Potential surgical wound infection due to colostomy leakage	(3) No s/s of local redness or swelling No leakage to incision	(3) √q 8°	(3) a. Chg colostomy drsg q 2° to prevent leakage to surgical incision (see instr problem [1] a-e) b. Remind pt to lie on rt side or sit up to keep drainage flowing away from incision M. Walker, RN

Analysis of Nursing Orders, Mrs. Mary R.   This patient's problem of embarrassment due to leakage of liquid bowel contents through the colostomy is designed to be solved by developing specific instructions about how to change and reinforce the dressing. The specific instructions would minimize trial and error and would facilitate meeting the goal.

On 4/15, or 24 hours after the plan is put into operation, a reevaluation is scheduled to be done. The nurse believes that after 12 changes (24 hours), it will be possible to observe whether or not the goal of "no smell or mess"—and therefore no embarrassment—has been met. If so, the nursing care will probably be continued. If not, the orders will be revised to be more effective.

The problem "emotionally upset" regarding the attitudes of the patient's children is designed to be met by problem solving with her. This has been delegated to one nurse to initiate and follow through. It is apparent that, if no one is delegated specifically to do this, several persons may make attempts, resulting in confusion. This kind of personal problem, which definitely requires a trust relationship and ongoing clear communication, can usually best be solved by delegating the responsibility to one person.

Case 3. Ralph L, Postoperative Right Hip Pinning and Active Pulmonary Tuberculosis.

Physician's expectations regarding course of treatment and convalescence:

( ) typical or routine

(√) atypical or complicated

If atypical or complicated, in what way? Malnourished, expect slow healing and slow progress regarding ambulation.

Identifying Information: _____

_____

Diagnosis: Dehydration, malnutrition, active pulmonary tbc, left hip fracture pinned, 3/20

_____

Nursing criteria for discharge or maintenance (overall expected outcomes):

(a) Will verbalize approval of convalescent facility or home care.

(b) Will demonstrate safe and efficient transfer and ambulation technique.

(c) Will verbalize understanding of and demonstrate safe isolation
    technique for tbc.

(d) Will verbalize appropriate understanding of medical care regimen and
    ability to follow up.   L. Pratt, RN

Home Care Coordination activities: HCC notified on 4/5.

Other relevant information (socioeconomic, etc.): On Medicare hospital insurance. Social worker notified on 4/5.

Date	Unusual Problems	Expected Outcomes	Deadlines	Nursing Orders
4/5	(1) Potential pulmonary hemorrhage or spontaneous pneumothorax due to active pulmonary tbc	(1) Prevention or early detection—pt to verbalize understanding of s/s and his need to report	(1) √daily	(1) Reinforce instructions to patient re reporting any streaking b. Check patient's disposal bag tissues for signs of streaking (wear glove) L. Pratt, RN
4/5	(2) Potential constipation due to immobility and liquid diet	(2) Soft, formed stool, at least qod	(2) √even days	(2) Offer (fracture) pan for BM every day after breakfast to establish habit L. Pratt, RN
4/5	(3) Severe pain upon moving and turning due to fr left hip and decubitis of sacrum	(3) Reports that he is reasonably comfortable	(3) √q 8°	(3) a. May lie on back, rt side, and prone—alternate positions q 2° during day, and q 3° at night b. Patient can assist c̄ turning by using trapeze and bed rail c. Patient will say when he is ready to assist c̄ turning, etc When he is "with you" there is less pain

Date	Unusual Problems	Expected Outcomes	Deadlines	Nursing Orders
				d. Make movements smoothly and quickly to avoid extreme pain e. Support well in side position—2 pillows along back, one pillow between knees, one thick pillow for left arm and hand f. See that pain Rx is given 30 min before AM bath and linen chg L. Pratt, RN
4/5	(4) Decubitus ulcer (sacrum) 2 inch diameter, ¼ inch deep due to immobility and poor tissue nutrition	(4) Continually ↓ size and depth	(4) √daily	(4) a. Turn q 2 hr during day and q 3 hr at night (see above instr) b. Keep a clean body-sized sheepskin in direct contact c̄ skin at all times L. Pratt, RN
4/5	(5) Dry, itchy skin due to dehydration and frequent bathing	(5) Minimum or no dryness No itching	(5) (4/10) √daily	(5) Total bath Monday and Thursday only Bathe face, neck, hands, axilla, and perineal area daily Total body rub c̄ hosp mss lotion daily L. Pratt, RN
4/5	(6) Potential joint contrac-tures due to immobility in bed	(6) Full range of motion, ankles	(6) √even days	(6) ROM of all joints except left hip and knee 10:00 AM and 4:00 PM (active and passive, as needed) L. Pratt, RN
4/5	(7) Dry, uncom-fortable mouth and nose due to nasogastric tube and dehydration	(7) Moist, clean mucous mem-branes States that mouth and nose are comfortable	(7) (4/7) √q 8°	(7) a. Cleanse nares c̄ warm soap and water 9 AM and 9 PM b. Apply hosp lubrica-tion cream to both nares q 2° (even hr) during day and when awake at night c. Offer mouth wash every 2° (even hours) during day and when awake at night L. Pratt, RN
4/5	(8) Feelings of loneliness, fear, and depression due to no family, hospital isola-	(8) Participates in planning day's activities Asks questions and initiates	(8) (4/10) √daily	(8) a. Encourage frequent visits to patient by other Spanish-speaking patients

Date	Unusual Problems	Expected Outcomes	Deadlines	Nursing Orders
	tion, and many unfamiliar procedures	conversations		Supervise isolation technique of visitors b. Use patient, S. Lopez, as interpreter to facilitate understanding of patient's feelings and needs c. Explain the plan for the day and any new procedures Encourage suggestions and questions from patient (use interpreter) d. Discuss and clarify patient's perceptions of his illness and his long-range plans (delegated to S. Brown, RN) L. Pratt, RN

Analysis of Nursing Orders, Mr. Ralph L.   Nursing order (1), a and b, specifies that the patient has been instructed to report any streaking, so the nurse's role is to reinforce that behavior. Additionally, the nurse would doublecheck the tissue before disposal.

Nursing order (2) requires offering the bedpan at the same time daily to establish a regular bowel habit. Other interventions, such as a laxative, are not mentioned because they would already be in the patient care system via the physician's orders.

The nursing care ordered in item (3) very specifically details six ways to minimize the patient's pain. Nursing orders must be this specific in order to result in consistently effective care.

Item (4) refers to the care ordered for the healing of the decubitus ulcer. A turning and cleaning routine is outlined. The medications or ointments to be used on the ulcer would not be mentioned because the doctor's orders already contain that information.

Nursing order (5) specifies how to manage skin care to reduce dryness and itching.

Orders (6), (7), and (8) continue to offer specific detailed nursing orders for good patient care.

Mr. L represents one of the more rare individuals who have many complex unusual problems. As a result, his care plan would require much more writing than is usually necessary for the average patient.

Case 4. Stephen F, Preoperative Cholecystectomy

Physician's expectations regarding course of treatment and convalescence:

    (√) typical or routine

    ( ) atypical or complicated

If atypical or complicated, in what way?

Identifying Information: _____

_____

Diagnosis: Cholecystectomy 3/29

_____

Nursing's criteria for discharge of maintenance (overall expected outcome):
See standard postoperative expected outcome.   J. Roth RN

Home Care Coordination Activities: _____

Other relevant information (socioeconomic, etc.): _____

Date	Unusual Problems	Expected Outcome	Deadlines	Nursing Orders
3/29	Appears to be coping satisfactorily, both physiologically and psychologically		3/31	Standard care, cholecystectomy

Analysis of Nursing Orders, Mr. Stephen F. On 3/29, the day before surgery, the nurse concludes that the patient "appears to be coping satisfactorily." Consequently, the nursing orders would refer to standard care plans, which in this case is standard preoperative care. The preoperative care plan contains such elements as certain observations and teaching, diet and liquid modifications, and certain base-line vital signs measurements.

Because the standard preoperative care plan is prewritten in detail, has been taught to the staff, and is readily available for reference, the nurse writing the order refers to it by title rather than tediously handwriting it.

After surgery, on the patient's first postoperative day (3/31), the patient will again be evaluated by the nurse. If at that time he appears to be coping as expected, the appropriate postoperative standard care plan will be ordered. If on 3/31 he has developed one or more unusual problems, his care plan would contain specific unusual problems, outcomes, deadlines, and nursing orders in addition to or instead of the standard care plan.

Case 5. Mrs. Helen H, Radical Mastectomy

Physician's expectations regarding   Identifying Information: _____
course of treatment of convales-
cence: _____
    (√) typical or routine   Diagnosis: Adenocarcinoma, rt
    ( ) atypical or complicated   breast c̄ metastasis to regional
If atypical or complicated, in what way?   lymph nodes.

Nursing's criteria for discharge or maintenance (overall expected outcomes):

(a) Will demonstrate ability to do arm exercises correctly and to manage

    any necessary self-care.

(b) Will verbalize correct understanding of what to do in case of swelling,

    fatigue, or other complications.

(c) Ongoing verbalization (c̄ associated congruent feelings) of ability to

    cope c̄ the changes in her life.

    —active plans for getting and using prosthesis.

    —active plans for getting back into normal life style.

(d) Ongoing verbalization (c̄ associated congruent feelings) by husband re:

    ability to give his wife the necessary support.   S. Hiskin, RN

Home Care Coordination Activities: _____

Other relevant information (socioeconomic, etc.): _____

Date	Unusual Problems	Expected Outcomes	Deadlines	Nursing Orders
6/4	(1) Severe incisional pain and aching of right arm 3 hr after each pain medication, due to surgical trauma and pressure (edema) of rt arm	(1) Statements by pt that arm is increasingly more comfortable	√q 8°	(1) a. Keep rt arm elevated on medium thickness pillow at all times b. Turn from back to left side q 2° when awake—prop arm when in side position c. Arrange for pt to watch TV, read, or converse c̄ roommate during hour prior to next pain medication to distract from discomfort d. See that pain Rx is always given right on time e. Do deep-breathing and coughing during intervals of comfort when analgesic is in effect S. Hiskin, RN

Date	Unusual Problems	Expected Outcomes	Deadlines	Nursing Orders
6/4	(2) Acute grief response and feelings of desperation due to loss of breast and associated changes in life style	(2) Verbalizes fears Looks at incision Asks questions and seeks information about recovery Actively plans for prosthesis	√daily	(2) a. Spend 30 min c̄ pt during time she is comfortable (q 8°) to allow verbalization Do active and supportive listening b. As readiness increases, introduce her to pt who has successfully adjusted and is back to normal life (Both a and b dele-gated to B. Joynes, AM shift and S. Haney, PM shift) S. Hiskin, RN
6/4	(3) Possible worry and concern by husband due to impact of diagnosis		√6/6	(3) Initiate discussion c̄ husband alone Ascertain his fears and concerns This may take several interviews Make specific appts. c̄ him (Delegated to S. Haney, RN S. Hiskin, RN
6/4	(4) Possible financial problems associated with unexpected surgery and long convales-cence		√6/6	(4) Discuss c̄ husband and make necessary referrals (Delegated to S. Haney, RN) S. Hiskin, RN

Analysis of Nursing Orders, Mrs. Helen H. Nursing order (1), a and b, specifies that the right arm is to be elevated on a medium thickness pillow at all times. In addition, it requires a change of position every two hours. The order also specifies the positions that are safe and comfortable. This combination of elevating the patient's arm and frequently changing her position in bed is designed to mini-mize edema of the arm and to minimize the generalized discomfort of pressure areas and stiffness associated with immobility.

The principle of distraction is utilized in nursing order (1)c. It requires that distracting types of activities be planned during the hour or two that intevene between the onset of pain and the next dosage of pain medication.

Nursing order (1)d reinforces the need to give pain medication on time so that anxiety over delayed administration of the analgesic is not added to Mrs. H's other worries.

The well-known, effective strategy of doing the deep-breathing and coughing procedure when the analgesic is at peak effect is utilized in nursing order (1)e.

For the problem of acute grief response, Miss Hiskin has appointed two nurses, B. Joynes on the morning shift and S. Haney on the evening shift, to establish a relationship with the patient, to spend extra time listening, and when appropriate, to begin actively working toward ways of helping the patient cope with her situation. The suggestion in the nursing order is to introduce Mrs. H to another woman who has had a mastectomy and who has managed a satisfactory adjustment. This kind of very personal emotional problem is much more effectively managed when specific nurses are delegated to follow through. If orders of this sort were written without specific delegation and if all staff persons subsequently interviewed the patient in their well-meaning but varying ways, it is doubtful that the patient would receive the real support she needs.

Nursing orders (3) and (4) require that further information be gathered from the patient's husband. This duty has also been delegated to one nurse.

SUMMARY

Nursing orders, the third and last major element of the nursing care plan, are statements of the specific nursing interventions that are required to solve the problem by the deadline.

Nursing actions, or nursing orders, must be clear and concise and must relate directly to the problem. Like physician's orders, they must say what, when, how, and under what circumstances. They must leave as little as possible to varying interpretations. They must be distinctively nursing actions—not a reiteration of the doctor's orders.

Nursing orders can be written clearly and in detail for actual and potential problems because expected outcomes are known. Since possible problems are those not yet identified as being actual or potential, nursing orders for them must be written so as to require that further data be gathered by a certain point in time.

All nursing orders must be signed by the nurse who writes them as indication that she, as a professional person, is assuming responsibility for them. Knowing which nurse has written an order also makes it easier for staff persons to share with her their ideas for changing, revising, or updating the care plan.

It is through the nursing orders that nurses reveal their unique and independent role in the prescription and delivery of health care.

REFERENCES

1. Little D, Carnevali D: Nursing Care Planning. Philadelphia, Lippincott, 1976
2. Bailey J, Claus K: Decision Making in Nursing: Tools for Change. St. Louis, Mosby, 1975, pp 68-90
3. Lewis L: Planning Patient Care. Dubuque Iowa, Wm C Brown, 1970, p 94

6

The Actual Outcome:
Test of Quality

EVALUATION OF PATIENTS' OUTCOMES

The patient's outcome is a written statement of his actual status in relation to a nursing care regimen. It is written with reference to the expected outcome as a criterion. When a nurse evaluates a patient in regard to a specific unusual problem, she utilizes the expected outcome as a guide for her assessment and for the resulting patient outcome notation.

For example, a patient with a decubitus ulcer 2 inches in diameter and ¼-inch deep has an expected outcome statement such as "continuously decreasing size and depth." The actual patient outcome statement should indicate the diameter and depth at the times called for in the deadlines column. If the patient's decubitus ulcer is smaller than it was at the last checking interval, the nurse is assured that the current plan of care is appropriate. The notation of a patient's response should be a reflection of the nurse's perceptions of the patient's status relative to the criteria listed in the expected outcome—his verbalizations, his competence, his clinical symptoms, or his environmental situation.

The statement of the patient's actual outcome is written on the patient's record, not on the care plan, because the purpose of the care plan is to provide the guide for care. The patient's chart is the document that must contain statements of the patient's actual status or condition. When the patient's actual status notations are entered on his chart at the required intervals, that record will contain a useful pertinent chronology of the patient's progress, since all the notes are written within the same frame of reference and with the same problems and expected outcomes in mind.

Actual or observed patient responses to the prescribed care provide the factual statements that are documented in the nurses' notes of the patient's record. When compared with the expected outcome statements, these actual outcome notations clearly indicate the success or failure of the prescribed nursing care. Patient outcome notations become a tool for evaluating the general success or failure of nursing care on a unit. They can, through the audit process, provide justification for more or different staffing, for policy changes, for staff education, or for whatever appears to be required to improve patient care.

ACTUAL OUTCOMES FOR USUAL PROBLEMS

Patients who are progressing within the expected norms, that is, those who have usual problems, will not have expected outcome statements handwritten on the care plan. The expected outcomes for these patients are the expected standards for the typical patient who is coping satisfactorily. Therefore, patient response notations should only include factual statements about the patient's status relative to the usually expected status for the given situation. This concept is discussed in more detail in Chapter 7.

The succeeding paragraphs give examples of how to record patient responses to standard care. The examples are derived from plans developed in Chapters 3, 4, and 5. The patient responses developed here will refer to the case examples in Chapter 5.

Case 1. Harry J, Emergency Appendectomy. Mr. J's care plan is illustrated in Table 5-1, page 87. Certain nurses' notes relating to it, as well as an analysis and explanation of them, follow.

Patient's record, excerpted nurse's notes:

> 2/20. Ambulating well and frequently. Taking dietary increments as expected. Requires no pain medication or sleeping medication. Anticipate no unusual problems with follow-up. J. Suchaki, RN

Analysis. The nurse evaluates and documents Harry J's status on 2/20 as required in the deadlines column. Her statements indicate that he continues to have no unusual problems. Since he will probably be going home on the third or fourth postoperative day, Miss Suchaki would update the deadlines column to require an evaluation upon discharge.

In any case, in any setting a patient must have a nursing evaluation and a statement of the patient's status upon discharge. A discharge evaluation must be done routinely to doublecheck that the patient has met the overall criteria for discharge. Standard care plans for appendectomy patients provide the interim and discharge expected outcomes which guide the nurse in her patient-outcome assessment and charting.

Case 2. Carol J, Acute Cystitis. Carol J's care plan is illustrated in Table 5-2, page 89. Excerpts from her record as well as an analysis of them are outlined below.

Patient's record, excerpted nurse's notes:

2/21. Is ambulating and taking diet and fluids well. Temperature is normal. Says she feels comfortable and well. Verbalizes appropriate understanding of medical treatment regimen and has appropriate plans for self-care and follow-up at home. B. Garrison, RN

Analysis. On 2/21, as scheduled, Mrs. J is reevaluated. The nurse documents specific observations regarding the patient's status. These reflect accomplishment of standard criteria (from the standard care plan for cystitis) for satisfactory progress. In this case the patient will be discharged very soon, so the nurse would update the deadlines column to require a discharge evaluation.

Case 3. James R, Lumbar Laminectomy. Mr. R's care plan is shown in Table 5-3, page 89. His nurse's notes and an analysis of them are given below.

Patient's record, excerpted nurse's notes:

2/20. Demonstrates good log-rolling technique. Verbalizes appropriate understanding of surgery and treatment regimen. Satisfactory demonstration of deep breathing and coughing routine. Some discomfort from flatulence but copes well with assistance of rectal tube for periodic discomfort. Taking prescribed diet and liquids well. L. Christian, RN

Analysis. On 2/20, as scheduled, Mr. R is reevaluated. The nurse documents specific findings regarding the patient's status. These reflect accomplishment of standard care plan criteria for satisfactory progress. In this case the nurse would update the deadlines column to 2/22. She believes that a two-day interval for reevaluation is appropriate at this point in his convalescence. In three days he will require further assessment of his progress.

Case 4. Alice M, A and P Repair.   In Table 5-4, page 89, Alice M's care plan is illustrated. Below are excerpts from her patient record, followed by an analysis.

Patient's record, excerpted nurse's notes:

2/22. Deep-breathing and coughing well. Ambulating with help. Requests analgesic every four to six hours. Urine clear through indwelling catheter. Alert and taking over own personal care needs. T. Bennett, RN

Analysis.   On 2/22, as scheduled, Mrs. M is reevaluated. The nurse documents specific findings concerning the patient's status. These refelect accomplishment of standard criteria for satisfactory progress. In this case the nurse would update the deadlines column to 2/25. She believes that a two-day interval for reevaluation is appropriate. In two days the catheter is likely to be removed. This could result in unusual problems that must not go undetected.

Case 5. Mrs. Joyce H, Abdominal Hysterectomy.   Mrs. H's care plan is shown in Table 5-5, page 89. Her nurse's notes, followed by an analysis, are outlined below.

Patient's record, excerpted nurse's notes:

4/23. Discharge evaluation. Voiding and ambulating well. Required no analgesia past 24 hours. Slept well past two nights without sedation. Verbalizes appropriate understanding of safe activity and rest pattern at home. Verbalizes appropriate plans for assistance with activities of daily living. Has made appointment with physician for first office visit. Verbalized satisfactory knowledge of medication schedule. Discharged from unit per wheel chair, accompanied by husband. C. Deming, RN

Analysis.   On 4/23, as scheduled, Mrs. H is evaluated for discharge. The nurse documents specific findings concerning the patient's status. These reflect accomplishment of standard criteria for discharge.

If upon discharge a patient does not meet one or more criteria for discharge, the nurse would specify the referrals to be made to insure appropriate follow-up.

ACTUAL OUTCOMES FOR UNUSUAL PROBLEMS

To continue with examples of how patient responses to nursing orders should be documented, examples from Chapters 3, 4, and 5 are developed and analyzed below.

Low Fluid Intake. Table 5-6 page 90, illustrates the care plan for a patient with low fluid intake. The nurses' notes and an analysis of them follow.

Patient's record, excerpted nurses' notes:

3/25. Intake-output sheet reveals that the required 1,200 ml of fluid was taken. Patient appears involved and motivated to maintain own intake schedule. I. Schulz, RN

3/26. Intake, 2,000 ml as scheduled. Patient appears to feel proud of accomplishment and will continue. L. Jones, RN

3/27. Intake, 2,500 ml as scheduled. Patient knows that this is maintenance intake and will continue his intake schedule accordingly. I. Schulz, RN

Analysis. The patient response statements on 3/25, 3/26, and 3/27 refer to the expected outcomes as defined on the care plan. They give a clear indication of the patient's success. Because the original problem, low fluid intake, is now obsolete, that problem and its nursing action can be discontinued. The nurse would therefore cross out and initial the old order, to indicate that it is discontinued. The nurse, however, believes that the patient is at unusually high risk for returning to his lifelong habit of not drinking much, so she would redesign the care plan as portrayed in Table 6-1.

TABLE 6-1. REVISED CARE PLAN FOR UNUSUAL PROBLEMS, LOW FLUID INTAKE

Date	Unusual Problems	Expected Outcomes	Deadlines	Nursing Orders
3/25	Potential low fluid intake due to lifelong habit of not drinking much	Maintain 2,500 ml daily intake	√daily	Give pt positive reinforcement in keeping and maintaining intake schedule I. Schulz, RN

Decubitus Ulcer. Table 5-7, page 91, shows the care plan for a patient with decubitus ulcer. Patient's record and nurse's notes are excerpted below:

3/27.   Decubitus ulcer, coccyx, 2¼ inch diameter, ¼ inch deep. Tissue soft around crater. Dr notified. Nursing care will be increased in vigor. S. Haney, RN

Analysis. The example cites a nurse's note made on 3/27. Since the deadline requires documentation of the size of the decubitus every day, an entry is made daily. However, for this example, only the notation of 3/27 is included.

On 3/27 the decubitus is larger with soft tissue around the crater, indicating a process of deterioration. The care plan would now be strengthened to prevent further breakdown and to meet the expected outcome of decreasing size and depth. The care plan can be updated by adding the new larger size (with date) under the original unusual problem and by increasing intervals of turning under nursing actions. This is done by crossing out the original intervals and adding the new ones. New nursing orders can also be added as needed. If the plan needs major revisions, the entire item can be discontinued, and a new unusual problem, expected outcomes, deadlines, and nursing orders can be written.

Extreme Anxiety. Table 5-8, page 91, shows the care plan for a patient who is experiencing extreme anxiety. The nurses' notes and an analysis follow.

Patient's record, excerpted nurses' notes:

3/25.   11 PM. Restless during most of PM. Talked with nurse at length about his worries and about his family, work, etc. Requested sedation for sleep. J. Canaris, RN
3/26.   3 PM. Busy with diagnostic routines. Continues restless when left alone. Verbalizes fears and concerns and the need to be patient until diagnosis is made. Slept poorly last night. L. Swanson, RN

Analysis. The nurse's notations will continue according to the schedule and will refer to such criteria as "expression of fears and questions" that are listed under the expected outcomes. When these criteria are consistently used it is possible to evaluate the success or failure of the nursing regimen.

Reluctance to Take Treatment. In Table 5-9, page 92, is illustrated the care plan for a patient who is having difficulty with his IPPB treatment. The associated charting and an analysis of it are given below.

Patient's record, excerpted nurse's notes:

3/26. Is now willing to use IPPB. Seems relaxed in using machine, laughs and is matter-of-fact about stress incontinence problem. States that the current way of coping with the problem is much better than before. B. Patterson, RN

Analysis.   At daily intervals before 3/26, as required by the deadlines column, entries are made regarding actual progress toward the expected outcome. The example shows the notation that was made on the deadline date, 3/26. This note reveals that the care has apparently been successful. Because the problem of reluctance to use the IPPB will recur if the care is not continued as outlined, the nurse would leave the care plan statement as it is except for crossing out 3/26 and entering a new deadline date. In this case the nurse has decided that weekly checking intervals are adequate, so the next deadline date will be 4/2. No daily checking intervals will be required.

Low Caloric Intake.   Table 5-10, page 92, portrays the care plan designed for a patient who is not eating well. His nurses' notes and an analysis of them follow.
    Patient's record, excerpted nurses' notes:

3/25. Took 1,600 calories past 24 hours. A. Hudson, RN
3/26. Took 1,950 calories past 24 hours. A. Hudson, RN
3/27. Took 2,400 calories past 24 hours. Should be able to take 2,500 calories next 24 hours and maintain with same level of nursing care. G. Barnaby, RN

Analysis.   In this case, notations regarding actual progress toward the expected outcome are made on schedule. On 3/27 the nurse indicates that the desired goal of 2,500 calories has been reasonably accomplished by virtue of the 2,400 calorie intake. The nurse believes that the nursing action must continue at the same level in order to maintain the 2,500 calorie intake. Therefore, she would leave the care plan as it is except for updating the deadlines column. In this case the nurse plans to evaluate again by making a calorie count in three days. To accomplish that, she would cross out 3/27 under the deadlines column and substitute 3/30.

Emotional Upset.   Table 5-11, page 93, is an illustration of the care plan that has been developed for a patient who is emotionally upset. The nurse recorded her response as shown below. It is followed by an analysis.
    Patient's record, excerpted nurse's notes:

3/30. Conversations with patient reveal many ambivalences and concerns about personal relationship with husband, mother-in-law, and children. Plan to continue talks with patient to assist with problem solving, particularly to assist patient to recognize need for counsellor. Still is emotionally upset but is able to discuss the situation openly. J. Landers, RN

Analysis. The nurse to whom the care was delegated documents follow-up on the required date. In this case she would indicate a need to continue the nursing action as outlined. She would update the deadlines column to a date which, in her judgment, is consistent with a reasonable interval of time for making progress. In this case the nurse sets 4/1 as the next checking interval.

Anxiety and Fear. Table 5-12, page 93, shows a care plan designed to help a patient cope with his anxiety and fear. The nurse's notes and an analysis of them are shown below.

Patient's record, excerpted nurse's notes:

3/15. 11 PM. Dyspnea decreasing throughout shift. Posture relaxed except for short periods. Talks about need to pace himself but still needs coaching and reminding. S. Sauer, RN

Analysis. The first eight-hourly interval notation reveals several facts about the patient's anxiety status. At each subsequent eight-hour interval, notations would be made, each utilizing the criteria listed under the expected outcomes column. In this way, the essential facts will be available for the ongoing assessment of the success or failure of the nursing care.

Feelings of Panic. Table 5-13, page 94, is an illustration of a care plan that has been designed for a patient who is experiencing feelings of panic due to memory loss. His nurse records his response as shown below.

Patient's record, excerpted nurse's notes:

3/28. Seems generally relaxed. Verbalizes frustration when can't remember. Laughs about problem at times and at other times seems impatient with inability to remember. Expresses hope that it will improve with time. B. Wolfe, RN

Analysis. Notations are made on the chart daily as required by the deadlines column. A sample patient outcome notation for 3/28 is cited in the example. The nurse would develop her statement to give an indication of the patient's coping mechanisms as referred to in the expected outcomes column.

ACTUAL OUTCOMES FOR OTHER PROBLEM CATEGORIES

The real, potential, and possible problems for Chapters 3, 4, and 5 are again presented to provide examples of how a patient's response to nursing care should be documented.

Real Problems

Depression and Withdrawal. Table 5-14, page 95, shows the care plan that has been set up for a patient who is experiencing depression and withdrawal. The associated charting and an analysis of it appear below.

Patient's record, excerpted nurse's notes:

3/15. Initiates some conversation c̄ staff. Talks openly c̄ family re: face and what to do until cosmetic surgery can be done. B. Walters, RN

3/20. Using cosmetics (approved by Dr) and has new wig c̄ hair that encroaches over forehead and cheeks. Smiles, laughs, handles hospital social situations well. Feels she can cope until further surgery is done. B. Watters, RN

Analysis. The preceding example contains two nurse's notations during the period of 3/10 to 3/20. The deadlines column requires a daily evaluation and notation; therefore, the nurse's notes would include a daily evaluative statement. For this example, on 3/15 the notation indicates some improvement of the patient's status since 3/10. On 3/20, the final deadline date, the notation indicates that the patient appears to be coping well. At this point the nursing orders related to depression and withdrawal would be discontinued. The problem is solved, and the patient is able to cope with the situation without specific additional intervention from staff nurses.

Pressure Areas. Table 5-15, page 96, shows the care plan that has been developed for a patient who is experiencing pressure areas over the thoracic spine. Below are nurses' notes, followed by an analysis.

Patient's record, excerpted nurses' notes:

3/12. No redness over thoracic spine. Reddened area over coccyx, 1 inch diameter. B. Valentine, RN

3/15. No reddened areas of thoracic or coccygeal areas. L. Swanson, RN

Analysis. On 3/12, two days after the problem was identified and a nursing care regimen was established, the reddened area over the thoracic spine has disappeared, and the area over the coccyx has decreased in size. By 3/15 no reddened areas are visible. Because the patient is still at high risk for pressure areas, the care in this case would be continued because it has proven to be successful.

Acute Grief. Table 5-16, page 97, is an illustration of a care plan that has been developed to assist a patient who is experiencing acute grief. The recording done by more than one nurse is shown below.

Patient's record, excerpted nurses' notes:

3/18. 11 PM. Will do own personal hygiene c̄ kindly encouragement. Slept 3 hours with sedation this afternoon. Verbalizes only, "Why?" L. Swanson, RN

3/20. 3 PM. Beginning to talk of memories of good time c̄ husband. Weeps openly now. Able to sleep 1 to 2 hours during day without sedative. S. Forsman, RN

3/22. 8 AM. Slept most of night c̄ sedative. Awoke to talk about loss for one hour during night. Does own personal care. Eats lightly with minimal urging. H. Brown, RN

Analysis.   Notations on 3/18, 3/20, and 3/22 reveal that progressive grief work is being accomplished. Because the care plan appears to be successful, it would be continued for a few more days until the responsible nurse believes that no further specific intervention is required from the nursing staff regarding the patient's grief response.

Multiple Decubiti.   The illustration in Table 5-17, page 97, is that of a care plan designed to help a patient who has multiple decubitus ulcers. The nurses' notes, as shown below, convey the principle of precise recording. An analysis follows.

Patient's record, excerpted nurses' notes:

3/15. Decubitus ulcers—Rt trochanter 3 inch diameter, ½ inch deep.
              Lt trochanter 4 inch diameter, ¾ inch deep.
              Sacrum and coccyx 5 inch diameter, ¼-½ inch deep.
    All areas appear to have firm tissue around craters. L. Swanson, RN

3/20. Decubitus ulcers—Rt trochanter 2¾ inch diameter, ½-¼ inch deep.
              Lt trochanter 4 inch diameter, ¾ inch deep.
              Sacrum and coccyx 4¾ inch diameter, ¼ inch deep.
    All areas have firm tissue around craters and are clean. L. Ramirez, RN

Analysis.   On 3/15, all areas either have remained the same or have improved slightly. By 3/20 more improvement is noted in all areas. Both times the nurse notes the presence of firm tissue around the craters, which tends to indicate that the areas are apparently not breaking down further. Because the ulcers seem to be improving at a satisfactory rate, the care plan as designed would continue.

Anxiety and Restlessness. Table 5-18, page 98, shows the care plan for a patient who is experiencing anxiety and restlessness. The charting of several nurses is illustrated below. An analysis follows.

Patient's record, excerpted nurses' notes:

3/10.   11 PM. Tense posture and restlessness when awake. Slept at ½ to 1 hour intervals during PM. J. Litizzetti, RN

3/11.   8 AM. Expressions of anxiety seem less. Relaxed posture and sleeping for 2 to 3-hour intervals during night. Less restless this AM. J. Cox, RN

3/11.   3 PM. More relaxed less dyspneic. Rests quietly and cooperates c̄ regimen to conserve energy. R. Hanson, RN

3/11.   11 PM. Dyspneic only upon exertion. Relaxed posture. Planned evening schedule and stopped activities before dyspnea occurred. No restlessness. J. Litizzetti, RN

Analysis. The nurses' notations at eight-hour intervals indicate consistent progress toward the expected outcomes, "relaxed posture and self-pacing." Because the care regimen appears to be successful and because the patient's underlying physiologic cause of dyspnea is still unstable, the nursing actions would be continued.

Potential Problems

Potential Postoperative Hemorrhage. The care plan for the patient with potential postoperative hemorrhage is illustrated in Table 5-19, page 99. The associated nurses' notes and an analysis follow.

Patient's record, excerpted nurses' notes:

3/2.   11 PM. Dark bleeding ¼ inch diameter at end of 1st hr postop. Drsg reinforced. Further checking as prescribed revealed no further incisional bleeding. No signs of hematoma. A. Dyman, RN

3/3.   8 AM. No further incisional bleeding since 1st hr po. No signs of hematoma. J. Hanson, RN

3/3.   3 PM. No further bleeding since 1st hr po. No signs of hematoma. B. Joynes, RN

Analysis. At the required eight-hour intervals for the first 24 hours, the nurse documents the bleeding status. No bleeding since one hour postoperative has occurred. Therefore, the nursing actions could be revised to less frequent checking for another 24 or 48 hours.

Potential Pressure Areas. Table 5-20, page 99, shows the care plan for a patient who is at high risk for pressure areas. Below are the nurse's notes followed by an analysis.

Patient's record, excerpted nurse's notes:

> 3/11. No redness over bony prominences—spine, sacrum, coccyx, and buttocks. M. Reynolds, RN

Analysis. On 3/11, one day after the potential problem is identified, the nurse evaluates the patient's skin and makes the notation that there is no redness of the areas indicated. Since, after 24 hours, the nursing action seems successful, it would be continued as long as the patient remains at high risk for pressure areas. If the nurse, at any of the required checking times, finds redness over one of the bony prominences, the prescribed nursing actions would have to be analyzed for efficiency of implementation or would have to be redesigned to be more effective for preventing circulatory stasis.

Potential Uncontrolled Diabetes. The care plan for a patient who is at high risk for uncontrolled diabetes is illustrated in Table 5-21, page 100. Below are the associated nurses' notes.

Patient's record, excerpted nurses' notes:

> 3/12. Negative Clinitest and Acetest past 24 hours. With help of interpreter, patient has expressed beginning understanding of pathophysiology of diabetes. Next two days will be spent discussing treatment in general and treatment specifically of his case. L. Swanson, RN
> 3/14. Clinitest and Acetest continue negative. Gives verbal response indicating basic understanding of his diet and insulin regimen and is actively interested in planning his own menu next two days. (Dietician will double-check menus.) Next two days will be spent practicing insulin injections. M. Ratekin, RN

Analysis. Every other day, as required by the deadlines column, M. Ratekin and L. Swanson make notations giving information regarding the patient's progress toward the expected outcome. This would be continued until the patient is ready for discharge.

Potential Injury. Table 5-22, page 100, illustrates the plan of care for a patient who is at high risk for falling. The charting and an analysis of it are given below.

Patient's record, excerpted nurse's notes:

> 3/11. No falls or near falls. Ambulated well c̄ prescribed assistance. A. Finch, RN

Analysis. Every day the nurse would document the patient's status regarding safety of ambulation. As the days go by and ambulation continues safely, the checking intervals may be more widely spaced.

If, during any 24-hour period, a fall or near fall should occur, the entire episode would be evaluated in order to ascertain the cause. If the fault is found to be with the nursing orders, they would be appropriately revised.

Potential Postpartum Hemorrhage. The care plan for a patient who is at high risk for vaginal bleeding is shown in Table 5-23, page 101. The nurse's charting is shown, followed by an analysis.

Patient's record, excerpted nurse's notes:

3/8.   11 PM. 3-8 PM. One pad per hour.
8-11 PM. One pad q 2 hr. Fundus firm c̄ prescribed massage schedule. P. Toney, RN

Analysis. At the prescribed eight-hourly intervals for the first 24 hours, the responsible nurse summarizes the patient's vaginal bleeding status.

At the end of the 24 hours the pad checking schedule would be revised to be less frequent if it appears that the patient is out of danger.

Possible Problems

Since possible problems have no expected outcome statements, there are no criteria for evaluating the patient's response. What must be done, however, is to indicate that the prescribed nursing action has occurred on or before the specified deadline. In addition, the rationale for ruling in or ruling out the possible problem should be briefly stated.

Following are examples of how to document nursing follow-up on possible problems.

Possible Financial Problem. In Table 5-24, page 102, is illustrated the care plan for a patient with possible financial problems. The documentation of follow-up and an analysis follow:

Patient's record, excerpted nurse's notes:

3/15.   Discussions c̄ patient and family reveal that the illness and convalescence are causing significant financial problems. R. Hanson, social worker, has been notified and will follow up today. Plan to check c̄ patient in one week. M. Dains, RN

Analysis. The nurse to whom the nursing action is delegated documents that she has ruled in a financial problem and that an appropriate referral has been made. However, in this case she feels her responsibility is not complete until she verifies at a later date that the patient and social worker are making progress toward the solution. To indicate this on the care plan, she would cross out 3/15 and enter 3/22, with the statement, "Recheck progress toward solving problem."

Possible Concern over Children. The care plan for a patient with possible concern over teenage children is shown in Table 5-25, page 102, and in Table 6-2. The associated nurse's notes and an analysis follow.

Patient's record, excerpted nurse's notes for Table 5-25, page 102:

3/15. Conversation with patient indicates that her teenage children (boy, age 17, girl, age 15) now have supervision. The patient's sister has come to live in until patient is home again. M. Daines, RN

Analysis. On 3/15, the deadline for ruling on the possible problem, M. Dains, RN, documents that the problem is solved. She would then discontinue that possible problem and nursing action on the care plan either by crossing it out or by superimposing the letters DC (discontinued). Table 6-2 illustrates how this would look on the care plan.

TABLE 6-2. FINISHED CARE PLAN FOR POSSIBLE PROBLEM, WORRY OVER CHILDREN

Date	Unusual Problems	Expected Outcomes	Deadlines	Nursing Orders
~~3/10~~ 3/15 DC P. McH.	~~Possible worry over teenage children at home~~		~~(3/15)~~	~~Initiate conversations c̄ pt to ascertain (Delegated to M. Dains, RN)~~ ~~P. McHugh, RN~~

Possible Lack of Understanding. Table 5-26, page 103, illustrates the plan of care for a patient who may not understand his diagnosis. The nurse's notes and an analysis are given below.

Patient's record, excerpted nurse's notes:

3/13. Several conversations with patient revealed a misunderstanding of the meaning of her diagnosis, with resulting unrealistic fears. The physician and nurse have talked with her and her family to clarify their questions and concerns. Patient now verbalizes understanding. Anxiety level is reduced, and patient and family are making realistic plans for the future. H. Moore, RN

Analysis. The nurse to whom responsibility is delegated documents the clarification and solution of the possible problem by the deadline date. Since the possible problem is an actual problem that is in the process of being solved, the problem and nursing action could be discontinued on the care plan. It could be crossed out and noted as discontinued, as in the previous example.

Possible Lack of Understanding of Treatment Regimen. Table 5-27, page 103, shows a patient's care plan for his possible lack of understanding of the doctor's treatment regimen. The associated nurse's notes are illustrated below.

Patient's record, excerpted nurse's notes:

3/15. Conversation with patient reveals that, with minor clarification, he does understand the rationale and purpose of the treatment regimen. He was made to feel welcome to ask questions of staff and physician at any time, if he has any new questions. S. Hoffman, RN

Analysis. In this case the nurse documents that the possible problem can be ruled out. That entry on the care plan could be crossed out and noted as discontinued, as cited in a previous example.

Possible Worry. Table 5-28, page 103, shows the nursing care plan for the patient subject to possible worry over job and family. Table 6-3 shows how the plan is updated after the problem is ruled in as an actual concern. The nurse's notes are included below.

Patient's record, excerpted nurse's notes:

3/21. Conversations with patient reveal that he is very concerned about losing his job if he has a long absence. He is also worried about his family and their fears for the future. He has not discussed these fears directly with anyone. Nurse discussed problem with the physician, who will support patient and family and will provide as much information as possible regarding the course of the illness so that realistic plans can be made. Nurse will continue to talk with patient and will assist in initiating discussions with family for problem solving. S. Hoffman, RN

Analysis. The nurse has documented that the possible problem is an actual problem and that further nursing intervention is necessary. The care plan would be revised as further shown in Table 6-3.

TABLE 6-3.   UPDATED CARE PLAN FOR PROBLEM, WORRY OVER JOB AND FAMILY

Date	Unusual Problems	Expected Outcomes	Deadlines	Nursing Orders
~~3/18~~ 3/21 DC L.H.	~~Possible worry over job and family adjustment to illness~~		~~(3/21)~~	~~Initiate conversation c̄ pt to ascertain and clarify (Delegated to S. Hoffman, RN) L. Harley, RN~~
3/21	Worry over job and family adjustment to illness	Making contacts to keep job Family involved in problem-solving discussions	(3/30) 3/26	Continue to problem solve c̄ pt and family (Delegated to S. Hoffman, RN) L. Harley, RN

CASE STUDY APPLICATIONS

To develop examples further for stating the patient's response when the nurse is evaluating care, the case studies from Chapters 3, 4, and 5 are continued here. Excerpts of nursing notes relating to each case are shown, followed by an analysis.

Case 1. Richard M, Multiple Traumatic Injury (Chap. 5, pp, 104-107). Patient's record, excerpted nurse's notes:

4/21. Beginning to learn how to plug trach for speaking. Hesitant and afraid, but did try and was successful in making a sound. Parents visited this PM, and they are interested in working on a visitor's schedule. Will bring patient's phonograph and records. Discussed treatment regimen and implications of illness. They plan to talk with physician re: certain questions that nurse cannot answer specifically. They then will plan their son's school program. Discussions will continue. L. Swanson, RN

4/23. Accepts tracheostomy suctioning without unusual anxiety. Has learned to plug tracheostomy for speaking and does so ad lib. Uses flash cards between times. Offers preferences regarding care. Will call nurse when he feels trach needs suctioning. Specific instructions for his trach care are posted at bedside. L. Swanson, RN

Analysis. On 4/21, the nurse evaluates and documents the patient's actual responses to the nursing orders that are prescribed in relation to problems (1) through (5).

On 4/23 she would evaluate the patient and document final outcomes regarding the patient's anxiety and fearfulness. She also will reevaluate his progress regarding all the other problems. At daily intervals she will assess the patient's frustration level and his potential feelings of loneliness and isolation.

Case 2. Mary R, Postoperative Celiotomy, Cecostomy, Double-Barreled Colostomy. (Chap 5, pp, 107-108). Patient's record, excerpted nurses' notes:

4/15. 3 PM. States that colostomy is more comfortable and less offensive. Is much more at ease discussing problem and having staff work with colostomy. No apprarent offensive odor in room. Dressing neat and clean. Surgical wound clean, no swelling or redness. Pt verbalized understanding of positioning to minimize leakage to incision. M. Walker, RN

4/17. Conversations with patient reveals considerable feelings of rejection and helplessness over her children and their apparent unwillingness to care for her. Anxiety level seems to be decreasing. Is beginning to think of constructive action. Will continue conversations. L. Krusche, RN

Analysis. The patient is evaluated by M. Walker, RN, on 4/15 as scheduled. She documents progress regarding the expected outcomes for problems (1) and (3). On 4/17, L. Krusche documents her appraisal of the patient's coping ability with respect to her family problems. Since she believes the expected outcomes are not yet reached, she would update the deadlines column by crossing out 4/17 and entering the next appropriate date for checking her progress. In this case she selects 4/21 as the next deadline date.

Case 3. Ralph L, Postoperative Right Hip Pinning and Active Pulmonary Tuberculosis (Chap 5, pp. 109-111). Patient's record, excerpted nurses' notes:

4/5.   11:00 PM. Still quite tense and experiences considerable pain when turning. Is starting to cooperate with staff to minimize pain. States nose and mouth are much more comfortable. R. Hudson, RN

4/6.   8:00 AM. Works with turning routine—pain less than previously. A. Jones, RN

4/6.   3:00 PM. No streaking past 24 hours. Says he will report any streaking immediately. Moderate amount soft, formed stool this AM. Decubitus ulcer 2 inch diameter, ¼ inch deep, clean. Skin still dry and itchy. All joints (rt hip and knee not tested) have full ROM. Mouth and nose continue comfortable with new care regimen. Unable to assess fear and loneliness due to patient's involvement with busy treatment schedule. L. Pratt, RN

4/7. 3:00 PM. Nasal and oral membranes continue comfortable with lubrication and mouthwash regimen. Continue same care. L. Pratt, RN

4/10. 3:00 PM. Skin more comfortable. Seems well lubricated and does not itch. All joints (rt hip and knee not tested) have full ROM. Oral and nasal mucous membranes moist and comfortable. Turns well with help and with minimal pain. Morale seems good. Pt Lopez visits daily. Beginning discussions of long-range plans. S. Brown, RN

Analysis. Two problems are required to be evaluated every eight hours. Referring to the care plan, a quick review would indicate to the nurse that problems (3) and (7) must be evaluated and documented during her shift. In addition, one of the AM or PM nurses also must evaluate those items that are required to be checked daily, such as problems (1), (4), (5), and (8). Every other day (even days) is the next level of frequency for checking, followed by ultimate deadline dates which require the patient's actual status to be re-evaluated.

Case 4. Stephen F. Preoperative Cholecystectomy (Chap. 5, p. 112). Patient's record, excerpted nurse's notes:

3/31. Dangles well with help. Doing deep-breathing and coughing on schedule. Requires analgesic every three to five hours during day. Voiding well. Appears to be progressing satisfactorily and coping well with the usual postoperative problems. J. Roth, RN

Analysis. On 3/31, the first postoperative day, the patient is reevaluated as scheduled, and is found to be progressing satisfactorily with no unusual problems. To update the care plan the nurse would cross out (3/31) and write in whatever date on which she believes the patient should again be evaluated. In the case of an uncomplicated postoperative cholecystectomy patient, this might be the third or fourth postoperative day.

Case 5. Mrs. Helen H, Radical Mastectomy (Chap 5, pp. 113-115). Patient's record, excerpted nurses' notes:

6/5. 3:00 PM. States that arm still aches a great deal, but is improving. Talks of her despair over loss of breast. Wonders if they "got it all." B. Joynes, RN

6/5. 11:00 PM. States that aching in arm is more tolerable. S. Haney, RN

6/6.   3:00 PM. States that arm is much more comfortable. Has learned to adjust pillows and position to maximize comfort. B. Joynes, RN

6/6.   11:00 PM. Talks of need to understand husband's feelings but is not sure she can face "really talking" with him about it yet. Seems to verbalize more easily. Seems more relaxed and less tense. Husband talks about the problem in terms of "I'm sure everything will work out ok." Seems hesitant to discuss his real feelings. Will talk c̄ him again tomorrow. S. Haney, RN

6/7.   3:00 PM. States that arm is quite comfortable now. Is easily able to wait four hours for pain Rx. Believes she can go even longer now. Manages her own comfort measures and calls for pain Rx when she needs it. Beginning to verbalize feelings of what she is going to do, such as a prosthesis, managing her home responsibilities, etc. Husband talks more freely of concerns. Says finances can be managed, but he is worried about his wife's life expectancy and her feelings of loss. Expressed need for more specific help in dealing c̄ problem. He and nurse will meet each evening when he comes to visit to think through his feelings and his role in supporting his wife. S. Haney, RN

Analysis. Entries in the nurse's notes on 6/5 refer directly to the patient's statements about her pain. In making the notations, B. Joynes, RN, refers directly to the expected outcome criterion, "statements by pt." Subsequent notes on 6/6 and 6/7 continue to refer to the patient's statements about her pain. It is apparent that by 6/7, as required by the deadlines column, the pain problem is under control. The orders can be discontinued as the nurse indicates on 6/7 that Mrs. H is now satisfactorily managing her own pain problem.

The problem of acute grief is referred to on 6/5 and indicates that the patient is verbalizing her feelings in a minimal way. On 6/7, B. Joynes writes that Mrs. H is beginning to talk of ways of coping with the problem (one of the expected outcome criteria).

The possible problems regarding her husband's feelings and the financial implications are referred to on 6/6 and 6/7. On 6/7, S. Haney indicates that the financial problem is under control. It can therefore be discontinued from the care plan.

On 6/6 Miss Haney mentioned an initial discussion with Mr. H, and on 6/7 she notes that he is beginning to talk of his concerns and that each evening the two will talk further. This would appear to be the beginning of a problem-solving relationship which the nurse will follow through. Since this has been ruled in as an actual problem, the care plan will be updated by the statement, "Worry and concern by husband over management of psychologic impact of dx." Also updated will be the expected outcome statement, "Verbalization by husband of sense of knowing his role in supporting wife," and the nursing orders statement, "Problem solve c̄ husband each evening."

Ongoing updates of the care plan would proceed as indicated by the changing circumstances in the situation.

Because the plan of care deals specifically with the apparent unusual problems, Mrs H and her husband are receiving relevant and helpful nursing care.

SUMMARY

The patient's outcomes are written on the chart and refer to the patient's actual status in relation to the expected outcomes. The statement of a patient's response to care should be a reflection of the nurse's perceptions of the patient's status relative to the criteria listed in the expected outcomes—his verbalizations, his competence, his clinical symptoms, his environmental situation.

When patient response statements are entered in the patient's record at the required intervals, that record will contain useful, relevant information about the patient's status. It will portray a concise chronology of his progress, because all of the entries will be written within the same frame of reference and with the same problems and expected outcomes in mind.

The actual or observed patient responses to care are factual statements which, when compared with the expected outcome statements, give a clear indication of the success of failure of the prescribed nursing care. They provide the rationale for ruling out a problem as solved, for revising nursing orders which are not meeting the expected outcomes, or for continuing the same approach.

As a result, the collective patient response statements provide a basis for evaluating the general success or failure of nursing care on a unit. Also, they can provide justification for more or different staffing, for new equipment, or for whatever else appears to be required for improved patient care. Chapter 13 explains how quality, assurance, and nursing audit processes are directly related to the expected versus the actual outcomes of care.

BIBLIOGRAPHY

Mayers M, Norby R, Watson A: *Quality Assurance for Patient Care: Nursing Perspectives.* New York, Appleton-Century-Crofts, 1977

Watson, A, Mayers M: *How to Write Nursing Care Plans.* Stockton Cal, KP Co Medical Systems, 1976

7

The Standard Care Plan:
Key to Quality

CONCEPT OF INDIVIDUALIZED CARE

Shortly after World War II, when behavioral science theories regarding the "whole person" and "individual differences" became prevalent, nursing accepted the concept of total, individualized care as the basic premise for effective therapeutic intervention. This concept resulted in progress from fragmented, disease-oriented nursing care to a more holistic approach for intervention.

A predictable result of the individualized care concept has been the conclusion that, if individualized care is to be accomplished, there must be respect for and adjustment to the individual wishes and needs of the patient. In effect, the conclusion was drawn that no two patients are identical, therefore no two plans of care can be identical.

CONCEPT OF STANDARDIZED CARE

Nursing professionals are coming to recognize that although persons have many differences, they also have many common characteristics, needs, and problems, and thus certain predictable responses whether they are well or ill. Nursing now considers similarities as well as differences among patients. The two concepts are mutually compatible, and when this is accepted as a basic premise, rational and systematic plans for care can be developed.

The individualized care approach to nursing practice has held that individualization requires a different plan of care for each patient. But because some patients have unusual problems and some have usual problems, the latter may require standard care plans. However, this distinction between patients cannot be made unless each patient has received an individual assessment. Thus, individualized assessment is critical in determining each patient's care. The resulting care plan is no less individualized if, after the patient's problems are determined as usual, standard care is prescribed. After thorough assessment, a nurse may well order for one patient a care plan that is essentially identical to that of another. The critical element for effective care is NOT the dissimilarity of care from patient to patient but rather the RELEVANCE of care based upon thorough, appropriately spaced nursing assessments. This is a key to quality.

DEFINITION OF STANDARD CARE

A standard care plan is a protocol for care that is likely to be applicable to most patients of a certain diagnostic or other category. The protocol is written in a format consistent with the agency's care planning form so that it can be easily put into operation in the day-by-day care planning process. The standard care plan protocol is carefully researched, written, and then ratified as the clinical standards for the designated group of patients. These protocols identify the usual, predictable problems, expected outcomes, and nursing orders. Combined with nurses' handwritten entries of unusual problems, a comprehensive plan of care is effectively composed. The combined plan attends to predetermined clinical standards and allows for the inclusion of atypical, nonstandard problems and interventions. An example of a standard care plan is shown in Figure 7-1.

Standards for care can and should be an integral part of every nursing care delivery system. It is a responsible and necessary function of an agency to identify the most frequently occurring kinds of patient problems that come to its attention and to develop standards of care relevant to them. Once the common, usually anticipated patient problems have been identified, expected outcomes and prescribed standards for nursing action can be formulated. Standard nursing orders can then be implemented appropriately for those patients whom the nurse assesses to be coping adequately with usual, predictable problems.

Basic standard care plans should be written in detail and should be updated periodically. The standard care plans can be listed by title on one portion of the Kardex or Rand so that a nurse developing a plan of care for a patient can check (√) the standard care plan that she wants to use. This checklist of standard plans is a time-saving and efficient way to institute an entire sequence of detailed standard care. The staff nurse, noting that a certain care plan has been checked (√), knows that a specified series of nursing activities has been ordered for her patients.

EXAMPLES OF STANDARD CARE PLANS

The problem-solving sequence is used for both usual and unusual problems. Thus, the method for developing a standard care plan is the same as for developing care plans for unusual problems. The standard care protocols, however, emphasize the usual, common, and predictable. Whereas the unusual problems described in Chapters 3, 4, 5, and 6 reflect the differences among patients, standard care plans reflect the similarities among patients.

To develop standard care plans, the following steps should be taken:

1. Compile a list of the most frequently occurring diagnosis— medical or nursing. This can be done most effectively by reviewing a sample of patient records. A list on a general surgical hospital unit might include standard care plans for abdominoperineal resection, for the early postoperative situations, or for potential pulmonary congestion.
2. Subdivide each of the diagnostic categories into specific, predictable (usual) problems. Include actual and potential problems. State all problems concisely and include their causes, just as suggested for unusual problems in Chapter 3.
3. For each usual problem, write an expected outcome statement. Follow the criteria for expected outcome statements as explained in Chapter 4. Include deadlines or checking intervals.
4. Write itemized, specific nursing orders for accomplishing the expected outcomes by the stated deadlines. Follow the criteria for nursing orders outlined in Chapter 5. These orders become the standard protocols for the agency or unit.
5. Review and revise the standard care plans at periodic intervals so that current scientific principles of care can be continuously incorporated.

Date	Usual Problems	Expected Outcomes	Deadlines	Nursing Orders
	1. Respiratory distress and coughing due to diagnosis	1. Normal respiratory rate between 16 and 20 per minute No cyanosis or dyspnea Verbalize reasonable comfort (breathing is easy)	day 5 √ q 8 hr	1A. Check temperature, pulse, blood pressure, and respirations every 4 hr B. Check lung sounds every 4 hr C. Intermittent positive pressure breathing as ordered D. Turn, cough, and deep breath every 2 hr E. Give cough medication F. Elevate head of bed to position conducive to easiest respiration
	2. Dehydration due to fever, inadequate intake, and anoexia	2. Taking 2000 ml liquid every 24 hr Moist mucous membranes Good skin turgor	√ q 8 hr	2A. Give 200 ml every 2 hr (even) while awake and 400 cc during night B. Record intake and output C. Give aspirin every 4 hr as ordered for temperature elevation D. Provide fluids patient prefers and tolerates
	3. Potential skin breakdown and thrombophlebitis due to immobility	3. Clear skin over all bony prominences Good pedal pulses No inflamed or tender veins	√ q 8 hr	3A. Air mattress or sheepskin in direct contact with patient's skin B. Four by fours or heel and elbow protectors C. Turn every 2 hr left side to back to right side and massage all bony prominences whenever turned D. Get order for antiemboli stockings or Ace bandages for legs and remove one hr per shift E. Unless contraindicated assist with isometric, isotonic and foot pedalling exercise to legs (10 AM, 2 PM, 7 PM, five times per session)

4. Chronic fatigue	4. Verbalize less fatigue Eating all meals and assisting with bath without undue fatigue	✓ daily	**4A.** Arrange patient schedule to allow 15 minute rest periods after meals, baths, treatments **B.** Don't begin stressful treatments until one hr after patient awakens **C.** Keep frequently used objects within easy reach of the patient **D.** Six small feedings per day may be helpful
5. Apprehension due to short-ness of breath	5. Relaxed facial expression Verbalize sense of optimism and less apprehension Verbalize under-standing of and recognition of role of apprehension in shortness of breath	day 5 ✓ q 8 hr	**5A.** Maintain calm, unhurried, appearance when in room **B.** Allow patient to verbalize fears and concerns **C.** Stay with patient during episodes of acute shortness of breath **D.** Delegate RN to explore with patient coping mechanisms to decrease apprehension

FIGURE 7-1. Standard care plan for patients with pneumonia. (Courtesy of Marlene Mayers and El Camino Hospital, used by permission)

Format for Standard Care Plans

An example of how a standard care plan might be developed is given below. The example is not intended to be comprehensive. Rather, it is intended to portray the process of problem solving as it relates to the development of standard plans.

Abdominoperineal Resection, Standard Care Plan

Usual Problems	Expected Outcomes	Deadlines	Nursing Orders
(1) Concern about how colostomy will alter life style (change of self-concept due to altered physiology and cosmetic effects)	(1) Verbalization of concerns and appropriate ideas for coping with and solving them	(hospital discharge) √ even days	(1) Initiate discussions with patient regarding what he knows about his diagnosis, the surgery, and the management of a colostomy Encourage verbalization of concerns Problem solve with patient Start before surgery and continue as patient shows readiness (Delegate one nurse to follow through with a patient)
(2) Lack of familiarity and skill with colostomy (Unfamiliar procedure and equipment due to no previous experience)	(2) Handles own equipment and describes use Inserts tube and regulates fluid flow c̄ nurse's help Inserts tube and regulates fluid flow independently Sets up equipment and solution and does irrigation independently (c̄ supervision) Changes own bag as needed Sets up, does irrigation, and	(po day 4) (po day 6) (po day 7) (po day 8) (po day 9)	(2) a. Po day 1—tell patient, if he feels able, that as soon as he feels ready the nurse will tell him about his care Review if this was done preoperatively b. Po day 2—have patient's equipment at bedside—look at it and discuss with patient how it is used c. Po day 3—demonstrate in detail how irrigation is done and how equipment is used If doctor has approved beginning the irrigations,

Usual Problems	Expected Outcomes	Deadlines	Nursing Orders
	puts away equipment independently (c̄ supervision)		demonstrate with the patient—if not, use model
			Use model if patient is not ready to look at his own stoma
			d. Po day 4—have patient demonstrate and describe irrigation either on self or model, but have nurse do actual procedure
			Give positive reinforcement for correct patient responses
			Clarify areas of doubt or misunderstanding
			e. Po days, 5, 6—have patient insert tube and regulate flow with nurse's help
			Nurse does remainder of procedure with patient's observation and discussion
			f. Po day 7—have patient insert tube and regulate fluid flow independently (with general supervision)
			g. Po day 9—have patient set up equipment, do irrigation, and put away equipment (with general supervision)
			h. Po day 10—same as po day 9
			Initiate discussion of what adaptation and assistance will be needed at home
			Give appropriate support in problem solving

Abdominoperineal Resection, Standard Care Plan (*cont.*)

Usual Problems	Expected Outcomes	Deadlines	Nursing Orders
			Get appropriate information, re-source persons, and make referrals for home care as needed

Analysis. This standard care plan has an ultimate deadline date of "discharge" for usual problem (1), with checking intervals of even days. This requires the nurse every other day to assess and document the patient's progress toward "verbalization of concerns and appropriate ideas for coping with and solving them." Upon discharge there should be a written evaluation of the patient's status and his response regarding this problem. In this case, standard care requires that one nurse be delegated to follow through with the assignment because the problem requires an ongoing trust relationship as a catalyst for its resolution.

Usual problem (2), that of "lack of familiarity and skill with colostomy procedure and equipment," has a very specific set of expected outcomes, or objectives, which are to be evaluated and documented on certain days. This particular colostomy irrigation teaching routine is set up for the average patient who is adequately prepared for surgery, who has adequate coping mechanisms, and who has a satisfactory potential for learning. This well-outlined teaching sequence provides the staff with a guide so that any qualified nurse on the staff can reinforce or continue the teaching based on this plan. When progress is documented on the days required by the deadlines column and is evaluated and written within the frame of reference of the expected outcome statements, a clear picture of the patient's progress results.

Early Postoperative Standard Care Plan

Unusual Problems	Expected Outcomes	Deadlines	Nursing Orders
(1) Potential shock due to hypovolemia or neurogenic causes	(1) Stable BP and pulse rate (near preoperative levels) and maintain	√q 2° first 12° postoperatively, then √q 8°	(1) a. BP and pulse q 15 min 1st and 2nd postoperative hours b. BP and pulse

Unusual Problems	Expected Outcomes	Deadlines	Nursing Orders
			q 30 min 3rd and 4th postoperative hours c. BP and pulse q 1° 4th to 8th post-operative hours d. BP and pulse q 2° 8th to 12th postoperative hours e. BP and pulse q 4° through po day 3 f. BP and pulse q 4° during day and at 2:00 AM until discharge
(2)Potential pul-monary congestion due to anesthesia and relative immo-bility	(2) Lungs clear to P and A (by Dr's evaluation) Patient to demonstrate ability to cough and deep-breathe correctly Verbalizes understanding of reason for coughing and deep-breathing routines	(po day 3) √q 8°	(2) a. Preopera-tively discuss c̄ patient the need to prevent pulmonary congestion, then demonstrate and have patient return demonstration Tease up a cough 10 times or to the point of fatigue Support incision with hands, pillow, or folded sheet during coughing Sit up (high or semifowler or dangling at edge of bed during cough-ing process unless contraindicated) Rest as needed between coughs (Teasing up a cough simultane-ously accom-plishes deep-breathing as well as coughing It is done by starting c̄ very gentle coughing expirations, gradu-ally increasing in depth and force to the patient's maxi-mum. Each gentle

Early Postoperative Standard Care Plan (*cont.*)

Unusual Problems	Expected Outcomes	Deadlines	Nursing Orders
			beginning to a full force cough is counted as one cough and is repeated 10 times or to the point of fatigue, whichever is first) b. Have patient deep-breathe and cough every 2° 8:00 AM to 8:00 PM and every 4° 8:00 PM to 8:00 AM
(3) Potential surgical wound or pulmonary infection due to possible wound contamination or immobility	Oral temperatures not over 99.6F	(3) √ q 8°	(3) √ and record oral temperature q 4° day of surgery and po day 1 √ and record oral temperature q 4° and at 2:00 AM thereafter
(4) Some lack of understanding of meaning of surgery and what to expect regarding nursing care, medical care, and home convalescent regimen due to lack of prior experience	(4) Verbal response that indicates appropriate understanding and ability to manage and to cope with follow-up regimen at home	(by discharge) √ even days	(4) a. Preoperatively initiate discussion with patient to ascertain understanding and to clarify possible misunderstanding Encourage continuing discussion of subject as patient needs and desires throughout hospitalization b. Clarify patient's understanding of patient's home care and medical follow-up regimen before discharge

Analysis. Usual problem (1), "potential shock," has an expected outcome of stable blood pressure and pulse rate maintained at or near normal preoperative levels. The deadlines column requires an evaluative summary at 12 hours postoperatively, every eight hours through postoperative day 1, and then daily.

Usual problem (2) is "potential pulmonary congestion." The expected outcome is for the lungs to remain clear, for the patient to demonstrate the ability to cough and deep-breathe correctly, and for him to verbalize an accurate understanding of the need for the care. The deadlines column requires that a summary evaluation be documented on the patient's record every eight hours and finally on postoperative day 3. On the third postoperative day, if the patient is progressing normally, the deep-breathing and coughing routine can be discontinued. The deep-breathing and coughing procedure is well outlined, leaving to no one's imagination just how or when it should be done.

Usual problem (3), referring to "potential wound or pulmonary infection," has as its expected outcome that the oral temperature not be over 99.6 F. The deadlines column requires evaluation and a summary statement that indicates whether or not the oral temperature has been below 99.6 F during the past eight hours.

Problem (4), referring to the common "lack of understanding of surgery," has as its expected outcome "verbal response that indicates . . . understanding and ability to . . . cope." Although one could make an expected outcome statement like "understands the . . . ," it would be hard to evaluate. When the expected outcome is written so that it can be more realistically evaluated, as in the notation "appropriate verbal responses," it becomes a more helpful criterion for measuring a patient's response to care.

The deadlines column indicates "by discharge" as the time for final evaluation of this problem, with interim evaluation and documentation every other day.

IMPLEMENTATION OF STANDARD CARE PLANS

Once standards of care for the common, expected patient problems have been developed, approved, and written, as in the previous examples, they can become vehicles for the effective delivery of consistently good care.

To accomplish this, the standards for care must be organized and written in a book or manual as a basic reference document. The various major categories of standard care plans can be copied into a card file or on a flip chart, to be readily available around the nurses' station, utility rooms, and nurses' conference rooms. Or they can be copied in sufficient numbers to be available to slip into the Kardex or Rand.

A part of every staff nurse's orientation should be the explanation and demonstration of the standard care plans. In-service education staff can provide continual review and reinforcement in order to facilitate maximum efficiency in the delivery of care.

Standard Care Plans—Case Examples

Further examples of how to use standard care plans are shown on the following pages. The typical cases developed in Chapters 3, 4, and 5 provide the basic data for the illustrations.

Part of the rationale for the system of care planning described in this volume is based upon a recognition of nursing's time pressures. To save time, standard care is not tediously written in detail every time it is ordered but rather is checked ($\sqrt{}$) on a list that is incorporated into the patient's total care plan. Each of the examples that follow includes a sample standard care checklist form to supplement the unusual problems section of the plan of care. None of the examples is intended to reflect a comprehensive treatment of the subject. They are intended to portray the problem-solving process as it applies to developing standards of care.

Mr. Harry J, Emergency Appendectomy. Table 7-1 illustrates the care plan developed for Mr. Harry J, who is experiencing an emergency appendectomy.

TABLE 7-1.   CARE PLAN

Date	Unusual Problems	Expected Outcomes	Deadlines	Nursing Orders
2/18	No apparent unusual problems at this time		(2/20)	See standard care plan

On an adjoining portion of this patient's total care plan, the checklist of standard and frequently ordered care reveals that certain items are checked ($\sqrt{}$). This form is illustrated in Table 7.2.

Analysis. The checklist indicates that the early postoperative standard care is checked ($\sqrt{}$). That particular plan includes the checking of vital signs at specific intervals, intake-output, and other relevant items. Nothing further is indicated for him except the type of bath

TABLE 7-2. CHECKLIST OF STANDARD AND FREQUENTLY ORDERED CARE FOR SURGICAL UNIT

Standard Care Plans	Frequently Ordered Items
__Preoperative	Vital Signs
2/18 ✓Early postoperative	__Oral temperature
__Late postoperative	__Rectal temperature
__Chest approach surgery	__Pulse, respiration
__Abdominoperineal resection	__Blood pressure
__Amputation, leg	__Neuro signs
__Masectomy, radical	__CVP
__Tracheostomy	__Sp gr (urine)
__Laryngectomy	Hygiene
__Skin care	2/18 ✓Bed bath
__Indwelling catheter care	__Tub bath
__Mouth care	2/18 ✓Shower
__Laminectomy	2/18 ✓With assistance
Activity:	__Self, total
Patient Preferences, Miscellaneous Information:	Intake
(1) Wants to wear own pajamas	__Intake-output
(2) Likes to read and watch TV	__Diet (type)
(3) Prefers bath in evening	2/18 ✓Surg liquid

and the diet, which are not included in the early postoperative standard care plan.

Notice that certain patient preferences have been listed in order to facilitate personalized care.

Carol J, Acute Cystitis. Tables 7-3 and 7-4 illustrate the standard care portions of the plan for Carol J, who has acute cystitis. Table 7-3 shows the care plan for her. The nursing orders section refers to the standard care plan. A checklist is illustrated in Table 7-4.

TABLE 7-3. CARE PLAN

Date	Unusual Problems	Expected Outcomes	Deadlines	Nursing Orders
2/19	Apparently coping satisfactorily at this time		(2/21)	Standard care plan

Analysis. Carol J's care checklist orders a medical standard care plan. This would include certain intervals for checking vital signs and

TABLE 7-4. CHECKLIST OF STANDARD AND FREQUENTLY ORDERED
CARE FOR MEDICAL UNIT

Standard Care Plans	Frequently Ordered Items
__Diagnostic workup	Vital Signs
__Diabetes	2/19 ✓Oral temperature
2/19 ✓Medical care	__Rectal temperature
__Hypertension	2/19 ✓Pulse, respiration
__Coronary insufficiency	__Blood pressure
__Dehydration malnutrition	__Neuro signs
__Acute CVA	__CVP
__Chronic post CVA	__Sp gr (urine)
Patient Preferences, Miscellaneous Information:	Hygiene
(1) Prefers own gown or pajamas	__Bed bath
(2) Don't awaken until 8:00 AM	__Tub bath
(3) Likes to nap and rest most of time	2/19 ✓Shower
	__With assistance
	2/19 ✓Self, total
	Intake
	2/19 ✓Intake-output
	2/19 ✓Diet (type)
	general

certain other signs and symptoms. Her checklist also indicates
that her temperature can be taken orally, that she may take a shower, and that she may have a general diet. Certain of her preferences
are also written.

James R, Lumbar Laminectomy. Tables 7-5 and 7-6 illustrate
how standard care is instituted for Mr. James R, who has had a
lumbar laminectormy. Table 7-5 shows that the nursing orders
column refers to the standard care checklist. Table 7-6 illustrates
the standard care checklist.

TABLE 7-5. CARE PLAN

Date	Unusual Problems	Expected Outcomes	Deadlines	Nursing Orders
2/17	No apparent unusual prob- lems at this time		(2/20)	See standard care plan

Analysis. The nurse has checked (√) postoperative laminectomy
care which would include certain turning, deep breathing, active and

TABLE 7-6. CHECKLIST OF STANDARD AND FREQUENTLY ORDERED
CARE FOR SURGICAL UNIT

Standard Care Plans	Frequently Ordered Items
__Preoperative	Vital Signs
__Early postoperative	__Oral temperature
__Late postoperative	__Rectal temperature
__Chest approach surgery	__Pulse, respiration
__Abdominoperineal resection	__Blood pressure
__Amputation, leg	__Neuro signs
__Mastectomy, radical	__CVP
__Tracheostomy	__Sp gr (urine)
__Laryngectomy	Hygiene
__Skin care	2/17 √Bed bath
__Indwelling catheter	__Tub bath
__Mouth care	__Shower
2/17 √Postoperative laminectomy	2/17 √With assistance
	__Self, total
	Intake
	2/17 √Intake-output
	2/17 √Diet (type)
	soft

passive exercises, vital signs at certain intervals, as well as other
relevant items. The only items not included in the postoperative
laminectomy standard care plan in this situation are the type of bath
and diet, as these are checked (√) separately.

Alice M, A and P Repair. In Tables 7-7 and 7-8 the initiation
of standard care for Mrs. Alice M is illustrated. Table 7-7 shows that
the nurse has referred to the standard care plan after stating that the
patient has "no apparent unusual problems at this time." Table 7-8
shows the checklist of standard care and indicates that the preoperative plan has been ordered by the nurse.

TABLE 7-7. CARE PLAN

Date	Unusual Problems	Expected Outcomes	Deadlines	Nursing Orders
2/20	No apparent unusual problems		(2/22)	See standard care plan

Analysis. The preoperative standard care plan would include
specific care items, such as vital signs at appropriate intervals, certain

TABLE 7-8. CHECKLIST OF STANDARD AND FREQUENTLY ORDERED CARE FOR GYNECOLOGY UNIT

Standard Care Plans	Frequently Ordered Items
2/20 ☑Preoperative	Vital Signs
__Early postoperative	__Oral temperature
__Late postoperative	__Rectal temperature
__D and C	__Pulse, respiration
__Vaginal hysterectomy	__Blood pressure
__Abdominal hysterectomy	__Neuro signs
__A and P repair	__CVP
Patient Preferences, Miscellaneous Information	__Sp gr (urine)
	Hygiene
	__Bed bath
	__Tub bath
	__Shower
	__With assistance
	__Self, total
	Intake
	__Intake-output
	2/20 ☑Diet (type)
	NPO after 12:00 midnight

observations, teaching, and nursing support for the usual and expected apprehension prior to surgery. The diet order states, "NPO after midnight."

After surgery, if Mrs. M is assessed by the nurse to be progressing satisfactorily, the preoperative standard will be discontinued and the early postoperative plan will be checked (√).

Joyce H, Abdominal Hysterectomy. Tables 7-9 and 7-10 illustrate how standard care for Mrs. Joyce H is instituted. Table 7-9 shows the nurse's statement that Mrs. H is "apparently coping and progressing well." Under nursing orders, standard care plans are referred to. Table 7-10 shows the standard care checklist. Since Mrs. H is now in her third postoperative day, the nurse has checked (√) the late postoperative standard of care.

TABLE 7-9. CARE PLAN

Date	Unusual Problems	Expected Outcomes	Deadlines	Nursing Orders
4/20	Apparently coping and pro-gressing well		(4/23)	See standard care plan

TABLE 7-10. CHECKLIST OF STANDARD AND FREQUENTLY ORDERED
CARE FOR GYNECOLOGY UNIT

Standard Care Plans	Frequetly Ordered Items
__Preoperative	Vital Signs
__Early postoperative	__Oral temperature
4/20 ✓Late postoperative	__Rectal temperature
__D and C	__Pulse, respiration
__Vaginal hysterectomy	__Blood pressure
__Abdominal hysterectomy	__Neuro signs
__A and P repair	__CVP
Patient Preferences, Miscellaneous Information:	__Sp gr (urine)
(1) Don't awaken until 8:30 AM	Hygiene
(2) Will bathe in evening	__Bed bath
(3) Wears own gown	__Tub bath
(4) Give hot tea at bedtime	4/20 ✓Shower
	__With assistance
	4/20 ✓Self, total
	Intake
	__Intake-output
	4/20 ✓Diet (type)
	general

Analysis.   A standard plan for the late postoperative phase would
include all of the relevant items of care—observations, teaching,
home care planning. In addition, the nurse has checked (✓) that the
patient may take showers and that she is on a general diet. Under
patient preferences, several items are listed. By the use of a few
checks (✓), the nurse has initiated an entire sequence of predetermined high quality standard care.

SUMMARY

Although people have many differences, they also have many
similarities. They have common needs, problems, strengths, and attitudes. They share cultural similarities, predictable responses, and
so on. This is true whether people are well or ill. Because nursing
recognizes the common elements as well as the differences among
its clients, nursing care planning reflects that recognition. Having a
system of specialized care for unusual problems (differences) and a
system of standard care for usual problems (common elements)
is a way to reflect and to act upon this realization.

Standard plans for nursing care should be a vital and basic part of
every care delivery system. The identification of common, frequently
encountered, predictable problems provides the basis for developing

standard care protocols. The problem-solving approach is used for usual problems, just as it is employed to develop care plans for unusual problems.

The content of standard plans should be specific but brief and should be kept as simple as possible. The total number of standard care plans a nursing unit uses should also be kept to a reasonable minimum.

Each standard care routine should have a title and should be included on a Checklist of Standard and Frequently Ordered Care. This allows a nurse, simply by checking ($\sqrt{}$), to initiate an entire sequence of predetermined standard care.

Standard care plans are justified for patients who have usual problems but not for those with unusual difficulties. This distinction between patients cannot be made unless each has received an individualized assessment at safe intervals. Thus, the individualized assessment is crucial to determining whether or not a patient's problems are usual, and, therefore, whether a standard care plan is appropriate.

BIBLIOGRAPHY

Anderson B: Nursing by trial and era—the standard misconception. Supervisor Nurse 7:35, July 1976

Holle M: Retrospective nursing audit—Is it enough? Supervisor Nurse 7:23, July 1976

Mayers M, El Camino Nursing Staff: Standard Care Plans. Stockton Cal, KP Co Medical Systems, 1975, Vol 1, Medical Surgical, Orthopedic

Mayers M, El Camino Nursing Staff: Standard Care Plans, Stockton Cal, KP Co Medical Systems 1976, Vol 2, Critical and Psychiatric Care

Mayers M, El Camino Nursing Staff: Standard Care Plans. Stockton Cal, KP Co Medical Systems, 1976, Vol 3, Maternal and Child Care

Nichols M, Wessells V (eds): Nursing Standards and Nursing Process. Wakefield Mass, Contemporary Publishing, 1977

Zimmer M: Guidelines for development of outcome criteria. Nurs Clin North Am 9 [No 2]:317, 1974

8

Diversified Care Settings: Adaptations

The system for patient care planning that has been explained in the previous chapters can, with minimum modification, be adapted to any nursing service situation.

Wherever nurses find patients, they also find a need for identifying problems and for setting up a strategy for care. The steps of the problem-solving process are equally applicable to short-term, long-term, and special service settings. Assessing, identifying problems, setting objectives, and planning nursing orders are universally appropriate. Only the specific content of the care plan varies from setting to setting. The framework remains the same.

This chapter provides examples of nursing care plans as they might be modified to meet the unique circumstances of various acute care settings. Case studies and sample care plan formats are discussed and developed for the emergency department, the operating room, acute medical-surgical, obstetrics, psychiatry, and extended care. For each of these nursing services areas, there is an example of how to develop standard care plans. After each example is a case study that provides a basis for applying the principles of patient care planning.

THE EMERGENCY DEPARTMENT

Nurses in rapid care settings have long felt a need for realistic ways to plan for the care of their patients. The relatively short duration of contact with each patient and preoccupation with the physician's services have militated against the formal planning of nursing care in emergency settings. In situations where rapid nursing action is necessary to save lives, the priorities for written plans on each patient clearly will be different from priorities in other nursing areas. However, systematic care planning can provide a good basic framework for realistic plans of care in emergency settings.

Development of Standard Plans

If a group of emergency department nurses wishes to establish systematic care planning, one of their first jobs is to identify the common presenting problems or diagnoses of the patients whom they see in the emergency setting. These problems provide the basis for the development of standard care protocols.

In the emergency care setting, frequently encountered or usual problems might be shock in both patient and family, emotional stress, fear of unknown consequences, pain, sense of disorganization, and so forth. When the major categories of common problems have been identified, they can be divided into subproblems and expected outcomes. Then standard nursing orders can be formulated.

A typical problem experienced by many patients in the emergency setting is illustrated as a standard care plan below.

Example of Standard Care Plan. In the following example, the problem "anxiety and fear due to interrupted life style and unfamiliar treatment" has been considered and a standard care plan has been developed.

Anxiety and Fear

Usual Problems	Expected Outcomes	Deadlines	Nursing Orders
Anxiety and fear due to interrupted life style and unfamiliar treatment	Verbalization of fears Asks questions	$\sqrt{}$q 2°	a. Explain progress and care in a relevant way b. Give general

Usual Problems	Expected Outcomes	Deadlines	Nursing Orders
			predictations about the expected course of care or treatment, such as special procedures, x-rays, hospital admission, length of time involved, and so forth c. Explain that nurses and Dr are always nearby— explain how to call Stay nearby so patient knows he can trust staff d. Give evidence of concern by appropriate physical contact (hand on arm, wiping brow) e. Be directive and supportive This is an appropriate time for the patient to be dependent

An emergency department can utilize two types of care plans: standard plans and transfer plans. The standard care plans are used for quick reference and review and for orientation of new staff. The transfer care plan is used when a person is admitted for inpatient care. The transfer plan is completed by an emergency department nurse, who sends it with the chart to the receiving unit. Nurses receiving the patient will refer to the transfer plan as part of the data base for formulating their own plan of care.

Figure 8-1 illustrates one hospital's example of a transfer care plan. Examples of diagnosis-related standard care plans are shown in Figures 8-2 and 8-3.

This standard care plan should have a title and should be listed among other protocols in the emergency department's checklist of standard and frequently ordered care. When checked ($\sqrt{}$), it would indicate that a patient is experiencing this particular problem and that the predetermined standard care is being implemented. Flow sheets incorporating standard expected outcomes aid in documenting the patient's response.

---

1. Present complaint: _____

2. Systems review:
   a. Cardiovascular-circulatory: Color_____ Edema site_____
      Hematoma bruises_____ other _____
   b. Gastrointestinal: nausea_____ vomiting_____ diarrhea _
      constipation_____ other _____
   c. Respiratory: dyspnea_____ irregular_____ shallow_____
      cough_____ wheezing_____ rales_____ congestion_____
      oral airway_____ nasal_____ ET_____ assisted _____
   d. Musculoskeletal: laceration site_____ deformity site _____
      fracture site_____ impaired movement_____ impaired sensitivity__
      other _____
   e. Neurologic: level of consciousness: _____
      level of orientation_____ paralysis, weakness, site of_____
      pupils R - L   reactive   nonreactive   equal   unequal
      pupils R - L   smaller   larger
      Mental state_____ calm, anxious, hysterical, nervous, crying,
      belligerent, restless, other_____
   f. Urinary: incontinent   retention   color_____ other _____

3. Pertinent medical and surgical history: _____
   _____

4. Pertinent family history: _____
   _____

5. Nursing history: Allergies: _____
   Visual problems_____glasses   contacts
   Hearing problems _____ hearing aid_____
   Dentures: upper   lower   partial   bridge   none
   Special diet:_____
   Previous hospitalizations_____ ECH _____
   Medication taken _____
   Other _____

FIGURE 8-1. Transfer care plan. (Courtesy of Marlene Mayers and El Camino
Hospital, used by permission)

Checklist for Standard Care, Emergency Room. The following
list contains phrases that are statements of some of the usual and
frequently encountered problems of patients experiencing acute
illness or injury. The problems are shown as they might appear on a
checklist form. The list is not intended to be comprehensive:

_____ Anxiety, patient
_____ Anxiety, family
_____ Shock due to emotional stress, patient
_____ Shock due to emotional stress, family

Date	Usual Problems	Expected Outcomes	Dead-lines	Nursing Orders
	1. Pain due to trauma	1. Verbalizes relief of pain	By trans-fer	1A. Obtain order for pain medication as needed B. Patch both eyes with two patches each to provide cushioning and tape loosely C. Keep room darkened
	2. Potential further injuries due to activity	2. Lies quietly at rest	By trans-fer	2A. Keep patient in bed with side rails up B. Instruct patient to lie still C. Keep call light in patient's hand and instruct in use
	3. Anxiety due to present visual impairment and fear of permanent damage	3. Verbalizes fears re vision loss or impairment	By trans-fer	3A. Reassure patient that everything possible is being done for him B. Explain all procedures as they are being performed C. Answer all patient's questions, directing questions to MD when necessary D. Visit patient q 15 minutes to ascertain needs and to support as needed
	4. Potential increased intraocular pressure due to edema or bleeding of laceration of penetrating foreign body	4. Early detection of signs/symptoms of increased intraocular pressure	By trans-fer	4A. Instruct patient to avoid straining (ie, sneezing, coughing) B. Check vital signs on admission and q 15 minutes C. Report immediately any signs/symptoms of increased intraocular pressure (severe pain, edema, darkening of eye color) D. Keep patient in high Fowler's position

FIGURE 8-2. Standard care plan for eye injury. (Courtesy of Marlene Mayers and El Camino Hospital, used by permission) (Continued on page 160.)

Date	Usual Problems	Expected Outcomes	Dead-lines	Nursing Orders
	5. IF APPLI- CABLE, SEE STANDARD CARE PLAN FOR HEAD INJURY			
	6. If laceration requiring sur- gery, potential anxiety due to abruptness of situation	6. Verbalizes knows what to expect now	By trans- fer	6A. As time and condition permit, prepare patient for what to expect after surgery **B.** Complete operating room checklist
	7. If chemical burn, potential further injury	7. Prevention of further injury	By trans- fer	7. Irrigate eyes with solution per ER protocol

FIGURE 8-2. Continued.

Date	Usual Problems	Expected Outcomes	Dead-lines	Nursing Orders
	1. Potential neurologic damage	**1.** Early detection of neurologic damage	By trans-fer	**1A.** On admission obtain from any available sources a history of injury **B.** Start intravenous fluid and keep open with slow drip **C.** Sandbag head and neck **D.** Administer O_2 **E.** Check at least q 5 minutes: Vital signs and report increase in blood pressure/decrease pulse Neuro signs Level of consciousness For restlessness and/or seizures (see standard care plan for seizures) For blood or cerebrospinal fluid drainage from ears and nose **F.** Apply armband identification
	2. Potential res-piratory diffi-culties due to cerebral edema and/or injury	**2.** Early detection of difficulties	By trans-fer	**2A.** Insert airway as needed **B.** Suction as needed **C.** At least every 5 minutes until stable, check: Respiratory rate and quality Breath sounds Pulse quality and rate Chest symmetry Level of consciousness **D.** At same time, check for and report: Cyanosis, pallor Signs of hyperventilation Adverse anxiety and apprehension

FIGURE 8-3. Standard care plan for head injury. For further care, see standard care plan for eye injury. (Courtesy of Marlene Mayers and El Camino Hospital, used by permission)

_____ Sense of disorganization, patient
_____ Sense of disorganization, family
_____ Eye injury
_____ Head injury

Priorities for Care

Many problems in emergency settings are primarily medical and are solved by physician's orders, such as the treatment of hemorhage, anaphylaxis, fractures, nausea and vomiting, and so on. Physician's orders are certainly of vital necessity and must be given highest priority in emergency situations. However, many nursing care problems, such as those listed above, can also be identified, and the indicated nursing care must be implemented. Adding the nursing component can greatly improve the total care which a patient receives.

As nurses know so well, many emergency problems are those experienced by the family or friends of the patient. Their fears and frustrations and their helplessness and disorganization are part of the patient's world; as such, they fall within nursing's domain. Because this is true, family member's problems should be considered.

Since most patients are under the care of the emergency department for only a few hours at the most, it is not realistic for nurses to have lengthy care plan and record-keeping systems. As much as possible, checklists should be used for standard nursing care and for frequently ordered medical care. Unusual problems, however, should be briefly documented. Because emergency care is rapid care, much of the nurse's problem solving of either usual or unusual problems is done mentally, is implemented immediately, and is recorded as soon as possible thereafter. If the nurse does her rapid, mental problem solving in the logical sequence described in this volume, the care she decides to give is most likely to be relevant and effective. To facilitate instantaneous problem solving and to minimize the risk of error or oversight, it is particularly critical for the nurse to have standard care protocols for ready reference.

Summary

Patient care planning in the emergency room is accomplished by making certain that the following criteria are met:

1. Identifying the most frequent patient-centered problems and developing expected outcomes, deadlines (or checking intervals), and nursing actions. These become the unit's standard care plans or protocols.
2. Listing the titles of the standard care plans on a checklist format for quick and efficient documentation of problems and care.
3. Orienting all staff to the meaning and magnitude of standard care plans.
4. Obtaining a statement of the physician's expectations of the patient's course of treatment or convalescence (routine or complicated).
5. Making statements of the overall nursing criteria for discharge.
6. Utilizing the agency's care plan format for the unusual, out of the ordinary problems of patients which require other than standard care.
7. Utilizing a transfer care plan when a patient is being admitted to the hospital.

THE OPERATING ROOM

In the operating room, effective nursing care standards have long been routine for maximizing patient safety during surgery. Most OR care routines are related primarily to the physical care of the patient from the time just prior to anesthesia to the time he leaves the operating suite.

Recently, however, surgery nursing staffs have been looking for, and finding, ways to do more comprehensive care planning. They have assumed more responsibility for the patient's care in surgery by identifying relevant usual and unusual problems in advance. This has become known as "preoperative assessment." An operating room nurse interviews each patient on the evening before surgery or earlier if indicated. She identifies usual problems and orders standard care. Also, she identifies any unusual problems and, for these, orders specialized nursing care.

Development of a Standard Care Plan

Usual problems commonly experienced by patients before and during surgery can be identified in a number of ways. Since patients' charts may not be too helpful for obtaining this information, it is suggested that OR nurses interview a sample of patients and thus identify the common core of usual problems.

Sample interviews might reveal some of the following usual problems: fear of helplessness about anesthesia induction and the like, fear of unexpected complications of surgery, anxiety about unknown surgical and recovery room procedures, a sense of ambiguity about the time element involved in surgical and recovery procedures, concern for the wellbeing, comfort, and availability of the family during and after surgery, and concern by the family regarding all of the previous items.

These are some of the usually expected problems of patients during the preoperative phase. Once problems have been identified and the relevant standard care plans implemented, the patient can probably cope satisfactorily with the experience of surgery.

Example of a Standard Preoperative Care Plan. Following is an example of how an operating room standard care routine may be developed. It is based upon one of the common problems previously enumerated.

Preoperative Care Plan

Usual Problems	Expected Outcomes	Deadlines	Nursing Orders
Anxiety regarding unknown surgical and recovery room procedures and a sense of ambiguity about the time elements involved	Ability to cope $\bar{c}$ anxiety ↓ expression of anxiety Asks questions and discusses concerns	(Anesthesia induction) $\sqrt{}$q 4°	a. Early during evening of hospital admission, show pt the videotape of OR and Recovery Room staff and procedures Answer his questions and discuss his concerns b. Give him appropriately specific information about his surgery

Analysis. The very common preoperative problems of anxiety about unknown surgical and recovery room procedures and a sense of ambiguity about the time elements involved are, in the preceding example, developed through to the expected outcomes and to the nursing actions designed to solve the problem. Each common or usual problem experienced by a patient preoperatively can in a similar fashion be solved. The resulting standard care policies help significantly to upgrade patient care during the preoperative and surgical phases of hospitalization.

A Case Study and Its Associated Care Plan

Mrs. Marilyn H is a 46-year-old housewife. She has just been admitted to a surgical unit and is scheduled for an abdominal hysterectomy the next morning. The hysterectomy has become necessary because of a large intrauterine fibroid tumor.

J. Jones, the OR nurse, stops by to talk with Mrs. H in order to ascertain what her concerns might be while she is under the care of the operating room staff the following morning.

Mrs. H is surprised and pleased to learn of the concern for her by the OR nurses. She says, "I've always thought of surgical nurses as efficient machines with deft hands and intense eyes peering over green masks. I had never thought of you as real people who care personally about the people who are wheeled in and out." She then goes on to say that her real fear is of taking the anesthetic and being completely "in the hands of someone else" for a short while. Just thinking about the moment of anesthetic induction appears to result in real feelings of anxiety. Her facial expressions are tense, and her voice sounds shaky and fearful. The feeling of "being out of control" in a strange environment is, apparently, unusually difficult for Mrs. H to cope with.

The nurse and Mrs. H talk for some time. Miss Jones is soon able to ascertain that the only unusual problem Mrs. H is likely to experience preoperatively is the anxiety related to being helpless for a period of time.

J. Jones discusses her findings with the patient's nurse on the unit. They agree that, in the morning, a nurse will be delegated to be a continuing source of familiarity and support pre- and postoperatively. J. Jones calls the physician to inform him of her findings and her plans. He says he will visit the patient this evening and will talk with her briefly in the morning before surgery. J. Jones also calls the family to assure them that they are welcome to be with Mrs. H as they wish. She tells them what to anticipate in the morning, where they can wait, and how they can be of most help to the patient.

The unit nurse makes notations under the unusual problems section of her care plan, and J. Jones makes the following statements on her OR care plan.

Unusual Problems	Expected Outcomes	Deadlines	Nursing Orders
Acute anxiety due to fear of unconsciousness and helplessness, and strange environment	Ability to cope Verbalizes fears and tensions ↓ facial expressions of anxiety and fear	$\sqrt{q}$ 2° when awake	a. One nurse establish rapport and provide ongoing support to increase familiarity of environment b. Include family and allow their presence and support at all possible times c. Include physician in the plan to facilitate his ability to provide a source of "a familiar person" to the patient d. Nurse delegated for ongoing care to accompany pt to surgery and stay until anesthesia induction Be available upon recovery to provide an ongoing sense of familiarity e. Be sure patient has opportunity to talk to physician in OR suite before anesthesia induction

Analysis.   The care plan for Mrs. H would be posted at the entrance to the designated operating room. In the morning, the circulating nurse who is in charge of that room reviews the care plans for the scheduled patients and assumes responsibility for implementing all the specialized care for unusual problems as well as for the prescribed ongoing standard care.

Summary

In operating room settings where nursing care planning is done, a nurse is delegated to visit preoperative patients on the afternoon or evening before surgery in order to assess and to identify their difficulties and concerns. If there is an unusual problem, it is documented as illustrated in the example of Mrs. H. The unusual problem is discussed with the responsible staff nurses on the unit, and a copy of the care plan is posted in the operating room where the patient is scheduled to have surgery. In the morning, the nurse responsible for the patients in certain operating rooms reviews the unusual problems and implements the required nursing follow-up or support. Care planning by operating room nurses can do much to ease the anxiety associated with surgical procedures.

THE MEDICAL-SURGICAL UNITS

Medical-surgical nursing units in the typical general hospital are perhaps the most diversified units. As a result, they are among the most challenging settings for nursing practice. Increasingly shorter hospitalizations with the resulting comparatively large number of patients acutely ill or disabled, coupled with a multiplicity of diagnoses and of diagnostic and surgical procedures, leaves the medical-surgical nurse with few complaints of boredom. She does, however, have an overriding concern about her constantly changing caseload. She recognizes that, in the absence of a viable and systematic method for assessment and care planning, all too many of her patients pass through her jurisdiction without the kind of nursing care they require.

Care Plans for Five Medical-Surgical Patients

To assist the medical-surgical nurse with this problem, many of the examples cited in this book relate to a medical-surgical care unit. More specifically, the five major cases from the previous chapters are included here to illustrate care planning as it applies to medical-surgical patients. Each of the five care plans is portrayed very much as it might be found in actual use and as it would be seen on a flip chart or in a care plan notebook. Each case begins with the overall care planning information, followed by the checklist of standard and frequently ordered care, and then medications, treatments, and diagnostic tests. Each would conclude with the unusual problems section. Because the unusual problems have already been elucidated, the reader will be referred to them in Chapter 5. Standard care plan checklists are now being incorporated for these patients to show how plans for unusual problems can be used in combination with standard care plans.

Each section of the care plan for each of the five patients is completed for a given point in time. Each plan may change subsequently as progress is made or as new problems develop.

Case 1. Richard M, Multiple Traumatic Injury

Patient Care Plan.

Physician's expectations regarding
course of treatment and convalescence:
( ) typical or routine
(√) atypical or complicated
If atypical or complicated, in what way?
Some possible unknown injuries,
delayed reduction of mandible. Keep
tracheostomy open for anesthesia for
mandible reduction.

Identifying Information: _____

_____

_____

Diagnosis: Multiple trauma, Fr zygoma,
mandible clavicle, basilar skull,
Intracranial clot. Facial lacerations,
Tracheostomy
_____

_____

Nursing criteria for discharge or maintenance (overall expected outcomes):
(a) Patient and family will verbalize appropriate understanding of course of convalescence and indicate ability to follow through.
(b) They will demonstrate ability to manage any necessary care.

M. Fullington, RN

Home Care Coordination activities: _____
Other relevant information (socioeconomic, etc): _____

Checklist of Standard and Frequently Ordered Care—Surgical Unit

Standard Care Plans

Frequently Ordered Items

__Preoperative
__Early postoperative
√Late postoperative
__Chest approach surgery
__Abdominoperineal resection
__Amputation, leg
__Mastectomy, radical
√Tracheostomy
__Laryngectomy
__Skin care
__Indwelling catheter care
2/18 √Mouth care
Activity
2/18—Ambulate with help ad lib
Patient Preferences, Miscellaneous Information
(1) Likes to read and watch TV
(2) Has own pajamas—prefers them
(3) Wants nurse nearby while eating

Vital Signs
__Oral temperature
2/18 √Rectal temperature
2/18 √Pulse, respiration
2/18 √Blood pressure
2/18 √Neuro signs
__CVP
__Sp gr (urine)
Hygiene
2/18 √Bed bath
__Tub bath
__Shower
2/18 √With assistance
__Self, total
Intake
2/18 √Intake-output
√Diet (type)
osterized diet

Medications, Treatments, Diagnostic Tests

Date—Medications	Date—Treatments	Date—Diagnostic Tests
2/10 Liquid ferrous sul- fate pc 300 mg tid 2/10 Valium 5 mg prn	2/10 Do not turn on rt side—patient has fractured clavicle	

Date—Medications	Date—Treatments	Date—Diagnostic Tests
2/10 Darvon, prn	2/10 Tighten clavicle braces q̄ AM 2/10 Tracheostomy —clean inner cannula q̄ shift —remove inner cannula and change q̄ day —suction prn —trach tube can be changed prn every few days	

Unusual Problems

Date	Unusual Problems	Expected Outcomes	Deadlines	Nursing Orders
	(See Chap 5, pp. 104-107)			

Mrs M's checklist of standard and frequently ordered care has certain standard care items checked (√) that are belived to be consistent with care at this time. The detailed standard care plans to which each of the checked (√) items refers would be slipped into the Kardex or would be easily available for reference or review. Examples of standard tracheostomy and late postoperative care plans are shown in Figures 8-4 and 8-5.

Case 2.   Mary R, Postoperative Celiotomy, Cestomy, Double-Barreled Colostomy

Patient Care Plan

Physician's expectations regarding course of treatment and convalescence:
   ( ) typical or routine
   (√) atypical or complicated
If atypical or complicated, in what way?
Obese—abdominal wound will heal slowly

Identifying Information: _____

Diagnosis: Celiotomy, cecostomy, double-barreled colostomy, 4/8.

Nursing criteria for discharge or maintenance (overall expected outcomes):
(a) Will verbalize appropriate understanding of medical regimen and follow-up.
(b) Will demonstrate satisfactory ability to irrigate own colostomy.
(c) Will verbalize feelings about colostomy, and state realistic plans for home care.
                                               Mrs. Walker, RN

Home Care Coordination activities: HCC notified on 4/14.
Other relevant information (socioeconomic, etc.): _____

Date	Usual Problems	Expected Outcomes	Dead-lines	Nursing Orders
	1. Anxiety due to suction procedure	1. Tolerates suctioning without becoming restless	1 day √ q 8 hr	1A. Frequent reassurance as needed B. Explain procedure before doing it C. Consistent personnel to care for patient
	2. Discomfort due to suctioning	2. Relates comfort	√ q 8 hr	2A. Give pain medication as needed for comfort B. Use good suctioning techniques
	3. Anxiety due to inability to verbalize	3. Communicates through alternate means	√ q 8 hr	3A. Provide paper and pen if able to write B. Make board with common phrases (in patient's language) if patient is able to point C. Use simple sign language D. Keep call light within patient's reach
	4. Potential post-op bleeding due to trauma during procedure	4. No bleeding	16 hr √ q 4 hr	4A. Only partially deflate cuff every hour for 3 to 4 minutes B. Suction gently without excessive pressure C. Instill 1 to 2 ml saline to avoid trauma to mucosa every suctioning
	5. Thick or tenacious secretions due to lack of humidification	5. Secretions can be easily removed	√ q 8 hr	5A. Instill 2 to 3 ml saline every suction B. Hyperinflate lungs with breathing bag or respirator 2 or 3 times and suction Have patient sigh after suctioning C. Continuous humidification via vaporizer or heated tracheostomy mist D. Push fluids to 3,000 ml per day
	6. Potential respiratory difficulties due to shallow respirations from bedrest	6. Normal rate and character of respirations	√ q 4 hr	6A. Encourage deep breathing B. Turn patient q 2 hr C. Percussion, vibration and coughing exercises q 4 hr

FIGURE 8-4. Standard care plan for tracheostomy. (Courtesy of Marlene Mayers and El Camino Hospital, used by permission)

Date	Usual Problems	Expected Outcomes	Deadlines	Nursing Orders
	1. Potential shock due to anesthesia or bleeding	1. Blood pressure stable for patient Pulse between 60 and 100 No blood-saturated dressing or linen No bright red bleeding	Day of surgery then q 8 hr	1A. Vital signs per hospital policy B. Check dressings with vital signs C. Note color and amount of drainage D. If shock occurs: —call MD —start oxygen —low shock block —get intravenous setups ready —have epinephrine ready
	2. Potential hypostatic pneumonia due to anesthesia and immobility	2. No obvious congestion Normal respiratory pattern Normal temperature (under 100 degrees)	√ q 8 hr	2A. Turn, cough, splint surgery area, and deep-breathe every 2 hr B. Activity as per orders
	3. Pain in surgical area due to pressure or spasms	3. Verbal or nonverbal expression of reasonable comfort	√ q 8 hr	3A. Offer and give pain medication every 3 to 4 hr first 2 to 3 days unless contraindicated B. Position comfortably, splint incision with pillows to maintain comfort
	4. Potential nausea and vomiting	4. Take and retain fluids	Day of surgery √ q 8 hr	4A. Start with sips of fluids B. Gradually increase amounts C. Give medication for nausea if it persists

FIGURE 8-5. Late postoperative standard care plan. (Courtesy of Marlene Mayers and El Camino Hospital, used by permission) (Continued on page 172)

Date	Usual Problems	Expected Outcomes	Dead-lines	Nursing Orders
	5. Potential oliguria or re-tention	5. Void satisfactor-ily at least 20 ml per hour	Day of surgery ⌄ q 8 hr	**5A.** Stand to void if not contraindicated **B.** Measure amounts **C.** Catheterize if ordered as needed **D.** Intake/output until voiding satisfactorily
	6. Potential fainting	6. No falls or near falls when ambu-latory No dizziness when up	Postop day 3 ⌄ daily	**6A.** Change from flat to vertical position slowly **B.** Assist when up as long as faintness persists
	7. Potential slow healing and/or infection	7. Clean wound No purulent drainage	By dis-charge ⌄ daily	**7A.** Use good aseptic techniques when changing dressings **B.** Inspect operative area at time of dressing change
	8. Potential ileus, gas pains, and/or constipation due to anes-thesia and sur-gical trauma	8. Soft abdomen Passing gas	Postop day 3 ⌄ daily	**8A.** Keep active in bed or ambulating **B.** Rectal tube for discomfort unless contraindicated **C.** Get order for enema or laxative if no bowel movement by third or fourth day **D.** Check daily and record amount and consistency of each bowel movement **E.** Check bowel sounds daily

FIGURE 8.5. Continued.

Checklist of Standard and Frequently Ordered Care—Surgical Unit

Standard Care Plans	Frequently Ordered Items
__Preoperative	Vital Signs
__Early postoperative	__Oral temperature
__Late postoperative	4/14 √Rectal temperature
__Chest approach surgery	4/14 √Pulse, respiration
√Abdominoperineal resection	__Blood pressure
__Amputation, leg	__Neuro signs
__Mastectomy, radical	__CVP
__Tracheostomy	__Sp gr (urine)
__Laryngectomy	Hygiene
__Skin care	__Bed bath
__Indwelling catheter care	4/14 √Tub bath
__Mouth care	__Shower
__Laminectomy	4/14 √With assistance
Activity: _____	__Self, total
4/14—Ambulate 10 min tid	Intake
Patient Preferences, Miscellaneous	__Intake-output
Information: _____	4/14 √Diet (type)
	Regular diet
	Hi pro, lo residue

Medications, Treatments, Diagnostic Tests

Date—Medications	Date—Treatments	Date—Diagnostic Tests
4/14 FeSo 300 mg po tid	4/14 Irrigate wound $\bar{c}$ H_2O_2 and NS and then pack $\bar{c}$ wet fine mesh gauze and 4 x 4's covering Change qid	4/14 CBC 4/14 Stool GUIAC 3-2-1
Librium 10 mg po tid		
Multivits po tid		
Colace 100 mg po		
Davron 65 mg po $\bar{q}$ 4° prn for pain	4/14 Teach patient colostomy care	
Chlortrimeton 4 mg po $\bar{q}$ 4° prn		

Unusual Problems

Date	Unusual Problems	Expected Outcomes	Deadlines	Nursing Orders
	(See chap 5, pp. 107-108)			

The standard care plan for abdominoperineal resection is illustrated in Figure 8-6.

Date	Usual Problems	Expected Outcomes	Deadlines	Nursing Orders
	PREOP			
	1. Standard	1. Standard		1. Standard
	2. Fear of cancer, colostomy and surgery	2. Verbalize understanding of situation	Day of surgery	**2A.** Follow through on MD's revelation to patient regarding colostomy and include family **B.** Describe function of a modern sigmoid colostomy Stress that colostomy will NOT be incontinent: —little care necessary —no odor after irrigation —no bags needed **C.** Possible cleansing enema, nasogastric tube, and Foley catheter preoperatively
	POSTOP			
	1. Standard	1. Standard		1. Standard
	2. Potential skin breakdown due to continuous perineal drainage	2. Clear skin around perineum	√ q 8 hr	**2A.** Change dressing as needed and record amounts, color, and number of times changed **B.** Cleanse area each time with soap and water **C.** Use fluffs and ABD's (not peripads) with T-binder or fuller shield
	3. Potential psychologic trauma from colostomy	3. Patient able to look at stoma Gradually able to care for own colostomy	√ q 8 hr	**3A.** Throughly explain and guide patient in his own care **B.** Encourage verbal ventilation of feelings

4. Potential abdominal trauma or excoriation of skin around stoma	4. Clear skin around stoma No bleeding around stoma	Dis-charge √ 8 hr	4A. Care not to disturb colostomy B. Later, change bags only when necessary and cleanse with PHisoHex and water around stoma each time bag is changed C. Protect skin around stoma with benzoin
5. Potential abdominal distention due to nasogastric tube not draining well	5. Nasogastric tube draining well No complaints or nausea	√ q 8 hr	5. Check for tube patency every 2 hr (even) and irrigated as needed per MD's orders
6. Potential complications at home due to inadequate understanding of colostomy irrigations	6. Patient verbalizes willingness and demonstrates ability to do own irrigations	Dis-charge √ daily	6A. Ascertain from patient most convenient time for irrigations at home and then do irrigations at same time each day B. Allow patient to do own care at his speed and as his ability to cope physically and mentally allows C. Keep instructions clear, simple, and concise D. Instruction to be delegated to same person each day
7. Potential difficulty with home management	7. Verbalizes satisfactory arrangement for home care	Dis-charge √ daily	7A. Discuss with patient his plans for care at home B. Ascertain if Public Health Nurse or Visiting Nurse Association referral needed and, if so, consult MD for approval

FIGURE 8-6. Standard care plan for abdominoperineal resection. (Courtesy of Marlene Mayers and El Camino Hospital, used by permission)

Case 3.   Mr. Ralph L, Postoperative Right Hip Pinning and Active Pulmonary Tuberculosis

Patient Care Plan

Physician's expectations regarding course of treatment and convalescence:
( ) typical or routine
(√) atypical or complicated
If atypical or complicated, in what way?
Malnourished, expect slow healing and slow progress regarding ambulation.

Identifying Information: _____

_____

Diagnosis: Dehydration, malnutrition, active pulmonary tbc, left hip fracture pinned 3/20.

_____

Nursing criteria for discharge or maintenance (overall expected outcomes):
(a) Will verbalize approval of convalescent facility or home care.

(b) Will demonstrate safe and efficient transfer and ambulation techniques.

(c) Will verbalize understanding of and demonstrate safe isolation technique for
    tbc.

(d) Will verbalize appropriate understanding of medical care regimen and ability to
    follow up.   L. Pratt, RN

Home Care Coordination activities: HCC notified on 4/5

Other relevant information (socioeconomic, etc): On Medicare hospital insurance.

Social worker notified on 4/5.

Checklist of Standard and Frequently Ordered Care—Surgical Unit

Standard Care Plan

__Preoperative
__Early postoperative
√ Late postoperative
__Chest approach surgery
__Abdominoperineal resection
__Amputation, leg
__Mastectomy, radical
__Tracheostomy
__Laryngectomy
__Skin care
__Indwelling catheter care
__Mouth care
__Laminectomy
√ Hip pinning

Activity: _____

_____

Patient Preferences, Miscellaneous
   Information: _____

Frequently Ordered Items

Vital Signs
      __Oral temperature
3/21 √ Rectal temperature
3/21 √ Pulse, respiration
3/21 √ Blood pressure
      __Neuro signs
      __CVP
      __Sp gr (urine)
   Hygiene
      __Bed bath
      __Tub bath
      __Shower
      __With assistance
      __Self, total
      Intake
3/21 √ Intake-output
3/21 √ Diet (type)
      Gavage feedings
      D/10/W 300 mg by dry
      NG—q 4°
      Skim milk 100 ml
      9-5 c̄ INH
      Bouillon 200 ml 9 AM
      daily

Medications, Treatments, Diagnostic Tests

Date—Medications	Date—Treatments	Date—Diagnostic Tests
3/20 Rainbow insulin coverage NPH insulin 15 U of U40 8:30 AM Thexforte 1 ml IM 9:00 AM daily Ethambutal 400 mg 9:00 AM daily Pyridoxine 100 mg 9:00 AM daily INH 100 mg c̄ 100 ml skim milk NG 905 KCL 20% tsp TT 9:00 AM daily Elase and neosporin to decubitus Tolwin prn hiccoughs	3/20 Do not get patient out of bed Weigh daily with bed scale Foot cradle Clinitest, Acetest 6:30-11:30-4:30- Hs IPPB c̄ NS 20 pressure q̄ 4° Cough qid Foley catheter clamp 9-1-5-9-1-5- unclamp 8:30- 12:30-4:30-etc Irrigate Foley c̄ ¼% Acetic acid 9-1-6 Clean decubitus c̄ Antiseptic soap uncovered	3/20 Sputum (Luken's tube) Tues and Fri

Unusual Problems

Date	Unusual Problems	Expected Outcomes	Deadlines	Nursing Orders
	(See Chap 5, pp 109-112)			

The standard care plan for hip pinning is illustrated in Figure 8-7.

Case 4. Mr. Stephen F, Preoperative Cholecystectomy

Patient Care Plan

Physician's expectations regarding course of treatment and convalescence:
 (√) typical or routine
 ( ) atypical or complicated

Identifying Information: _____
_____
_____
Diagnosis: Cholecystectomy 3/29

Nursing criteria for discharge or maintenance (overall expected outcomes):
See standard postoperative expected outcomes.   J. Roth, RN

Home Care Coordination activities: _____
Other relevant information (socioeconomic, etc): _____ _____

Date	Usual Problems	Expected Outcomes	Deadlines	Nursing Orders
	PREOP			
	1. Standard	1. Standard		1. Standard—expect to be up in wheel chair by postop day 2—no weight-bearing on affected extremity for three months
	2. Severe muscle spasms with increased pain due to injury	2. Verbalizes reasonable comfort	Day of surgery $\sqrt{}$ q 8 hr	2A. Position of comfort unless contraindicated B. Traction adjusted properly, if in traction C. Medicate as needed for spasm and pain
	POSTOP			
	1. Standard	1. Standard		1. Standard
	2. Potential surgical complications and pain due to poor alignment of affected extremity	2. Affected extremity always in good alignment	$\sqrt{}$ q 8 hr	2A. When turning to either side, keep pillow between legs B. Keep sandbag or pillow against outer aspect of legs to prevent external rotation
	IMMOBILIZED PATIENT			
	3. Standard	3. Standard		3. Standard
	4. Potential impairment of circulation, movement, and sensation	4. Able to move toes Toes warm and pink No complaint of numbness or tingling in toes No edema	$\sqrt{}$ q 8 hr	4. Observe toes every 2 hours (even) for 24 hours, then every 4 hours (12-4-8) for warmth, sensation, movement, blanching, and swelling

Potential problem	Expected outcome		Nursing orders
5. Potential edema and discoloration after getting out of bed	5. No edema No discoloration	✓ q 8 hr	5. Elevate leg whenever patient is in chair
6. Potential confusion due to senility and/or medication	6. Oriented to home place and person Not lethargic Participates actively in self-care	Discharge ✓ q 8 hr	6A. Introduce self whenever entering room and mention time of day B. Medication for pain as needed, but do not oversedate C. Restraints only if absolutely necessary D. Develop with patient diversion activities and encourage visitors and TV set E. Encourage to participate in care (bath, meals, turning) and praise for steps in that direction
7. Potential unsafe ambulations due to improper crutch-walking or use of walker	7. No falls Proper crutch-walking with no weight-bearing on affected extremity	daily	7A. Get order for physical therapy B. Observe ambulation at least first 2 times ambulates for: —proper crutch-walking techniques or use of walker and —no weightbearing
8. Concern over management after discharge	8. Verbalizes satisfactory plans for care after discharge	Discharge ✓ daily	8A. Ascertain from MD if patient to return home or to convalescent home B. Talk with family regarding their feelings and concerns C. Encourage patient to ventilate feelings and wishes but reinforce MD's plans
9. If hip prosthesis, potential dislodging of prosthesis due to improper positioning of affected extremity	9. No sudden development of severe pain No extreme external rotation	Discharge ✓ daily	9A. Keep leg abducted and remove splint (if used) only for bath B. Avoid flexion beyond what MD specifies C. When turning onto side place 3 pillows between legs and support with pillows in front and behind legs D. Do NOT turn to affected side (too painful)

FIGURE 8-7. Standard care plan for hip pinning. (Courtesy of Marlene Mayers and El Camino Hospital, used by permission)

Checklist of Standard and Frequently Ordered Care—Surgical Unit

Standard Care Plans	Frequently Ordered Items
3/29 √ Preoperative	Vital Signs
__Early postoperative	__Oral temperature
__Late postoperative	__Rectal temperature
__Chest approach surgery	__Pulse, respiration
__ Abdominoperineal resection	__Blood pressure
__Amputation, leg	__Neuro signs
__Mastectomy, radical	__CVP
__Tracheostomy	__Sp gr (urine)
__Laryngectomy	Hygiene
__Skin care	__Bed bath
__Indwelling catheter care	__Tub bath
__Mouth care	__Shower
__Laminectomy	__With assistance
Activity: _____	__Self, total
	Intake
Patient Preferences, Miscellaneous Information:	__Intake-output
(1) Walks c̄ cane due to old CVA	3/29 √ Diet (type)
Left-sided weakness.	NPO after midnight
(2) Likes hot drink before bedtime (as diet allows.)	

Medications, Treatments, Diagnostic Tests

Date—Medications	Date—Treatments	Date—Diagnostic Tests

(In this space are written any current medical orders for medication, treatments, and diagnostic tests)

Unusual Problems

Date	Unusual Problems	Expected Outcomes	Deadlines	Nursing Orders
3/29	Appears to be coping satisfactorily, both physiologically and psychologically		(3/31)	See standard care plan J. Roth, RN

Mr. F's preoperative cholecystectomy is illustrated in Figure 8.8.

Date	Usual Problems	Expected Outcomes	Deadlines	Nursing Orders
	1. Anxiety due to impending surgery and unfamiliar environment	1. Verbalizes questions and concerns Verbalizes: "I know what to expect now," Good preop night	AM day of surgery	1A. Evening or afternoon before surgery, explain unit routines and postop routines B. Explain specific procedures relating to patient's type of surgery —prep —sleeping medication —preop medication —time of surgery —visitor's policy —time in recovery room and what to expect —general postop management —nothing by mouth
	2. Potential complications or injury while medicated and anesthetized	2. No injuries, falls, or accidents No physical complications	AM day of surgery	2A. Complete preop checklist before preop medication given B. Patient to void before preop medication is given C. Stay in bed after preop medication—side rails up
	3. Short term admissions: potential injuries due to going home unassisted	3. Will have assistance going home	Discharge	3. Explain to patient that he must have someone drive him home after having general anesthesia

FIGURE 8-8. Standard preoperative care plan. (Courtesy of Marlene Mayers and El Camino Hospital, used by permission)

Case 5. Mrs. Helen H, Radical Mastectomy

Patient Care Plan

Physician's expectations regarding
course of treatment and convalescence:
  (√) typical or routine
  ( ) atypical or complicated

Identifying Information: _____
_____
_____

If atypical or complicated, in what way?

Diagnosis: Adenocarcinoma, rt breast
c̄ metastasis to regional lymph nodes.

Nursing criteria for discharge or maintenance (overall expected outcomes):

(a) Will demonstrate ability to correctly do arm exercises and to manage any
    necessary self-care.

(b) Will verbalize correct understanding of what to do in case of swelling, fatigue,
    or other complications.

(c) Ongoing verbalization (c̄ associated congruent feelings) of ability to cope c̄ the
    changes in her life. (1) active plans for getting and using prothesis. (2) active
    plans for getting back into normal life style.

(d) Ongoing verbalization (c̄ associated congruent feelings) by husband re ability
    to give his wife the necessary support.   S. Hiskin, RN

Home Care Coordination activities: _____
Other relevant information (socioeconomic, etc): _____

Checklist of Standard and Frequently Ordered Care—Surgical Care

Standard Care Plans

Frequently Ordered Items

	Standard Care Plans		Frequently Ordered Items
	__Preoperative		Vital Signs
	__Early postoperative	6/4	√Oral temperature
	__Late postoperative		__Rectal temperature
	__Chest approach surgery	6/4	√Pulse, respiration
	__Abdominoperineal resection	6/4	√Blood pressure
	__Amputation, leg		__Neuro signs
6/4	√Mastectomy, radical		__CVP
	__Tracheostomy		__Sp gr (urine)
	__Laryngectomy		Hygiene
	__Skin care	6/4	√Bed bath
	__Indwelling catheter care		__Tub bath
	__Mouth care		__Shower
	__Laminectomy	6/4	√With assistance
	Activity: _____		__Self, total
			Intake
	Patient Preferences, Miscellaneous		__Intake-output
	Information: _____	6/4	__Diet (type)
			Surg liquids

Medications, Treatments, Diagnostic Tests

Date—Medications	Date—Treatments	Date—Diagnostic Tests
6/4 Demerol, 100 mg prn q 4° for pain Seconal, 100 mg prn at hs	6/4 Connect drain to suction machine Catheterize q 8° if necessary	

Unusual Problems

Date	Unusual Problems	Expected Outcomes	Deadlines	Nursing Orders

(See Chap 5, pp. 113-114)

Mrs. Helen H's standard plan for radical mastectomy is illustrated in Figure 8-9.

Summary

Each of the five case studies illustrates how a plan might appear in actual usage on a medical-surgical unit. If it is assumed that a unit has a flip chart system for data storage and retrieval, each of the care plans would require two sides of an 8½ by 11 inch sheet of paper or card. Each of the four major sections of the care plan, (1) overall planning information, (2) unusual problems, (3) checklist of standard care, and (4) medication, treatments, and diagnostic tests, would appear on one half of each side of the care plan page. The 8½ by 11 inch page can be folded and inserted into the Kardex or Rand in various ways to meet the requirements of the nurses involved. For unusual problems sections, which in some cases are quite long and extend beyond half a page, additional half-pages can be added and attached by using adhesive or staples. Many agencies are obtaining larger flip charts to accommodate more information.

As each unit nurse or other responsible nurse comes on duty, she reviews the Kardex or Rand. Very quickly she is able to ascertain which of her patients are coping well and which have unusual problems. For those with usual problems, she will indicate by checking (√) or by writing on the care plan "see standard care" such-and-such. These standard care plans are available for reference in books on the unit or in Xeroxed form in a file so that a nurse can have a copy for her personal reference. For those with unusual problems, she will delegate to her staff the appropriate specialized care, and she will note for herself the intervals at which she must assess and record the patient's response to that care.

When all of the important abstracted patient care information is filed together, as in a flip chart, it is possible to very quickly obtain a clear picture of the status of the individual patients, as well as of an entire group.

Entries on the checklist of standard or frequently ordered care

Date	Usual Problems	Expected Outcomes	Deadlines	Nursing Orders
	PREOP **1. Anxiety and fear due to unknown results**	1. Verbal and non-verbal expression: "I can cope with what will happen"	Preop	1A. Listen Let patient verbalize own feelings, hopes, fears, and questions B. If surgery is known to be extensive, demonstrate arm exercises preoperatively C. One nurse to establish a one-to-one relationship for duration of hospitalization
	EARLY POSTOP **1. Grief due to loss of breast**	1. Verbalizes feelings Sleeps all night without sleep medications	✓ daily	1A. Listen and clarify concerns B. Reply with honesty C. Be direct in encouraging interest in getting up, grooming, self-care, etc
	2. Potential hypostatic pneumonia due to shallow respiration	2. No respiratory distress Temperature under 101F	✓ q 8 hr	2A. Be especially thorough with breathing and coughing exercises B. Give pain medication before deep-breathing and coughing C. Ambulate vigorously and frequently

LATE POSTOP			
1. Limited movement and edema of arm and hand due to surgical trauma	1. Able to close hand Able to comb own hair	Postop day 4 √ daily	1A. Exercise and positioning per MD's orders B. Get orders if there are none
2. Altered self-concept due to surgical procedure	2. Verbal and non-verbal expression: "I can cope with this situation" Do own makeup Have specific plans for prosthesis and grooming Verbalize concern re close personal relationships	By discharge	2A. Listen Let patient express feelings and fears B. Check with MD regarding Mastectomy, Club or Public Health Nurse, and information regarding clothes and stores for mastectomy patients C. Give specific ideas and information regarding clothes and stores for mastectomy patients D. Allow husband to express concerns Problem solve with him and help him to see his role

FIGURE 8-9. Standard care plan for radical mastectomy. (Courtesy of Marlene Mayers and El Camino Hospital, used by permission)

may be made in pencil because they are likely to change. If an agency does not want erasures, a system of pen-and-ink entries with crossing out or a superimposed "DC" can be easily implemented.

When medical-surgical nurses use a systematic method of care planning and when they actively follow it through, their growing feelings of satisfaction that patient problems are identified and solved and that excellent standard nursing care is being done will reward them for their efforts.

THE OBSTETRIC UNIT

Obstetrics is a specialized variation of an acute medical-surgical unit. In addition, it has the labor and delivery components, which have many of the elements of rapid care settings. As a result, the basic medical-surgical care plan format is very satisfactory for the postpartum setting. The rapid care variations are applicable to labor and delivery.

Development of a Standard Care Plan

In any specialized care area, such as obstetrics, orthopedics, and neurology, it is relatively easy to identify a manageable core of predictable patient problems and, therefore, to develop a set of standard care plans for them.

Some typical problems that postpartum patients experience are potential hemorrhage, uterine cramping and pain, uncomfortable breast tissue, lack of knowledge about infant care, fatigue, lack of knowledge about self-care after hospital discharge, lack of knowledge about how to manage sexual intercourse, what to do about contraception before the six-week checkup, and so forth.

Some of the items that might appear on an obstetric unit's checklist of standard care plans are portrayed in the example below. A nurse checking ( ) any specific item would automatically be ordering a detailed sequence of predetermined standard care.

Sample Standard Care Checklist

Postpartum bleeding
Infant care teaching
Contraception teaching
Self-care teaching

Medical follow-up teaching (mother and infant)
Breast-feeding teaching
Bottle-feeding teaching
Uncomplicated postpartum
Caesarean section

If a nurse indicates that contraception teaching is necessary, the sequence of care to be implemented would be based upon a predetermined standard care plan for that topic, much like the one that follows.

Contraception, Standard Care Plan

Usual Problems	Expected Outcomes	Deadlines	Nursing Orders
Lack of specific knowledge of how to manage fertility regulation, postpartum	Reiteration of correct understanding of use of interim birth control method	(Before discharge)	a. On first or second postpartum day, initiate discussion of birth control Ascertain pt's feelings, knowledge and preferences b. Answer questions and clarify misunderstandings re: —lactation and fertility —pros and cons of sexual intercourse first 6 weeks postpartum —use of birth control foam as an interim method c. If foam is the method of preference, discuss in detail Have pt reiterate instructions for use d. Clarify need for a more reliable method to be determined at time of 6 week checkup e. If another method is desired, obtain specific

Contraception, Standard Care Plan (*cont.*)

Usual Problems	Expected Outcomes	Deadlines	Nursing Orders
			order from physician and instruct carefully f. Allow to verbalize her concern regarding feasibility and therefore the reliability of any method that is ordered g. Be sure pt knows about 6 week checkup appointment and ascertain that she will be able to keep it

A Case Study and Its Associated Care Plan

Mrs. Janie J is admitted to the postpartum unit after delivering a premature infant girl. The baby weighs 4 pounds and is progressing satisfactorily for her size. She is in the premature nursery and is receiving a specialized regimen of care.

Mrs. J is recovering satisfactorily. She had been planning to breastfeed but is now undergoing a breast-drying routine. She is trying to adjust to a revised life style based upon the fact that the infant will remain in the hospital for some time.

The nurse reviews her situation and initiates the following standard care plans: postpartum bleeding, child spacing teaching, mother-infant bonding, and self-care teaching. In addition she makes an entry under the unusual problems section of the patient care plan. Mrs. J's care plan follows:

Patient Care Plan, Mrs. Janie J

Physician's expectations regarding
course of treatment and convalescence:

(√) typical or routine

(   ) atypical or complicated

If atypical or complicated, in what way?

Diagnosis: _____

Vaginal delivery of premature infant

(No episiotomy) gr T, para T

_____

_____

Nursing criteria for discharge or maintenance (overall expected outcomes):
(a) Will verbalize ability to cope c̄ frequent hospital visits
(b) Will demonstrate clear evidence of maternal—infant bonding.
(c) Will correctly reiterate information regarding medical follow-up for self and indicate willingness to follow through.
(d) Will correctly reiterate information regarding use of interim birth control method.
Home Care Coordination Activities: 6/28 Referred to Public Health Dept for premature infant home evaluation, within two weeks.
Other relevant information: _____

Standard Care Plans

√ Postpartum bleeding
__ Infant care teaching
√ Child spacing teaching
√ Self-care teaching
__ Medical follow-up teaching
    (mother and infant)
__ Breast-feeding teaching
__ Bottle-feeding teaching
Activity: _____
Patient Preferences, Miscellaneous
Information: _____

__ Perineal care routine
__ Breast drying routine
__ Breast pump
√ Mother-infant bonding

Bathing:
√ Shower
__ Bed Bath

Diet: Regular

Unusual Problems

Date	Unusual Problems	Expected Outcomes	Deadlines	Nursing Orders
6/28	Frustration and anxiety due to thwarted maternal instinct because of premature infant	↓ frustration and feelings of anxiety ↑ maternal-infant relationship	√qod	a. Arrange with nursery for mother to hold infant and to assist c̄ feeding 2 or 3 times daily while in hospital b. Arrange for daily visits of mother to nursery to assist c̄ feeding or to be with infant, after mother's discharge from hospital c. Assist mother c̄ planning transportation and scheduling of home activities to accommodate daily hospital visits

Unusual Problems (*cont.*)

Date	Unusual Problems	Expected Outcomes	Deadlines	Nursing Orders
				d. Arrange c̄ nursery to do follow-up teaching of infant care and feeding as well as necessary medical follow-up after infant's discharge

Analysis. With the special nursing assistance outlined for Mrs. J by the nurse, her feelings of frustration and anxiety should gradually diminish, and a growing mother–infant relationship should begin. The nursery nurses will have an even more specifically designed care plan to guide their activities to facilitate the bonding process between the mother and her infant.

Other kinds of unusual problems that an obstetric patient might experience are high risk for hemorrhage due to atonic uterus, frustration and tension due to difficult breast feeding that results from infant's poor sucking reflex, and apparent disinterest in infant care due to emotional and physical fatigue from long, difficult labor.

Summary

Because of its specialized nature, obstetric nursing lends itself well to the concept of standard care for patients with usual problems. The spectrum of usual problems is not difficult to identify. Much obstetric nursing tends to be standardized into protocols for care, whether or not formal policies are written. However, informal protocols can be significantly improved if standard plans for usual problems are formulated, ratified, and systematically implemented.

As in any other patient care situation, unusual obstetric problems are handwritten, criteria (expected outcomes) for measuring success or failure are stated, and specialized, nonstandard nursing orders are implemented.

THE PSYCHIATRIC UNIT

Psychiatric nurses work daily with clients who experience a wide range of behavioral disorders. These nurses have become expert in individualized care planning. They are accustomed to working closely with psychiatrists, psychologists, and social workers to assess patients' progress and in designing plans for therapy. These plans are written either in charts or on other forms that are accessible to all so that there will be consistency of approach and intervention methods among all the staff. On psychiatric units, care plans can provide most useful guidelines for all members of the health care team.

Formulation of a Standard Care Plan

Applying standard care policies for a psychiatric unit warrants a great deal of discussion. At first thought, psychiatric nurses generally tend to believe that there can be no standard care applicable to many patients. Upon closer investigation they find that, as in other patient care settings, some common predictable problems do seem to be identifiable. For example, when formulating care plans for all the patients on a given psychiatric unit, nurses find that they are continually writing certain problems, such as withdrawal, mistrust of staff, disorientation to time and place, depression, and agitation. As they write expected outcomes and nursing actions, they find they are ordering the same basic intervention methodologies for a large number of patients. As a result, psychiatric nurses interested in developing a systematic approach to care planning find it helpful to commit to writing those standard nursing plans they believe essential for good patient care. In addition, they specifically hand-write the unusual problems, expected outcomes, and specialized nursing interventions that apply when a patient experiences difficulties and concerns outside a predictable range.

Sample Standard Care Checklist.   Here are some of the items that might appear on the patient care plan checklist* for a psychiatric unit:

Unawareness of genesis of present problems
  Self and others
  Emotional/somatic
Dangerous to others
Dangerous to self
Dependence on drugs or alcohol
Disorientation to time and place
Environment, impaired contact

*This list is adapted from Mayers and El Camino Hospital Nursing Staff: *Standard Care Plans*, 1975, Vol. 2.

Escape needs
Inability to control impulses
Impaired self-care abilities
Seizures
Impaired self-preception
Sleeping problems

When one or more titles are checked, a detailed sequence of standard care is automatically initiated. For example, if dangerous to self is checked ($\sqrt{}$), the staff knows that certain specific care is ordered. The standard care plan for disorientation to time and place might be developed as follows. This care would be expected to be implemented whenever the specific item is noted.

Disorientation to Time and Place

Usual Problems	Expected Outcomes	Deadlines	Nursing Orders
Disorientation to time and place	Sense of knowing time and place Responds correctly to queries re time and place	Weekly	a. When talking with patient, state where he is and the general or specific time of day Repeat as appropriate b. Reinforce by saying "This is your room," "This is my office." At mealtimes, say, "It is 8:00 o'clock, breakfast time," and the like c. At appropriate intervals, ask the patient, "Do you know where you are?" or "Do you know what time it is?" Clarify misconceptions d. Show pt how to read signs or how to recognize a room Show him the clock Give him a calendar and refer to it frequently

Date	Usual Problems	Expected Outcomes	Deadlines	Nursing Orders
	Potential inadequate awareness of own contributions to present problems: **—profound** **—considerable** **—some**	Verbalizes or demonstrates adequate awareness of own contribution to present problem(s)	Day of discharge daily 5 to 7 days	**A.** Have patient participate in a primary process group: much/moderate/some **B.** Have patient participate in group therapy: much/moderate/some **C.** Staff to establish verbal contact with patient: much/moderate/some **D.** Staff to establish touch contact with patient: much/moderate/some **E.** Help patient establish daily structure: much/moderate/some **F.** Encourage patient to interact with other patients and staff: **much/moderate/some** **G.** Make behavioral contracts with patient: much/moderate/some **H.** Offer interpretations of behavior to patient: much/moderate/some **J.** Encourage/demonstrate mechanics of problem solving: much/moderate/some **J.** Explore grief work with patient: much/moderate/some **K.** Help patient establish normal sleep patterns: much/moderate/some
	LEVEL OF IMPAIRMENT PROFOUND IMPAIRMENT occurs when there is *inability* to function in the area CONSIDERABLE IMPAIRMENT occurs when there is *disability* in or restriction of function in the area SOME IMPAIRMENT occurs when there is *disturbance* in function in the area LEVEL OF INTERVENTION MUCH—almost *constant* nursing interaction with patient in dependent state MODERATE—*frequent* nursing interaction with patient achieving some independence SOME—*intermittent* nursing interaction with patient basically independent ADEQUATE—patient exhibits *no* significant *impairment* in the given problem area			
	Potential inadequate awareness of others contributions to present problems: **—profound** **—considerable** **—some**	Verbalizes or demonstrates adequate awareness of others' contribution to present problem(s)	Day of discharge daily 5 to 7 days	**L.** Encourage patient to interact with other patients and with staff: **much/moderate/some**

FIGURE 8-10. Standard care plan for unawareness. (Courtesy of Marlene Mayers and El Camino Hospital, used by permission)

Another example of a psychiatric standard care plan is shown in Figure 8-10.

A Case Study and Its Associated Care Plan

James R is 48 years old. He has a recent history of depression and inability both to keep a job and to cope with the pressures of daily life. He is withdrawn and verbalizes very little. He is hospitalized because of acute withdrawal and depression. In addition to noting certain usual problems, the responsible psychiatric nurse would write a statement of the patient's unusual problem and her orders for specialized care. Mr. R's care plan is illustrated below.

Patient Care Plan, James R

Physicians expectations regarding course of treatment and convalescence

Diagnosis: _____
  Depressive reaction

( ) typical or routine
(√) atypical or complicated
If atypical or complicated, in what way?
6/10 deferred, re √ on (6/25)

Nursing's criteria for discharge or maintenance (overall expected outcomes):
6/10 Deferred until more data can be obtained re √ on (6/25)

Home Care Coordination Activities: _____
Other Relevant Information: _____

Standard Care Plans

√ Interpersonal contact impaired
__Mistrust of staff
__Disorientation to time and place
√ Depression
__Agitation
__Compulsive behavior

__Group therapy
__Occupational therapy
__Recreational therapy

Diet: _____
_____

Patient Preferences, Miscellaneous Information: _____
Likes to play volleyball outdoors

Enjoys television and reading

Likes cleansing shower in AM, sedative bath in PM

Medications, Treatments, Diagnostic Tests

Date—Medications   Date—Treatments   Date—Diagnostic Tests

(In this space are written the current medical orders for James R for medications, treatments, and diagnostic tests.)

Unusual Problems

Date	Unusual Problems	Expected Outcomes	Deadlines	Nursing Orders
6/10	Unable to sleep at night Paces the floor due to anxiety and depression	Increasing length of intervals of sleep at night	√qod	a. Provide warm sedative bath at 9:30 PM and follow c̄ warm milk b. Assist to bed and give sedative backrub c. If he awakens and can't get back to sleep, make him comfortable in day room Turn on TV and offer warm drink—not coffee Repeat sedative if sufficient time lapses d. Sit c̄ patient and talk if he desires, then assist back to bed Repeat as necessary e. If sleeping in AM do not awaken before 9:00 AM f. Encourage activity during daytime to create normal fatigue

Mr. James R's standard care plan for impaired interpersonal contact is shown in Figure 8-11.

Summary

Systematic care planning can be applied in the psychiatric setting in a fashion similar to that applied in other patient care areas. Both standard and specialized care plans can be successfully implemented. A resultant upgrading and consistency of patient care will be realized when specific nursing actions are committed to writing. The care plans will also be an invaluable reference to the other therapeutic disciplines.

When criteria for discharge are written, all members of the team should consult with the psychiatrist and psychiatric social worker so as to maximize the possibility of formulating meaningful and realistic goals.

Date	Usual problems	Expected outcomes	Dead-lines	Nursing Orders
	Potential impaired inter-personal contact: **—profound** **—considerable** **—some**	Continually increas-ing ability to initiate or not withdraw from interpersonal contact	Day of dis-charge daily 5 to 7 days	**A.** Have patient participate in a primary process group: much/moderate/some **B.** Have patient participate in group therapy: much/moderate/some **C.** Staff to establish verbal contact with patient: much/moderate/some **D.** Staff to establish touch contact with patient: much/moderate/some **E.** Help patient establish daily structure: much/moderate/some **F.** Encourage patient to interact with other patients and staff: much/moderate/some **G.** Make behavioral contracts with patient: much/moderate/some **H.** Offer interpretations of behavior to patient: much/moderate/some **I.** Encourage/demonstrate mechanics of problem solving: much/moderate/some **J.** Explore grief work with patient: much/moderate/some **K.** Help patient establish normal sleep patterns: much/moderate/some

FIGURE 8-11. Standard care plan for impaired personal contact. (Courtesy of Marlene Mayers and El Camino Hospital, used by permission)

EXTENDED CARE FACILITIES

The convalescent or extended care setting has many elements of a typical medical-surgical nursing unit. In addition, it has long-term components more characteristic of community health and home nursing. The care of the elderly, who tend to be in the majority in convalescent hospitals, is a challenge that many nurses have found to offer great satisfaction. Care planning for extended care patients provides many possibilities for improving the quality and consistency of care for the elderly. Particularly when criteria for maintenance or discharge are committed to writing via the care plan, the processes of problem identification and strategy planning gain real meaning and relevance. The resultant attention and enthusiasm from the staff have a multitude of beneficial side effects.

The same principles of systematic care planning utilized in other nursing situations can just as easily be applied to the extended care setting. Designing standard care plans has many possibilities for good care. So, of course, does defining unusual problems and developing associated specialized care.

Development of a Standard Care Plan

Standard care plans for an extended care unit or hospital can be developed only after a core of difficulties or concerns commonly experienced by patients in that setting is identified. Some usual problems likely to be identified are frustration and depression due to long-term illness, sense of isolation from accustomed surroundings and life sytle, and disorientation due to unaccustomed surroundings. Typical physical problems are likely to be poor nutrition, constipation, sleeplessness, slow mentation, lethargy, and skin breakdown.

Sample Checklist.   A checklist of standard care plans on an extended care unit might include:

Post CVA (hemiplegia)
Transfer and ambulation techniques
Socialization milieu therapy
Dietary intake, assist
Dietary intake, feed
Bowel care routine
Sleep routine
Skin care

Oral hygiene
Decubitus care
Nail care

If one or more of the standard care items are checked (√), the staff nurses know that an entire sequence of nursing care has been ordered. If, for instance, mouth care is checked (√), a nurse knows that certain detailed standard mouth care has been ordered, as in the following.

Standard Care Plan for Oral Hygiene

Usual Problems	Expected Outcomes	Deadlines	Nursing Orders
Unclean teeth and dry oral mucosa Foul breath	Clean teeth Moist, comfortable mucosa Clean breath	√daily	a. Brush dentures and teeth c̄ dentrifice q AM and after every meal b. In the case of dentures, have pt rinse mouth c̄ mouthwash or other approved solution c. Massage gums lightly with gloved finger dipped in glycerin and lemon d. Assist pt in attaining recommended fluid intake e. Involve pt in own mouth care as much as possible Assist as needed to assure that care is thoroughly done

Thus, each item implies a completely detailed strategy for care.

A Case Study and Its Associated Care Plan

Mrs. Mildred O, age 74, is newly admitted to an extended care facility. Six weeks ago she had surgery for an abdominal obstruction. She was discharged to the home of her son and daughter-in-law. This has been her only home for two years, since the death of her husband. Unfortunately, the physiologic stress of major surgery left her weak, debilitated, and mentally irritable. Her volatile emotions and unpredictable mood swings have caused her son and daughter-in-law to request her admission to an ECF until she is significantly improved. The decision and her subsequent admission to the extended care facility have left Mrs. O feeling depressed, angry, abandoned, and rejected.

The nurse responsible for Mrs. O's care interviews her and her family and identifies both usual and unusual problems. Her care plan, when complete, provides a clear summary of the nurses' and physicians' perceptions of her status relative to long-range therapeutic goals.

A quick review of Mrs. O's care plan gives a comprehensive idea of her problems, the overall goals, and the necessary standard care. In addition, it provides a clear picture of her unusual problems and associated nursing care orders. It follows:

Patient Care Plan, Mrs. O

Physician's expectations regarding
course of treatment and convalescence:
( ) typical or routine
($\sqrt{}$) atypical or complicated
If atypical or complicated, in what way?
Progress will be slow due to emotional
upset over admission to hospital.
Wants to be at home.

Identifying Information:
_____
_____
Diagnosis: Malnutrition, postoperative
laparotomy, 3/2
_____
_____
_____

Nursing criteria for discharge or maintenance (overall expected outcomes):
(a) Will show pattern of emotional stability for a minimum of two weeks.
(b) Will have a pattern of regular and adequate dietary intake c̄ steady weight gain.
(c) Will radiate a sense of comfort with and ability to express feelings about
    hospital and family.
(d) Family will verbalize satisfactory plans for coping c̄ home care.
Home Care Coordination Activities: _____
Other relevant information: _____

Standard Care Plans

    __Post CVA (hemiplegia)
    __Transfer and ambulation technique
4/10 $\sqrt{}$ Socialization milieu therapy
4/10 $\sqrt{}$ Dietary intake, assist
4/10 $\sqrt{}$ Bowel care routine
    __Sleep routine
    __Skin care

__Physical therapy
__Range of motion
__Catheter care
__Bladder irrigation
__Colostomy care
__Vaginal douche
__Oral temperature

Standard Care Plans (*cont.*)

4/10 √Oral hygiene	__Rectal temperature
__Decubitus care	4/10 √Blood pressure
__Nail care	__Pulse, respiration
Activity: _____	Hygiene
	__Bed bath
Patient Preferences, Miscellaneous Information:	__Self, total
Has own pillow and comforter for bed	__Tub bath
	4/10 √Shower
	4/10 √With assistance
	__Self, total
	4/10 √Diet: Regular, c̄ between
	meal snacks

Medications, Treatments, Diagnostic Tests

Date—Medications	Date—Treatments	Date—Diagnostic Tests
4/10 Multivitamins po, 9 AM daily	4/10 K pad to lower abdomen ad lib	
4/10 Milk of magnesia, 9 PM		

Unusual Problems

Date	Unusual Problems	Expected Outcomes	Deadlines	Nursing Orders
4/10	Severe feelings of rejection and abandonment due to admission against wishes	↑ verbalization of feelings ↓ verbal and nonverbal expressions of rejection ↑ expressions of comfort and well-being	qod	a. Spend extra time c̄ patient Listen b. One nurse to develop ongoing trust relationship (Delegated to J. White LVN) Find out what makes her feel happy and comfortable and obtain those items as possible Arrange for frequent family visits and outings c. Maintain a positive attitude about getting well and going home d. Allow family to verbalize feelings of guilt over the forced admission

Unusual Problems	Expected Outcomes	Deadlines	Nursing Orders
			Assist them in making satisfactory and realistic plans for home care e. Actively assist pt in socializing to find compatible acquaintances among patient groups

Summary

The criteria for discharge or maintenance are of particular importance in the extended care setting. The long-term nature of the majority of disease processes predisposes toward open-ended thinking among staff, that is, an inability to think in terms of wellness goals or criteria for discharge. For many patients in the convalescent care setting it is unrealistic to consider discharge plans, *but it is absolutely necessary to establish criteria for maintenance*. In the absence of written criteria or overall expected outcomes, the patient's care lacks meaning and focus, and care is unlikely to result in any real progress toward any desired or intended outcomes. The lack of established criteria for discharge or maintenance is at the root of much of the hopelessness, lethargy, and deterioration among patients. Aged persons with debilitating long-term illnesses are particularly vulnerable unless aggressive, meaningful, well-directed care is given by a staff that knows why the care is given and what its overall goals are.

SUMMARY

The basic approach to systematic care planning can be utilized in any patient care setting. Only the clinical content differs from one area to another. The sequence of assessment, problem identification, goal setting, and writing nursing orders is appropriate—it is, in fact, necessary—in any nursing service unit.

In acute care settings, such as emergency room and operating room, certain streamlined versions of the basic care plan are suggested. The use of more checklist items that call for standard care plans is a practical way of achieving brevity and clarity.

Medical-surgical units, with their wide range of problems and rapid patient turnover, can easily utilize a well-balanced combination of standard care plans and specialized care programs for patients with unusual problems. Obstetric and other clinical specialty units are likely to be able to easily identify a core of usual problems. Standard care plans for these problems are generally already well known; therefore it is relatively simple to commit them to writing. Systematic care planning can be applied to the psychiatric setting in a manner similar to that for other patient care areas. Both standard and specialized care plans can be successfully utilized. Extended care nursing services include both acute medical-surgical and long-term care strategies. Hence, extended care can easily utilize a well-balanced combination of standard and specialized care.

With only minor internal variations, the basic problem-solving approach, which utilizes the concept of usual and unusual problems, is a viable and workable system for any patient care setting.

BIBLIOGRAPHY

Cady J, Freshman D, Norby L: Taking the Pain Out of Care Planning. Chicago, Medicus Corp, 1975

Mayers M, El Camino Nursing Staff: Standard Care Plans. Stockton Cal, KP Co Medical Systems, 1975, 1976, 1977, Vol 1, 2, 3

Watson A, Mayers M: How To Write Nursing Care Plans. Stockton Cal, KP Co Medical Systems, 1976

9

Community Health: Adaptations

GENERAL COMMUNITY HEALTH DEPARTMENTS

Community nurses, whether they work in home nursing, school nursing, or generalized public health, have long been accustomed to thinking in terms of plans of care for their patients or families. Although under general medical supervision, community health nurses are generally without specific medical orders for most situations. They must independently assess patients and make judgments about the care that is needed. Their comparative independence has been a factor in causing community nurses to think in terms of plans of care as a way of documenting their judgments and actions.

Community health nurses often find themselves planning care for whole families instead of for a single individual. The difficulties of setting goals for a family group are great. The variations of growth or progress among family members and the changing composition of families make it difficult to develop objectives applicable to the whole family. Until that difficulty can be resolved satisfactorily, this system of patient care planning focuses on care plans for individuals. Nevertheless, family dynamics and their influence upon individual family members do alter a nurse's assessments, expected outcomes, and nursing orders for individual family members.

This chapter shows how patient care planning can be applied to generalized community health, home nursing, and office nursing. Standard care plans for each area are illustrated, and presentations are made of case studies with their associated plans for care.

Generalized public health, or community health nursing, has in recent years become infamous for the large amount of paperwork it involves. Innumerable pages of tediously written longhand narratives are recorded day after day. Nurses wonder about its real value. Yet, the large amounts of information generated in the field must somehow be accounted for and documented. Numerous conversations, teaching sessions, and negotiations, as well as family health problems and responses to care, are recorded. It is not surprising that increasing amounts of a public health nurse's time are devoted to record keeping. Surely there is an answer to this dilemma! Is it not possible to abbreviate and systematize public health record keeping without compromising content?

One answer has been the Problem-oriented Medical Record system (POMR).[1] Its problem list and subjective-, objective-, assessment-, and plan- (SOAP) recording format lend themselves well to the pace and to the large amounts of information in a community agency's charts. Systematic care planning is similar in principle to the POMR system: a listing of problems, plans of care, and outcome-oriented documentation. In some respects, systematic care planning may be less cumbersome and repetitious than POMR.

Development of Standard Care Plans

A major strategy for streamlining record keeping is, of course, the concept of standard care plans. Much of what nurses write over and over again is the same words and the same phrases that apply to a large number of persons. Such frequently recurring problems and interventions can become part of an agency's standard care protocols. When problem identification and intervention directions are managed by use of a checklist and protocols, a great deal of handwriting can be eliminated.

To begin development of standard care protocols, a review of sample nursing records will yield information from which a core of frequently occurring, usual problems can be abstracted. The following problems appear to be some of the common, usual, and frequently occurring ones among public health nursing clients:

1. Inability to follow prescribed medical routine
2. At high risk for prenatal complications

3. At high risk for difficulty with infant care
4. Inability to stay on prescribed diet
5. At high risk for spreading a communicable disease
6. Difficulty coping with multiple problems associated with chronic illness
7. At high risk for unwanted pregnancy
8. Overwhelming threats to preferred life style

Several of these problems cut across diagnostic or other categories. The problem "inability to stay on prescribed diet" applies equally to a child with nephrosis, an expectant mother, a patient with heart disease, or a diabetic. Only the content of the nursing orders is different.

When an agency has a list of standard care plans, nurses can assess which plans or which elements of several prewritten plans will best assist a patient or family. Whenever a usual or common problem on the list is checked (√), it means that a certain predetermined sequence of planned care is to be implemented. For instance, if a standard care routine for "high risk for unwanted pregnancy" is checked (√), it indicates that certain policies for nursing action are to be put into effect. An example of a standard care plan for "high risk for unwanted pregnancy" is illustrated in the following model.

High Risk for Unwanted Pregnancy, Standard Care Plan

Usual Problems	Expected Outcomes	Deadlines	Nursing Orders
(1) Potential unwanted pregnancy due to inaccessability to knowledge about or source of birth control methods	(1) Reiteration of correct information about relevant birth control methods Acquisition and use of appropriate method	(3 weeks)	(1) a. Initiate discussion of child spacing Ascertain patient's knowledge, misunderstandings, and feelings b. Show various birth control devices by use of demonstration kit Review of pros and cons of each c. Problem-solve c̄ pt regarding which might be best for her, pending physician's advice d. Ascertain appropriate source of care, assist pt if

High Risk for Unwanted Pregnancy, Standard Care Plan (*cont.*)

Usual Problems	Expected Outcomes	Deadlines	Nursing Orders
			necessary in making appointment
			e. Ascertain ability to meet appointment and assist $\bar{c}$ transportation arrangements as needed
(2) Potential unwanted pregnancy due to personal, cultural, or other factors that cause incorrect usage of available method	(2) Correct use of a personally acceptable method (Ascertain by interview)	(3 weeks)	(2) a. Initiate discussion of feasibility of current birth control method b. Listen to patient's feelings and concerns Clarify misunderstandings c. Refer to physician for review of method if clarification does not resolve problem

Analysis. When each usual problem has been taken through to the standard nursing orders a public health agency will have the documentation of the standards it advocates and sponsors. All staff must be oriented to these care standards and should evaluate their nursing practice in relation to them. The very process of identifying usual problems, deciding upon intended outcomes, and designing nursing actions becomes a learning experience which cannot help but result in better care. Furthermore, the time saved by the use of standard care protocols will free nurses for more direct care. Only concise notations that primarily document patient's responses to specialized care for unusual problems need be written on the narrative notes. A checklist can quickly and simply document a patient's usual problems and the nursing actions that are in progress to deal with them.

As recommended for other nursing settings, the patient care plan should contain four basic sections: overall care planning information, medications, treatments, and diagnostic tests, checklist of standard and frequently ordered care, and unusual problems and specialized nursing orders. Separate from the care plan per se is the narrative, or nurse's notes, section of the patient's record. In public health nursing it seems logical to keep the care plan filed with the patient's record rather than to keep it separate in a flip chart or other holder.

A Case Study and Its Associated Care Plan

The Smith family have been referred to Public Health Nursing by the Social Welfare Department. They are on welfare, have poor housing, and are of an ethnic minority group. They have been referred because Mrs. Smith is expecting her third child. She is in her fourth month of pregnancy. The other children, both boys, are two and three years old. Mr. Smith works sporadically as a laborer, most often in the seasonal agricultural industry.

A public health nurse visits, makes an assessment, and starts a plan of care.

The following example illustrates the elements of the care plan and the associated nurse's narrative for the Smith family over a one-month period.

Patient Care Plan, Mary Smith

Physician's expectations regarding course of treatment and convalescence.
  (√) typical or routine
  ( ) atypical or complicated
If atypical or complicated, in what way?

Identifying Information: _____
_____
_____
_____
Diagnosis: _____

Nursing criteria for discharge or maintenance (overall expected outcomes):

(a) Continually verbalize understanding of progress of pregnancy and self-care
    implications.

(b) Demonstrate ability to feed and care for infant safely, including medical
    follow-up.

(c) Demonstrate satisfactory development of mother-infant relationship.

(d) Demonstrate ability to manage family responsibilities.

(e) Verbalize satisfactory resolution or management of marital problem.

                                                                  B. Anderson, PHN

Other relevant information: _____

Checklist of Standard and Frequently Ordered Care and Medications

___Inability to follow prescribed medical regimen
___At high risk for prenatal complications
___At high risk for difficulty with infant care
___Inability to stay on prescribed diet
___At high risk for spreading a CD

√ Prenatal
___Postpartum
___Infant
___Preschool
___School

Checklist of Standard and Frequently Ordered Care and Medications (*cont.*)

__Difficulty coping with problems associated
   with chronic disease
__At high risk for unwanted pregnancy

Medications: <u>Multivitamins</u>

__Crippled Children's Service
__Tbc case
__Tbc suspect
__Tbc contact
__Other CD
__Chronic disease
__Short-term illness

Patient preferences, miscellaneous information: <u>Prefers visit on Tuesday afternoons</u>

Unusual Problems

Date	Unusual Problems	Expected Outcomes	Deadlines	Nursing Orders
4/18	Apparent dissatisfaction c̄ her marriage due to "he stays out late and drinks a lot"	Verbalizes insight into problem and development of her own ideas for a solution To cope constructively c̄ problem while it still exists	(6/15) √ q 2 weeks	a. Initiate and continue discussions regarding problem b. Actively listen and guide with problem solving c. Provide support and allow dependence at moments of crisis d. Give active support to patient's decisions regarding resolving problem B. Anderson, PHN

Narrative

Initial Assessment: 4/18. Well-groomed, courteous, responsive. Home neat and sparsely furnished. Responds with warmth and firmness to the two preschool boys. Says she has seen Dr J at the neighborhood clinic. Says he said she is "fine" and that he prescribed vitamins for her pregnancy. Says she was very unhappy about the pregnancy at first but now accepts it and is beginning to be involved with planning ahead for the baby. Verbalizes understanding of the general medical care routine and need for good prenatal supervision. With clarification, she has basic understanding of the current physiologic aspects of pregnancy. Expresses concern over her marriage. Says husband works sporadically, "stays out late a lot and drinks too much." Expresses feelings of helplessness, depression, anger, and disappointment over husband's behavior. B. Anderson, PHN

4/18. Telephone call to Dr J. States that patient was found to be physically within norms at the time of his examination on 4/2. Next appointment is 5/6. Expects her progress to be within norms, based upon current data. He prescribed multivitamins. Wants PHN to follow routine prenatal nursing teaching and counseling. B. Anderson, PHN

5/3. Home visit. Verbalized at length about her continued concern over her husband's behavior. With guidance of PHN, began to consider some possible reasons for husband's behavior, including some of her own which could be contributory. Expressed desire to explore further at next visit in two weeks.

5/20. Met last appointment with doctor. Says next appointment is 6/4. Continued to verbalize about marital problems. Says she has been thinking a lot about it since last visit. She is trying to understand it better. Continued verbalizing further ideas about reasons for problem. Now beginning to say, "What shall I do about it?" Says she'll think about that, and we'll talk further at next visit in two weeks. B. Anderson, PHN

Analysis. The excerpts from the Smith family's public health nursing record demonstrate certain principles in care planning.

The plan of care and narrative for Mary Smith, the mother, illustrates documentation, by checkmark ($\sqrt{}$), that the doctor believes she will probably experience a normal prenatal course. This information helps the nurse then to set a priority for care and she implemented the standard prenatal care protocol. The standard care protocol would include certain observations, teaching, and supporting medical follow-up at appropriate intervals throughout pregnancy. At four months gestation, monthly checking intervals are set. Therefore, every month a brief narrative note will be written to document the patient's progress in relation to the expected outcomes of the standard care plan.

Under the unusual problems section of the plan of care is the statement, "Apparent dissatisfaction with her marriage. . . ." It is followed by written criteria for measuring the expected outcome, the checking intervals (every two weeks), and the itemized nursing actions (orders). The narrative portion is used to record both the patient's response to specially designed nursing interventions and, at designated intervals, her response to standard care.

Each time a visit is made, the nurse assesses and intervenes according to the plan (standard and unusual). She would record the patient's response by utilizing the expected outcomes criteria as her frame of reference.

A very important part of the plan of care is the nursing criteria for discharge or maintenance. As soon as relevant data are gathered, the overall criteria, or long-term objectives, should be written. In the case of Mary Smith, the nurse indicated that five major long-term criteria, or goals, should be met before she closes the patient to care. Four of the criteria, items a through d, might be expected of the average prenatal-postpartum patient. However, item e refers specifically to the patient's unusual problem and would not ordinarily be found on another prenatal patient's record. Before Mary Smith is closed to public health nursing service, the summary recording would document that the patient has met all five criteria.

Patient Care Plan, David Smith

Physician's expectations regarding course of treatment and convalescence.
( ) typical or routine
( ) atypical or complicated
If atypical or complicated, in what way?

Identifying information: _____
_____
_____
Diagnosis: _____
_____

Nursing criteria for discharge or maintenance (overall expected outcomes):

(a) Immunizations current and kept current for sample period of one year.

(b) Demonstration of normal growth and development pattern for sample period
    of one year.

(c) Demonstration and verbalization by mother regarding needs of child and ability
    to meet them.

(d) Demonstration of pattern of satisfactory well-child and sick-child medical and
    dental care for sample period of one year.   B. Anderson, PHN

Other relevant information: _____

Standard Care Protocols

—Inability to follow prescribed medical regimen
—At high risk for prenatal complications
—At high risk for difficulty with infant care
—Inability to stay on prescribed diet
—At high risk for spreading a CD
—Difficulty coping with problems associated
  with chronic disease
—At high risk for unwanted pregnancy
Medications: _____

Patient Preferences, Miscellaneous
Information: _____

—Prenatal
—Postpartum
—Infant
√ Preschool
—School
—Crippled Children's Service
—Tbc case
—Tbc suspect
—Tbc contact
—Other CD
—Chronic disease
—Short-term illness

Unusual Problems

Date	Unusual Problems	Expected Outcomes	Deadlines	Nursing Orders
4/18	No apparent unusual problems		√ q 2 months for 1 year	See checklist B. Anderson, PHN

Narrative

Initial Assessment: 4/18. Appears to be within norms physically and mentally, based upon PHN's observation of child playing, talking, and relating with mother and nurse for 1½ hours in the home setting. Recommend preschool standard care. B. Anderson, PHN

Analysis.   The excerpts for 3-year-old David Smith follow the same format as those of his mother's record.

First it is noted that the child is not under medical care. The nursing criteria for discharge are specified in items a through d and reflect the overall criteria or objectives that might be typical of any apparently normal preschooler. The criteria are written so that if family and child demonstrate compliance with safe standards of care for a one-year sample of time, the child will be closed to nursing service. Not all agencies would agree on a one-year period as an adequate sample of time. This example merely demonstrates the concept of establishing deadlines, or time priorities, for standard care objectives. The assumption in this case is that, if for one year the family demonstrates compliance without significant assistance from the nurse, it is reasonable to predict that they will continue to do so. If the nurse is in reasonable doubt at the end of the specified time period, the sample time period could be extended.

Following the checklist section is the unusual problems section, where the nurse has noted that there apparently are no special problems, and the nurse has referred to the standard care checklist. The checklist indicates that the usual problems, expected outcomes, and standard care are appropriate for David. The nurse has briefly documented two evaluative visits that were made at a two-month interval, as required by the standard care protocol.

Because the preschool standard care protocol automatically documents by a check (√) that certain nursing orders are being employed, it is unnecessary to rewrite the actions again in the narrative. Only very brief notations of patient response are made at the required intervals.

Patient care plan, John Smith

Physician's expectations regarding course of treatment and convalescence.	Identifying Information: _____
( ) typical or routine	_____
( ) atypical or complicated	Diagnosis: _____
If atypical or complicated, in what way?	_____
Deferred re √ 5/15	_____

Nursing criteria for discharge or maintenance (overall expected outcomes):

(a) Immunization current and kept current for sample period of one year.

(b) Demonstration of normal growth and development pattern for sample period of one year.

(c) Demonstration and verbalization by mother regarding needs of child and ability to meet them.

Patient Care Plan, John Smith (*cont.*)

(d) Demonstration of pattern of satisfactory well- and sick-child medical care and
dental care for sample period of one year.

(e) Current medical care and follow-up by family for apparent orthopedic problem
(right leg shorter than left) for sample period of two years without significant
assistance, or until corrected.   B. Anderson, PHN

Other relevant information: _____

Standard Care Protocols

__Inability to follow prescribed medical regimen	__Prenatal
__At high risk for prenatal complications	__Postpartum
__At high risk for difficulty with infant care	__Infant
__Inability to stay on prescribed diet	∨_Preschool
__At high risk for spreading a CD	__School
__Difficulty coping with problems associated	∨_Crippled Children's Services
with chronic disease	__Tbc case
__At high risk for unwanted pregnancy	__Tbc suspect
Medications: _____	__Tbc contact
_____	__Other CD
Patient Preferences, Miscellaneous	_Chronic disease
Information: _____	__Short-term illness

Unusual Problems

Date	Unusual Problems	Expected Outcomes	Deadlines	Nursing Orders
4/18	(1) Possible lack of under- standing by parents of con- sequences of untreated orthopedic problem		(5/3)	(1) Discuss problem c̄ mother Get background and feelings regarding problem Ascertain why no care Assist mother in making arrangements for care B. Anderson, PHN
5/3	(2) None at this time			(2) See checklist B. Anderson, PHN

Narrative

Initial assessment: 4/18. Appears to be within norms physically and mentally except for slight limp. Measurement reveals right leg ¼ inch shorter than left. Mother did not respond to questioning about problem, due to her own anxiety over marital problem.

Just said she hasn't taken him to a doctor yet. PHN will discuss in-depth at next visit in two weeks. B. Anderson, PHN

5/3. Mother states that financial and marital problems have kept her from seeing doctor regarding John's limp. Also states she hasn't been aware of it very long, as it was difficult to detect limp in early stages of walking. Wishes to make a Crippled Children's Services application for care. Now verbalizes an understanding of the need for care. CCS fact sheet completed. B. Anderson, PHN

Analysis. In the case of 2-year-old John Smith, his plan of care, as with the others, begins with the physician's statement of his expectations of the course of treatment or convalescence. In John's case the nurse entered the word "deferred," to indicate that this item would be completed at a later date. Once the child is diagnosed and under care for his apparent orthopedic problem, this item can be completed.

At the time of the initial assessment, the nurse was able to gather enough information to develop and write the nursing criteria for discharge. In the case of John, she wrote the same criteria (items a through d) as for his brother, David, because they are standard for preschoolers. However, in addition she added item e, which requires that there be current medical care and follow-up by the family for the apparent orthopedic problem. Before this child is closed to public health nursing service, it must be well demonstrated that the family can independently maintain a current medical care and follow-up regimen for this problem.

Under unusual problems, the nurse entered, "Possible lack of understanding by parents of consequences of untreated orthopedic problem." She did not write an expected outcome because an actual or potential problem had not yet been identified. She did, however, give herself a deadline of two weeks to rule in or rule out the possible problem.

Reference to the narrative notes clarifies why the nurse was unable to rule the problems in or out at the initial visit and shows the decision she made at the subsequent visit. After the second visit, on 5/3, the nurse could discontinue the possible problem and nursing action by drawing a diagonal line and noting in red ink the date and the letters DC. This would be necessary because the nurse had ruled out the problem as an unusual one. Because, at the second visit, the mother verbalized a desire to follow-up through Crippled Children's Services, the nurse would continue the child's care via the standard care routine for Crippled Children's Services. A quick review of the standard care checklist reveals that John Smith has the standard nursing care protocol ordered for preschool and Crippled Children's Services.

Care Plan, Joel Smith. If the nurse does an assessment of the husband, Joel, she will follow a similar format for his record.

Summary

Patient care planning in generalized community health is accomplished by:

1. Identifying the major categories of service
2. Identifying the usual, expected, typical patient problems in each category and following through each problem with expected outcomes, deadlines (or checking intervals), and standard nursing actions
3. Listing all of the major categories for usual problems and standard care on a checklist format
4. Orienting all staff to the meaning and content of the standard care protocols
5. Obtaining a statement of the physician's expectations of the patient's course of treatment or convalescence (routine or complicated)
6. Making statements of overall nursing criteria for discharge
7. Utilizing the unusual problems format for the unusual, out-of-the-ordinary patient problems which require other than standard care

A quick review of the nursing care plans for Mary, David, and John Smith provides the reader with a clear perception of the problems, care, and patient progress toward overall goals. After the unusual problems care plan has been established, a minimal amount of writing in the narrative notes is required, except for necessary updates. However, the writing that is done has particular meaning and relevance, because the notations are always made relative to the established expected outcomes criteria.

When a nurse or agency staff wishes to evaluate the effectiveness of nursing practice, it is relatively easy for them to review a sample of records and to match documentation of patient progress or response against the overall expected outcomes.

HOME NURSING AGENCIES

Home nursing, although similar in many ways to generalized community health nursing, is at the same time quite different in several basic ways. The similarities related to the setting for care, which in both instances is the patient's home, are the very family-centered approach that needs to be taken and the significant utilization of family and community resources for care which both require. The differences have evolved through the years. Home nursing focuses on direct physical care. It depends significantly upon, and is limited by, physician's orders. Generalized public health nursing, though, has become considerably less bound to specific medical orders and is more self-directive.

Perhaps as a result of home nursing's focus on direct physical care prescribed by doctor's orders, home nursing records are normally quite different from those of a generalized public health nursing department. Home nursing charts for many years have included checklists or code systems either to indicate that certain nursing care is being done or to document patient responses. Home nursing narrative notes are usually brief, confined to the patient's response to the ordered care.

As emphasis upon nursing care planning has accelerated, home nursing staffs in recent years have begun to feel that care planning systems and guides should reflect more than simply the scheduling and implementation of physician's orders. Home nursing staffs are looking for ways to enhance nursing assessment skills and to provide a vehicle for documenting care planned by the nurse as a complement to the physician's orders.

The system described in this book provides an excellent basis for accomplishing nursing care planning in the home setting.

Developing Standard Care Plans

To use this system the home nursing staff must, just as other agencies do, first identify the most frequently encountered problems of their patients. This can be done by reviewing a sample of records. Problems can be listed by primary diagnosis or by identifying physiologic or emotional difficulties. Agencies frequently find that using a combination of the two categories is the most functional method. The following list is a sample of common patient problems identified by one home nursing staff:

1. Postoperative cataract removal
2. Colostomy management
3. Inability to meet all or some of own personal care needs
4. Decubitus ulcers
5. Delayed wound healing
6. Postpartum and infant care

7. Urinary incontinence—indwelling catheter
8. Ambulation difficulties
9. Feelings of hopelessness and depression
10. Feelings of isolation and boredom
11. Decreased mentation and decreased involvement with life activities
12. New diabetic with insulin injections

After major problem areas have been identified, subproblems can be defined. Then the expected outcomes or objectives, the deadlines or checking intervals, and the standard nursing orders can be developed. When approved by the appropriate policy group, these standard care plans can become an effective basis for care. A further advantage to having a written selection of standard care is this: When physicians realize that well-designed, rational, standard nursing care protocols are available, they will consistently order the agency's standard care for their patients.

As nursing experience, research, and expertise in identifying patient problems and designing care increase, nursing as a profession can offer significantly more content to the body of knowledge for patient care. This is particularly true for home nursing because of the close patient contact and frequent visits of nurses to patients in the home setting. Physician observations are generally limited to less frequently spaced office visits.

A further challenge to home nursing is to develop increased skills, and to make more time, for assessing problems and planning care for the total family. The direct care role of home nursing can be significantly improved by incorporating more of the community nursing philosophy and skills into its own armamentarium for care.

In any case, once the major problem categories have been formulated as standard care plans, they can be printed on a checklist format for quick, easy, and effective documentation of nursing care. Some of the common or unusual problems of home nursing patients are related to postoperative cataract removal, colostomy management, healing of decubitus ulcers, wound healing, postpartum convalescence, infant care, joint contractures, bowel and bladder problems, and others.

If the preceding items, or others, are included in a checklist of standard care plans, a nurse would have a quick, effective method for ordering the specific standard care she wishes. Every item on a checklist would, of course, be backed up by a prewritten detailed sequence of care.

An example of how one checklist item, "new diabetic," can be developed for a standard care plan is provided in the following example.

Standard Care for New Diabetic

Usual Problems	Expected Outcomes	Deadlines	Nursing Orders
(1) Potential hyperglycemia	(1) Receives insulin before 11:00 AM Negative urine	√ daily	(1) a. Make home visit before 11:00 AM b. Check urine before each insulin administration (Urine—freshly voided half hour after emptying bladder) All teaching by one nurse to minimize confusion
(2) Inexperience with injection technique	(2) Demonstrates progressive ability to do own injection safely	(3 weeks)	(2) a. Assemble all equipment in one area (box) b. Instruct sterile technique of injection c. Observe and rotate sites of injection (lower abdomen, right and left; anterior and outer thighs, right and left)
(3) Potential insulin reaction or diabetic coma or infection of injection site	(3) Verbalizes correct recall of s/s of each and what to do in case of each No s/s of infection	√ weekly	(3) a. Day 1, teach about insulin reaction Have written information Day 2, review insulin reaction Day 3, ask patient to reiterate s/s and what to do for insulin reaction— clarify incorrect perceptions Day 4, again ask patient to reiterate b. Day 5, as in day 3 Teach about diabetic coma (Follow same schedule as for

Standard Care for New Diabetic (*cont.*)

Usual Problems	Expected Outcomes	Deadlines	Nursing Orders
			insulin reaction) c. Day 9, review both insulin reaction and diabetic coma d. Day 10, review both insulin reaction and diabetic coma e. Day 11, repeat Quiz patient on both problems, clarify any misconceptions f. Day 12, quiz patient on both problems, clarify any misconceptions g. Review weekly to reinforce and to maintain recall
(4) Potential dietary misman-agement	(4) Verbalizes correct understanding of diet management Periodically demonstrates satisfactory dietary intake by sample daily menu diary	√ weekly	(4) a. Day 1, give overview of diet Meaning and reason for its being ordered for patient b. Day 2, discuss food exchanges c. Day 3, review d. Day 4, ask patient to reiterate major principle of diet management Clarify misconceptions e. Explain how to keep a diet diary one day per week for evaluation Set schedule
(5) Potential skin breakdown of legs and feet	(5) Clean, clear skin Well manicured feet No breakdown	√ weekly	(5) a. Teach regarding skin and feet care concurrently with insulin and dietary teaching however, reserve in-depth teaching for after major emphasis on other is completed

Analysis. The standard care plan for a new diabetic has been subdivided into five problems that are typical of the difficulties of a patient with a new diagnosis of diabetes mellitus. Each of the five problems is followed through with a statement of expected outcomes, deadlines, and nursing orders. The nursing orders have been designed to be implemented on a chronologic basis. The nurses who developed these nursing actions and their associated time table studied many new diabetics. As a result of their research, certain norms for learning progress emerged. The norms are used as a basis for the time table for care. This kind of clinical nursing research could be done on many kinds of patient problems, ascertaining norms for patient responses to care. These norms could then be utilized effectively as a basis for standard care. They could also be an excellent source of information against which to make judgments about usual or unusual problems.

Following is another example of the evolution of a standard care plan in the home nursing setting.

Standard Care for Colostomy Management

Usual Problems	Expected Outcomes	Deadlines	Nursing Orders
(1) Potential irregular evacuation due to inconstancy of irrigation and diet	(1) Daily evacuation between 8 and 10 AM No major evacuation in the interim	√ weekly	(1) a. Do irrigation between 8 and 10 AM daily
(2) Potential resistance to self-care due to altered self-concept	(2) Gradual involvement in self-care	(2 weeks) √ weekly	(2) a. Day 1, do procedure for patient Explain steps Do not persist beyond patient's fatigue and readiness levels b. Day 2 and 3, repeat previous day c. Day 4, do procedure. Let patient assist as wishes d. Day 5, repeat above e. Day 6, let patient do procedure with assistance of nurse f. Day 7, repeat g. Day 8, review and discuss proce-

Standard Care for Colostomy Management *(cont.)*

Usual Problems	Expected Outcomes	Deadlines	Nursing Orders
			dures, questions, and problems h. Day 9 to 14, provide support Resolve problems and concerns
(3) Potential confusion if taught by different nurses in different ways	(3) Verbalizes and demonstrate progressively clear understanding and ability for self-care	√ weekly	(3) Irrigation procedure to be taught as follows: a. Assemble equipment b. Seat patient in front of toilet c. Hang irrigation bag level with patient's shoulders d. If no specific orders, use 500 ml tap water Repeat once if necessary e. Care of equipment: Bucket of soapy water to soak and cleanse Clothes hanger with clothes pins to clip sleeve up to dry
(4) Potential skin excoriation around stoma due to adhesive and drainage	(4) Clear nonirritated skin around stoma	√ weekly	(4) a. Observe skin daily, cleanse with warm water and antibacterial soap, soft cloth, and gently friction Pat dry b. Teach pt to keep to a reasonable minimum the number of times he changes adhesive bag Each change irritates skin Cleanse skin each time changed
(5) Potential infection or deep tissue sloughing from perineal area due to deep wound	(5) Gradually ↓ serosangineous exudate No foul odor	√ daily	(5) Check perineal wound daily Gently part buttocks and observe with aid of flashlight

Usual Problems	Expected Outcomes	Deadlines	Nursing Orders
			Note and record amount and type of drainage on perineal dressing
(6) Potential constipation or diarrhea due to irregular dietary patterns	(6) Soft, formed stool	√ weekly	(6) Teach regarding diet: a. No roughage or fresh fruit b. Force fluids, 2,000 ml daily if no contraindication

Analysis. The preceding colostomy management protocol is subdivided into six problems. Each has a written statement of the progressive problem-solving steps. All of the problems are listed as potential rather than actual. If in the course of convalescence one of these potential problems becomes an actual difficulty, it then would be rephrased and entered as an unusual problem in the appropriate section of the care plan. Specialized objectives and nursing actions would then be developed.

In the example, each potential problem is stated precisely, incorporating the reason why it is a potential problem. The expected outcomes clearly tell what specific phenomena to observe during the ongoing appraisals of progress. Deadlines for documenting progress are indicated.

The nursing orders are specifically written and are in chronologic sequence. This sequence delineates the pattern of progress an average patient is likely to follow. Significant deviations by a patient from the expected pattern of progress warn that he has an unusual problem which needs to be identified and managed in a specialized way.

In the absence of unusual problems, a visiting nurse need only check (√) colostomy management on the checklist and then make brief notations on the progress notes at the deadline intervals to indicate the patient's response.

A Case Study and Its Associated Care Plan

Mrs. Emma H is 76 years old and lives alone in a three-room second floor apartment. She has been referred to the Visiting Nurse Association for postcataract-removal care. The following care plan format reflects the care as planned by the nurse after her initial assessment visit.

Patient Care Plan, Mrs. Emma H

Physician's expectations regarding course of treatment and convalescence.
(√) typical or routine
( ) atypical or complicated
If atypical or complicated, in what way?

Identifying Information: _____

_____

Diagnosis: Cataract removal, right eye,
7/10 _____

Nursing criteria for discharge or maintenance (overall expected outcomes):
(a) Verbalize understanding of and the ability to follow physician's follow-up
    regimen.
(b) Demonstrate ability to manage own life style in a way that is realistic and yet
    satisfactory to patient.
(c) Verbalize satisfactory plans for assistance quickly in case of emergency.
(d) Give specific indication of having available resources for assistance, support, or
    comfort when needed.   B. Baker, RN
Other relevant information: _____

Standard Care Protocols

Standard Care Protocols	Frequently Ordered Care
√ Cataract, postoperative	__Bath, with help in bathroom
__Colostomy care	__Bed bath
__Decubitus care	__Oral hygiene
__Wound healing	__Weekly shampoo
__Postpartum	√ Blood pressure
__Infant care	√ Pulse, respiration
__Foley catheter care	__Temperature
__Poor motivation	__Ambulate with help
__Skin care	
__Joint care	

Activity: _____

Patient preferences, miscellaneous information: Pt prefers home visit about
11:00 AM _____

Diet: _____

Medications, Treatments, Diagnostic Tests

(In this space are written any current or ongoing medications orders, whether administered by the patient or by the nurse. Treatment orders for bladder irrigations, catheter changes, wound care, and the like are entered on this form. Any periodic laboratory examinations are documented under diagnostic tests.)

Unusual Problems

Date	Unusual Problems	Expected Outcomes	Deadlines	Nursing Orders
7/14	None apparent at this time		(7/21)	See checklist B. Baker, RN

Analysis. Mrs. Emma H has experienced surgery for cataract removal. Her physician prognosticates that the surgery should heal well with no complications. The nurse also judges that the patient is coping well with her recovery and that she has no unusual problems at this time. The nurse enters four overall expected outcomes which indicate the level of progress to be expected by the time the nurse closes the case. Hence, at the time of closure or before, the nurse documents her perception of the patient's status relative to the four criteria. If one or more of the four criteria have not, in the nurse's judgment, been met, either the case is continued or a referral is made to another agency for follow-up.

Summary

In review, it can be said that the basic methodology for planning patient care in home nursing agencies is the same as that used in other care settings. Developing predetermined standard care plans, to be implemented by a check ($\sqrt{}$) on a list, is a time-saving yet care-improving activity by home nursing staffs. The unusual problems section, for patient difficulties which are not within normal ranges or with which the patient is not coping, is used very nearly the same way as in other care settings. The differences lie mainly in the kinds and intensity of patient problems and in the content of nursing actions. The basic general system for managing patient care information remains precisely the same from setting to setting.

A method of care planning that encourages good assessment and sound problem solving for independent nursing action can provide unparalleled opportunity for visiting nurses to make significant contributions to total patient care.

OFFICE NURSING

A nurse whose domain is the physician's office has unique possibilities for planning patient care. She becomes well acquainted with the individuals and families who see the physician over long periods of time. She and the physician work closely and can share concerns and ideas about their patients. They experience a camaraderie as colleagues that is rare in more other areas of nursing. The doctor, his office, and his staff are, in most people's minds, the primary resource for help with health problems. The doctor's patients look to him and his nurses for therapy, advice, counselling, and support. During periods of diminished stress they often share a relationship of reciprocal friendship.

Because the doctor's office is a patient's most common source of medical care, the nurse can play a major role in facilitating a client's acceptance of, and adjustment to, the various therapeutic regimens which may be needed. For instance, a patient instructed by his physician to get himself admitted to a hospital usually needs specific information about what to expect there, what to ask about, what to take along, what his rights as a patient are, how he can make his stay more pleasant, and so forth. If a patient is referred to another physician because of a special problem or for diagnostic tests, the office nurse can anticipate his problems and assist him in advance by providing relevant information. Patients receiving prescriptions almost always need clarification or reinforcement of the physician's instructions. A patient with a newly diagnosed health problem who is facing new and unexpected difficulties or a person feeling hopeless about chronic illness can be aided immeasurably by an office nurse who takes the time to talk it through with him.

Because of the multiplicity of her regular duties, the office nurse rarely has the time to devote to keeping long, detailed nursing records and do extensive care planning. And because her time and skills are valuable, it is essential that the type and pattern of her activities reflect the best use of her abilities. An effective patient care planning system can significantly help her provide a basis for facilitating and documenting good nursing care in the physician's office setting.

Developing Standard Care Plans

Like nurses in other settings, the office nurse can review a sample of patient records and identify the problems most frequently encountered by her clients. They can be described in terms of diagnosis, by physical or emotional symptoms, or by a combination of each. Office nurses will find some typical problems of patients in a general practitioner's caseload to be:

1. Worry over the unknown implications of an acute illness
2. Confusion about medications, diagnostic reports, and medical terminology
3. Anxiety due to lack of information about the predictable duration of medical care, the cost of care, length of disability, and so forth
4. Grief and a sense of loss (altered self-concept) due to debilitating injury or illness
5. Guilt over inability to pay the doctor's bills or to follow the doctor's orders

The basic problems of specialist's patients are very much like those of general practitioner's patients. But for specialists' patients there is an added focus, or core, of physical and emotional problems associated with the specialty area.

When the most frequently encountered usual patient problems have been identified, they can be divided into more specific sub-problems. Each usual problem provides a basis for the nurse to develop expected outcomes, deadlines or checking intervals, and nursing orders or standard care plans for that problem. These guides can be followed for patients who, in the nurse's judgment, are experiencing one of the usual problems.

Some standard care plans a nurse in the office of a general practitioner might develop are:

1. Acute temporary illness
2. Medications
3. New diagnosis
4. Altered self-concept
5. Diabetic control
6. Heart disease
7. Hypertension
8. Peripheral vascular disease
9. Constipation
10. Peptic ulcer
11. Colostomy
12. Inability to follow doctor's orders

Several of these short titles refer to the usual problems mentioned earlier and illustrate how short phrases can be used to refer to complex usual problems. Each of the standard care plans would have a detailed sequence of care developed and prewritten for easy reference.

When a standard care plan is well detailed and written into an approved manual or book, the nurse can, by use of a checklist or brief notation, refer to a certain protocol and thereby document that that specified series of nursing actions is in operation. It is a questionable use of nursing time to write in detail every item of standard care for patients with anticipated, usual problems. Nursing has wasted uncounted sums of money, energy, and skill in its over-dedication to recording in tedious longhand the same notations about patient after patient, all of whom had standard care and who responded within a normal range. Just as nurses can in other settings, the office nurse can abbreviate standard care titles and encapsulate response notations.

In order to demonstrate how an office nurse might design a set of standard care plans, anxiety due to lack of information will be developed in the following example.

Standard Care, Information Regarding Length and Cost of Care

Usual Problems	Expected Outcomes	Deadlines	Nursing Orders
(1) Anxiety due to lack of information regarding length of medical care and any associated disability	(1) Verbal expressions of correct understanding and realistic plans for coping	(at time of first visit)	(1) a. After pt has seen physician, ascertain his understanding of predictable length of illness and medical care If this understanding seems incorrect, clarify with physician and explain to pt b. Ascertain if pt expects any unusual difficulties in managing the required care Assist in solving difficulties, or refer to other agencies for assistance as needed
(2) Anxiety due to lack of knowledge of cost of projected medical care	(2) Verbal expressions of knowledge of predictable cost and ability to cope with it	(at time of first visit)	(2) a. Ascertain pt's understanding of costs of projected care Clarify misconceptions

Usual Problems	Expected Outcomes	Deadlines	Nursing Orders
			b. Ascertain his concerns regarding ability to pay Problem solve $\bar{c}$ pt re options for solving any real financial difficulty

Analysis. The foregoing model of a standard nursing care plan, to be used in the physician's office setting, sets forth two subproblems. Then it follows each of them through to the development of standard nursing orders. When a protocol such as this one becomes specifically identified as part of an office nurse's responsibility, each patient is more likely to benefit from appropriate intervention. When the nurse notes that this protocol is in effect, she implies that all details of the sequence are being implemented. A brief subsequent note regarding the patient's response is all that is needed to document an entire care sequence.

Standard Care, Peripheral Vascular Disease

Usual Problems	Expected Outcomes	Deadlines	Nursing Orders
(1) Pain in extremities due to tissue anoxia	(1) Verbalizes sense of reasonable comfort	√q visit	(1) a. Interview patient regarding type and amount of pain Be sure Dr knows and that patient understands physician's recommendations b. Verify at each visit the patient's perceptions of the success or failure of the doctor's recommendations c. Be sure physician is informed of patient's current pain problem
(2) Difficulty with work and life style due to limited am-	(2) Verbalization that he is able to meet own life style	√q visit	(2) a. Interview patient regarding how he manages his

Standard Care, Peripheral Vascular Disease (*cont.*)

Usual Problems	Expected Outcomes	Deadlines	Nursing Orders
bulatory ability	needs to his reasonable satisfaction		work, etc How much can he walk? Has he obtained or does he need help with some activities? b. Be sure doctor is informed of patient's current ambulatory status c. Provide suggestions and ideas for solving daily ambulation problems
(3) Lack of ability to do good foot care due to no previous experience, or carelessness	(3) Clean, well-manicured feet Evidence of maintenance of at least current status (no deterioration) of peripheral circulation	√q visit	(3) a. Interview patient regarding his perceptions of what to observe and how to care for feet and legs: cleaning and dressing, medication, exercises, support activity b. Clarify and supplement patient's perceptions Discuss one or two items each visit Review at next visit c. Keep doctor informed of patient's problems with foot care d. When goals have been met, do maintenance interviews at 4 to 6 month intervals Give continued positive reinforcement

Analysis. The standard care model just illustrated incorporates three problems that are typical for patients experiencing peripheral vascular disease. Each problem is followed by expected outcomes which include specific criteria for the subsequent evaluation of progress. On each required checking date, a nurse evaluates and documents the patient's status and compares it with the expected outcome. Any significant variance from the expected outcome on the checking date would warn the nurse to reevaluate the plan of care for that item and to design specialized care as necessary. A well-detailed guide for standard care provides predetermined, high quality nursing care. When care is prescribed and implemented by a nurse, it can appreciably improve the quality of standard care.

Standard Care, Acute Temporary Illness

Usual Problems	Expected Outcomes	Deadlines	Nursing Orders
(1) Limited ability to meet personal care and life style needs	(1) Verbalization of satisfactory arrangements for meals, bathing, shopping, and work	(at time of first visit)	(1) a. Interview and clarify realistic plans for personal care for expected duration of illness b. Be sure patient knows physician's prediction of duration of acute s/s so patient can plan accordingly
(2) Acute discomfort and weakness	(2) Reasonable comfort and low energy output	(at time of first visit)	(2) a. Ascertain severity of patient's s/s Obtain physician's advice regarding analgesia and rest Reinforce physician's instructions regarding analgesia Suggest appropriate comfort measures b. Be directive about instructions and suggestions
(3) Misinformation regarding medication and follow-up due to poor attention span associated c̄ acute discomfort	(3) Reiteration of accurate information regarding Rx's and follow-up care and appointment	(at time of first visit)	(3) a. Clarify patient's perception of doctor's instructions Write them if patient has difficulty concentrat-

Standard Care, Acute Temporary Illness (*cont.*)

Unusual Problems	Expected Outcomes	Deadlines	Nursing Orders
			ing or remember- ing b. Call patient to check on his well-being if he misses his follow-up appointment

Analysis. Many patients who see a physician in his office are experiencing the problem of acute temporary illness. The preceding example lists three subproblems commonly experienced by people who are acutely ill. The expected outcomes provide the standards against which to measure the patient's responses to nursing care. The nursing orders clearly outline the interventions considered basic to the standard nursing care of acutely ill patients. On the patient's record (not illustrated here), the sample entry of "acute care protocol" would indicate that the entire sequence of care has been instituted. Of course, much of that sequence is completed at the time of the patient's first visit. Therefore, at the time of the first visit—as required by the deadline—the nurse will record the patient's response to her care.

Unusual Problems

For unusual problems, a format like that recommended for other nursing settings can be used. Each unusual problem should be written concisely with expected outcomes, deadlines, and specialized nursing orders. For the office setting, a form sheet for assembling these data might be included in the patient's chart rather than kept in a flip chart or notebook. A tickler file for deadlines would remind the nurse when to pull a particular chart for the required follow-up.

A Case Study and Its Associated Care Plan

A demonstration of the use of systematic care planning in the office setting follows.

Mr. Henry W is 64 years old. He and his wife have been patients of Dr J for several years. Mr. Henry W has had three minor coronaries during the past 4½ years. Since the most recent coronary two months ago, he has developed signs and symptoms of congestive heart failure. Dr J has added a diuretic to the patient's medications regimen and is checking him more frequently than before. Both Mr W and his wife became quite frightened at the time of his last coronary episode.

The office nurse starts a plan of care that is illustrated on the following pages. Following the care plan are associated excerpts from the nurse's notes and an analysis.

Patient Care Plan, Henry W

Physician's expectations regarding course of treatment and convalescence.
  (√) typical or routine
  ( ) atypical or complicated
If atypical or complicated, in what way?

Identifying information: _____
_____
_____

Diagnosis: Coronary artery disease
CHF, compensated

Nursing criteria for maintenance or discharge (overall expected outcomes):
(a) Ability to verbalize fears and concerns. Achieve sense of equanimity.
(b) Verbalize satisfactory knowledge of medications, diet, and activity orders.

B. Watson, RN

Other relevant information: Lives c̄ wife. Retired engineer. Has lived in community for 30 years.

Unusual Problems

Date	Unusual Problems	Expected Outcomes	Deadlines	Nursing Orders
6/28	Tense and anxious with fear of possible "fatal attack next time"	Copes c̄ anxiety by learning to relax and enjoy each day. Verbalizes knowledge that, c̄ care, his life expectancy need not be shortened	(√ q 2 weeks)	a. Initiate discussion c̄ patient to clarify his perceptions of his wife's concerns b. With patient's considered agreement, involve both in conversations about their feelings, management of the health problems, and their life style. Clarify misunderstandings. Assist in problem solving. Be a phone resource as needed

Unusual Problems (*cont.*)

Date	Unusual Problems	Expected Outcomes	Deadlines	Nursing Orders
				c. Hold conversations in nurse's office Sit down Take necessary time B. Ritter, RN

Excerpted Nurse's Progress Notes

6/28. Standard care "medications" and "heart disease" are in operation. Verbalizes good understanding of Rx regimen. Progressing well c̄ heart disease information. Re tension and anxiety over possible fatal attack, says he and wife have not talked much. They try to avoid it because "What good will it do?" Also, he doesn't want to alarm his wife unduly. Says he'll "wait and see how things go in next couple of weeks." B. Ritter, RN

7/15. Says they've started talking about their fears, but they're getting more relaxed progressively as he feels better. Says they have asked their son to come and assist in getting some "business affairs in order" so, if he becomes seriously ill, his wife won't be left with it. B. Ritter, RN

8/15. Both Mr and Mrs W seem relaxed and happy. Planning small trip c̄ doctor's approval. Seem to feel free to bring up questions and concerns as they arise. Both husband and wife verbalize safe understanding of medications, diet, and activity as ordered. (DC unusual problem) B. Ritter, RN

Analysis.   The office nurse's care plan transmits a significant amount of information. The notations "medications" and "heart disease" on the progress notes reveal that Mr Henry W has the usual problem of learning a new medication schedule and that he is experiencing certain problems associated with a recent diagnosis of heart disease. Implied also is the information that the nurse is implementing the standard teaching care for each of these problems. Depending upon how often each standard care plan requires an assessment and its associated evaluative statement—that is, at the designated checking intervals—the narrative notes would contain references to those items. The nurse's notes indicate that, after six weeks, the objectives have been met: the patient and his wife show every indication of coping satisfactorily with the illness and of knowing how to get assistance if a crisis should arise. Because they have reached this point, the nurse would discontinue her specialized intervention for the "unusual anxiety and tension" problem, which has, for the moment, been solved.

The entire care plan, including standard and specialized care, requires minimum writing but results in the delivery of excellent care—care that has justification and purpose. The progress notes and care plan data serve as ongoing reminders to both the nurse and physician of the patient's progress.

Care plan information also provides good summary information for referrals to other agencies. For example, a patient entering a hospital will have more relevant and appropriate nursing care designed for him by the hospital nurse if the office nurse communicates summary referral information. A written summary referral can follow a telephone transmission of nursing care planning information. Similarly, after a patient's discharge from the hospital, a liaison nurse can communicate relevant information back to the office nurse for her further care planning and follow-up.

The office nurse can indeed significantly facilitate patient care in many ways. Her close working relationship with the physician gives her a unique opportunity for consistent and effective intervention.

THE NURSE PRACTITIONER

The nurse practitioner who functions either independently or on a colleague basis with a physician can formulate plans of care that would be similar to any of those illustrated in this chapter. The nurse practitioner's clients' problems may be quite specialized, such as in pediatric practice, or her clients may be quite diverse, representing some home care problems, some children, some adults, and so forth.

Whatever the client population, a nurse practitioner can devise, in consultation with her client, a plan of care that assists both of them in achieving the patient's goals.

SUMMARY

Systematic care planning is as adaptable to community health nursing practice as it is to acute care nursing. Minor modifications of content are the only real differences. Community health nursing, devoted as it is to the whole family, develops standard or specialized care plans for each family member being given service.

Developing standard care plans or protocols proceeds, just as it does in other settings, by the identification of a core of common, usual patient problems, followed by a problem-solving approach to the development of standard nursing orders. For unusual problems, specialized nursing care is defined and ordered. Notations made on progress charts are kept brief and specifically relevant to the patient's responses to nursing actions.

The same principles apply to nursing care planning in any community agency, whether that agency is a public health department, a home nursing agency, a school, a work site, a clinic, or a physician's office.

REFERENCE

1. Weed L: Medical Records, Medical Education, and Patient Care. Cleveland, Case Western Press, 1971

BIBLIOGRAPHY

Bjorn JC, Cross HD: Problem-oriented Private Practice of Medicine. Chicago, Modern Hospital Press, 1970

Bonkowsky M: Adapting the POMR to community child health care. Nursing Outlook 20:515, August 1972

Cross HD: The problem-oriented system in private practice in a small town. In Hurst JW, Walker, HK (eds): The Problem-oriented System. New York, Medcom Press, 1972, p 167

Field FW: Communication between community nurse and physician. Nurs Outlook 19:722, Nov 1971

Hurst JW: Instructions for the use of the problem-oriented concept and record in the "nonappointment" clinic. In Hurst JW, Walker HK (eds): The Problem-oriented System. New York, Medcom Press, 1972, 137-138

10

Nursing Education: Adaptations

It is in the educational setting that a nurse first learns how to use the formal method of problem solving. Most educational institutions teach the problem-solving process from the first day onward. Students are taught to identify and to define a problem, to gather and analyze data about it, and to devise methods for solving it. They are taught to test their methods by a further process of data gathering and analysis. They learn that the degree of accuracy and specificty with which a problem is defined can affect the attainment of a valid solution for it.

Care plans are used as a medium for applying the problem-solving process to nursing practice. The teaching tools generally referred to as care plans vary in format from instructor to instructor and from student to student. However, in spite of their varying terminology and format, care plans should follow the basic principles of the problem-solving process.

ELEMENTS OF AN EDUCATIONAL CARE PLAN

A systematic approach to care planning provides a minimum basic framework upon which nursing education can build a teaching tool. The sequence of problem, expected outcome, deadline, and nursing orders has been found to facilitate a student's grasp of the problem-solving process as it applies to care planning. In addition to the basic framework, an educational care plan should also provide for the inclusion of scientific principles and rationale. A nursing education care plan format should contain at least the following elements in approximately the following order:

1. Identify and define the patient's problems, whether they are usual or unusual, one at a time
2. State the scientific facts and principles relating to the problem, including its cause
3. State the expected outcomes or objectives, including deadlines and checking intervals
4. Write the specific nursing orders—the methods to be used—that are designed to solve the problem
5. Document the rationale and the scientific principles that justify the recommended care
6. Indicate the patient's responses to care
7. Evaluate the success or failure of the recommended nursing actions by analyzing the patient's response
8. Make recommendations pertaining to maintaining or revising the nursing actions

If students consistently follow the steps of the problem-solving process as outlined, they will develop care-planning skills which will be invaluable in the service setting.

While still students, nurses learn which problems are usual and expected and which are not. For care planning, they should identify and include both categories of problems but should state which are usual and which are unusual. The process of continually gathering data to make these kinds of decisions will aid immeasurably in improving their critical thinking skills.

TRANSITION FROM EDUCATION TO SERVICE

One of the disappointments a graduate finds after being employed by a service agency is that what she has known as a care plan in the educational setting is unrealistic to use as a care plan in the service setting. She feels committed to care planning and wants to implement it, but her only experience with care planning has been the educational model. The educational care plan is an excellent teaching-learning tool, but it has a very different primary purpose from that of the care plan in the service setting. In education, the care plan is used to facilitate the student's learning of basic principles, concepts, and facts about people's health problems. For this reason it is highly detailed, and it contains all of the conceivable relevant problems the nursing student is able to identify. In this way the student sees and learns in a comprehensive way about a health problem situation. The principles that she learns, the nursing care skills she develops and tests, and the broad spectrum of problems she identifies and analyzes result in an intellectual approach to life and to nursing care that is invaluable.

On the other hand, the service-oriented care plan has quite a different primary purpose. It is a care delivery tool. It is a medium for the quick and efficient communication of relevant data about a patient's care. A detailed scholarly approach is neither quick nor efficient. The care delivery tool must be streamlined—an abstract of relevant data that is easy to read and use. It must have a commonly known format and operational definitions, and it must be used in the same way by all staff. It must require a minimum of time to use per unit of information gleaned.

Although the purposes and uses of the educational and service care plans are very different, they are both based upon the problem-solving method. This basic intellectual process is a common thread throughout. The educational model prepares a student for the intellectual processes required for care planning in the service setting.

EXAMPLES OF CARE PLANS IN NURSING EDUCATION

Following are several examples of student care-planning formats.

Example 1, Mr JH, Age 69

History 10/23: The patient was admitted to the emergency room with a large infected lesion of an old fracture of the patella. He was malnourished and dehydrated. Mentation was poor (thought to be secondary to chronic brain syndrome). He progressed well, the infection cleared and he was sent to an extended care facility, where he has continued under care for healing of the patellar lesion. It has cleared, and he has had no unusual problems with the infection. However, the tissue will not fill in adequately. The skin that has filled in is primarily scar tissue and is of very poor quality.

The patient is cooperative, walks around, but speaks very little. His mentation is difficult to evaluate but would appear to be low.

Plastic surgeons have seen the patient recently and have decided that a flap procedure must be done. The patient is now being transferred to the acute unit to go to the plastic surgery division for repair of the patellar lesion.

Physician's admission note: Sixty-nine-year old male with chronic brain syndrome transferred from ECF for an elective cross leg skin flap to cover a necrotic ulcer over the left patellar region. Patient is a very poor historian, and only history known is that which can be obtained from his old chart. He has no family or friends. Apparently this ulcer is the result of an old fracture of his left patella which he has had for a number of years. Patient was in the hospital last year for six months with repeated debridements and split-thickness skin grafts to the area. However, grafts did not heal, and patient was sent to ECF to allow lesion to granulate. There has been very little epithelialization over patella, and patient is now left with a 2 cm defect going down to bone with a surrounding area of 7 to 8 cm diameter, poor, red, indurated skin. Although patient has essentially no personality and does not converse, he is ambulatory.

Patient was born in Greece, but no further history known.

Physician's diagnosis: Left prepatellar infected open lesion improved
General arteriosclerosis c̄ chronic brain syndrome
Old fracture of patella

Treatments: Surgical debridement left knee, 3/24 (flap right leg to left knee)
Wound isolation (gown, mask, etc.)
VS and temp q 4°
Irrigate Foley catheter c̄ GU irrigant (Neosporin in saline)
Wash penis c̄ antiseptic soap
IPPB 5 minutes q 4° 20 ml H_2O
Suction through nose and cough
Wet to dry soaks c̄ fine mesh gauze c̄ saline
Change dressing q 4°, 2 ulcers left leg, 1 ulcer right leg
Cover c̄ fine mesh gauze c̄ dry Curity wrap, 4 by 4s and Kerlix
Flap to be kept flush against defect, DSD over flap
Legs on pillow
K pad to wound

Medications: Vitamin C, 250 mg po 9-5
Multivits 1 po 9 PM

Care Plan. Mr. JH

1. *Problem* (usual—open wound): Potential spread of infection left patella due to contamination or poor condition of tissue.
   Reason: Poor cleaning technique combined with poor quality tissue can result in spread of infection. Granulation tissue has few functional cells, is comprised primarily of connective tissue; therefore, poor local circulation of antibodies and phagocytes.
   Expected outcome (objective): No increase in size of ulcer—2 cm diameter. No signs of local swelling, redness, pain. Temperature within normal limits.
   Deadlines: Check and document daily.

Nursing orders:

a. Check vital signs q 4°

b. Every time dressing is changed observe wound for swelling, redness, and pain.

c. Use extreme care with cleansing techniques.

Rationale: Temperature will rise as part of body's defense mechanism. Frequent careful observation will increase possibility of early detection and therefore early treatment of any further infection. Strict sterile cleansing techniques will minimize chance of secondary infection.

2. *Problem* (usual—chronic disease): Potential discouragement due to chronic nature of illness.

Reason: History of poor results of treatment result in loss of hope for improvement in future. Principle of negative reinforcement.

Expected outcome (objective): Verbalize feelings. Expression of hope and sense of optimism.

Deadlines: Check and document q 2 days.

Nursing orders:

a. Initiate subject of illness and possible feelings.

b. Listen actively, allow verbalization.

c. Clarify patient's misunderstandings about illness and treatment to facilitate sense of reality as well as of optimism.

d. Reinforce positive information about progress.

Rationale: Initating subject will bring feelings to patient's consciousness so that he can express them if he wishes. Active listening creates a milieu of safety for the patient to express himself. Verbalization reduces tension. A hopeful feeling combined with a sense of reality creates a psychologic climate that facilitates physiologic process.

3. *Problem* (unusual): Difficulty breathing with IPPB due to misunderstanding of how to work with it.

Reason: How to breathe with IPPB is not simple nor apparent. A patient is unlikely to learn without specific, directive assistance.

Expected outcome (objective): Demonstrate ability to breathe successfully with machine, without assistance.

Deadline: Check every eight hours. Accomplish in two days.

Nursing orders:

a. Explain reason for using breathing machine and how it operates.

b. Demonstrate procedure with another mask.

c. Have patient try with his mask. Coach him. Say, "Breathe now, relax. Work with the machine, in, out, in, out, that's good. Rest a minute. Now let's start again."

d. Repeat coaching every time treatment is scheduled. Give positive reinforcement. Invite his questions and problems. Solve them.

f. Include patient in goal of independent use of machine by the end of the second day.

Rationale: When a mechanical skill must be learned, a visual mental perception of the skill is needed. This can be achieved by demonstrations and explanations. Secondly, physical coordination skills must be developed by establishing new neuromotor pathways. This is accomplished by successful repetition of the skill. To maximize the potential for the repetitive functions being successful, direct coaching is required. Positive reinforcement establishes a psychologic climate that will motivate the person to devote energy to "trying again." The patient's understanding and acceptance of the same goal as the nurse's will result in teamwork and a sense of accomplishment and satisfaction.

4. *Problem* (unusual): Severe feelings of isolation, loneliness, and dehumanization due to no family and friends, and due to the label of "No personality."

Reason: When one is in an environment of "no closeness or caring" by significant others, one has feelings of low self-worth, of aloneness, and of life's having no purpose. These feelings cause a person to become introverted, nonverbal, and nontrusting, which compounds the isolation and the negative labeling by others.

Expected outcome (objective): Increased self-esteem and trust. The criteria for evaluation would be: verbalizing more, initiating conversations, smiling, and relaxed body posture.

Deadline: Evaluate and document every day.

Nursing orders:

a. Delegate to one nurse, who feels she cares, to establish a trust relationship, and gradually extend it to other persons.

b. Talk to him even though he does not respond.

c. Be directive and supportive. Use physical contact to communicate support.

d. Follow through with promises.

e. Give positive reinforcements even to small steps toward progress.

f. Through case conferences, involve staff in a feeling of hopefulness and concern so that their care will be positively reinforcing.

Rationale: The creation of an environment of caring, consistency, support, and encouragement will assist in bringing to the patient's awareness heretofore repressed emotions of response to human kindness. Positive reinforcement to the small responses will make it safe and nonthreatening to respond again. One nurse who makes a special effort to develop a trust relationship will serve as an experience model for the patient to use as a guide for relating to other people.

Example 2, Mrs. IB

Background: Mrs. B is an 88-year-old widow. She lives alone but has children who visit her. She has been taking digitalis for some time, has arthritis, has poor nutritional status, and is legally blind. She was admitted to the hospital and was diagnosed as having acute cholelithiasis. She soon had a cholecystectomy performed and now is making a poor postoperative recovery. Two weeks after surgery a student cared for her and developed a care plan. Excerpts from the student nursing care plan are portrayed in the subsequent paragraphs.

Physician's orders: Metahydrin 4 mg po, 9 AM
Digoxin 0.25 mg qod (odd days), 9 AM
Intake-output
Push 2,500 ml fluid intake daily
Daily weight (standing scale)
Vital signs every 4°
Change dressing tid
IPPB, 20 cm 1:4 Mucomist qid
Clamp T tube for one-half hour at 10:30 AM and 2:00 PM daily
Ambulate to door daily
Up in chair tid
Diet (per nasogastric tube): Mix 200 ml formula with 75 ml bile and gavage feed q 2°

Care Plan

1. *Problem* (unusual): Unable to meet own personal care needs due to weakness and blindness.
   Reason: No energy reserves are available for extra exertion. The postoperative metabolic requirements drain all available resources. The frustration of blindness in an unfamiliar environment results in greater energy requirement per task accomplished, thus reducing the feasibility of the patient doing any of her own care at this time.
   Expected outcome (objective): Minimum energy output above that required for therapeutic activities.
   Deadline: Evaluate and document daily.
   Nursing orders:
   a. Discuss with patient the need for rest and minimum energy output. Clarify and listen to her feelings regarding dependency. Support in her an understanding that physical dependency is necessary and appropriate at this time.
   b. Maximize patient's independence in other ways. Let her decide, let her be in charge about timing activities and so forth. Initiate discussions regarding patient's remarkable independence prior to surgery and, therefore, the good potential for becoming quite independent again.
   c. Plan and organize care ahead of time so that each activity can be accomplished quickly and smoothly, and with a minimum of exertion by the patient.
   d. Plan care activities in blocks, leaving longer periods of uninterrupted rest.
   Rationale: Discussion, clarification, and agreement reduce anxiety and tension, thereby reducing energy requirements. Psychologic compensation for feelings of dependency can be promoted by maximized independence, which helps the patient in her coping process, and reduces tension. Fast, smooth movements require less energy than the same movements done slowly according to principle relating to overcoming inertia.

2. *Problem* (unusual): Red, excoriated buttocks, 2 inch diameter each buttock due to poor tissue turgor, secretions, and friction.
Reason: Secretions containing irritating chemicals, destruction of epithelium by rubbing against linens, and poor tissue resistance due to malnutrition and metabolic drain of surgery; these combine to cause erosion and inflammation of the skin.
Expected outcome (objective): Continual decrease in size and redness of areas.
Deadlines: Check every eight hours.
Nursing orders:
a. Cleanse area with soft cloth, warm water, and germicidal soap qid and more frequently as needed. Pat dry. Apply cornstarch.
b. Keep clean square of sheepskin under hips and buttocks at all times.
c. Enlist patient's involvement in avoiding supine position except for short periods, no more than one-half hour at a time.
Rationale: Cleansing, mechanically and by dilution, removes irritating secretions. Sheepskin provides flexible airspace which levels or spreads pressure over greater area. Cornstarch adsorbs moisture, preventing its penetration through to the skin. Avoiding supine position reduces the length of time that there is pressure against the already damaged tissue area.

3. *Problem* (usual): Potential potassium depletion due to diarrhea.
Reason: Gastrointestinal secretions have a high potassium content. When these secretions are not reabsorbed at the usual rate, such as in gastrointestinal hypermotility, the overall body content of potassium is depleted.
Expected outcome (objective): No signs and symptoms of potassium depletion. No s/s of slow weak pulse, weakness, tingling of fingers, poor tissue turgor, low K blood values.
Deadlines: Check every eight hours.
Nursing orders: Observe for symptoms listed above. Since many of the symptoms are those of the patient's other multiple problems, the symptoms which are a more reliable index of potassium depletion would be weak pulse or a tingling sensation of the fingers. The physician is having daily blood chemistries done to assess more accurately the electrolyte balance. Under the circumstances, the daily blood chemistries are the most efficient and reliable method of monitoring potassium (and other electrolytes).
Rationale: The tissue symptoms of potassium depletion are related to the fact that intracellular potassium is normally in greater percentage. It is vital to the structure and metabolism of body cells. In potassium depletion cells are weakened and are less viable, causing the symptoms of weakness, poor tissue turgor, weak heart beat, and so forth. When blood chemistries are done at appropriate intervals, electrolyte imbalances can be detected and remedied early. When done at appropriate frequent intervals blood chemistries provide the only reliable guide and will warn of impending deficits before other symptoms develop.

The preceding two examples of nursing education care plans did not include the patient's responses to nursing actions. In the actual teaching–learning setting, however, recording and evaluating actual patient outcomes are a vital and integral part of the educational experience.

INCORPORATING CARE PLANNING INTO THE CURRICULUM

Introducing the elements of the nursing process into one of the early sequences of the curriculum is as important as introducing other fundamentals of patient care. Providing the learner with such a tool as a care plan format for putting the process into operation aids in translating an abstract concept into understandable and applicable elements of learning.

The next section of this chapter will suggest an overall curriculum design for the nursing process. It is followed by a more detailed description of a suggested teaching–learning process.

Curriculum Planning Design

Most nursing curricula are organized according to a conceptual framework which encompasses at least four elements[1]: the individual, society, health, and nursing. Whatever conceptual framework is adopted, a person's basic needs, his motivational systems, his growth and development patterns, and how these elements influence his proactive and reactive responses are considered. Society is studied in terms of social systems that impress the individual in a myriad of ways. The family, social groups, work groups, work, social norms, and political, regulatory, and economic systems are studied and analyzed. Hypotheses are generated regarding the effects of individual–social system interactions. Health as a certain state of being is defined. Various definitions of health from minimal to optimal are explored. Students gain beginning insight into the implications of health, both as a definition and as a value that varies not only from person to person and group to group but from one point in time or situation to another.

The nursing component of a curriculum defines nursing: its philosophy, its belief systems, its history and traditions, its biases, and its current responsibility as a health care discipline. Nurse practice acts are explored and discussed. Within this context, the nursing process is defined and is put into operation as part of the practice of nursing in the early learning phases of a student's development.

Although the nursing process can be described in various ways, it includes several sequential yet interrelated and recycling phases: data gathering (assessment), problem identification (diagnosing), goal determination (predicted patient outcomes), intervention planning (prescribing), plan implementation (direct or indirect care), and evaluation (concurrent and retrospective).

Early Curriculum Content

For beginning courses, the nursing process is introduced and is discussed in terms of its application to individual patients. The nursing care plan is explained as a tool for assisting one in methodically applying the nursing process. One can illustrate how the nursing process is applied by showing a standard care plan for one of the kinds of health problems the students are studying. Individualized adaptations to a standard care plan can be made, depending upon the variables associated with the individual, his social systems, and his values about health. This early learning phase focuses on comprehending and applying the nursing process to relatively simple situations.

Intermediate Curriculum Content

Later nursing courses add complexity. Health problems are more complex, and technical skills are more advanced. The nursing process is learned and applied in greater depth. Intermediate courses reinforce the nursing process as learned in earlier phases, but now the learners are ready to formulate their own standard care plans and to analyze and criticize them for comprehensiveness and potential effectiveness. This intermediate phase reinforces comprehension and application. It also adds prediction, analysis, and evaluation as additional cognitive steps.

Advanced Curriculum Content

Advanced nursing courses add new dimensions in terms of health-illness complexities, in terms of individual professional responsibility for planning and decision making, and in terms of leading, guiding, or facilitating the efforts of other health team members. Advanced courses focus on the nursing process within a theoretical frame of reference and require that the students formulate standard care plans that reflect differing theories of health and illness. Students also analyze individual patient situations from several theoretical perspectives. They develop a plan of care based upon the theory that is most relevant to the situation. Thus, the advanced courses in nursing focus on discrimination and the synthesis of data to make the most relevant application of plans of care to individuals or groups.

This general progression of nursing process content follows a simple-to-complex order of learning. It integrates comprehension, application, prediction, analysis, evaluation, discrimination, and synthesis in a continually reinforced sequence of curriculum design themes.[2]

SUGGESTED TEACHING—LEARNING PROCESSES*

Early Courses

Suggested learner objectives for early learning phases are:

1. Correctly associate examples of application of the nursing process with the element which it exemplifies.
2. Given a descriptive patient situation, select a standard care plan, among several, that best applies.
3. Make at least one important adaptation to a standard care plan so as to demonstrate recognition of an unusual problem.
4. Using expected outcomes, correctly assess and document a patient's status over a period of three or more days.
5. Select a data-gathering guide and demonstrate that at least minimum baseline data were collected via interview, observation, inspection, and history review.
6. Correctly discriminate between usual and unusual situations for a selected number of descriptive patient situations.
7. Identify well-written elements of a patient care plan by successfully discriminating 9 or 10 choices each for problems, expected outcomes, and nursing orders.

To accomplish these objectives:

1. Review, explain, and provide examples of each element of the nursing process.

*Adapted from suggestions made by A. Watson, Professor of Nursing, California State University, Sacramento.

2. Provide an example of a standard care plan explaining each component and showing its relationship to one or more elements of the nursing process.
3. Explain how the nursing care plan will be a learning tool and how a more streamlined version is used in the service setting.
4. Role play (two instructors) or show videotape of the nursing process in action with a real or simulated patient. Criticize and reinforce important points.
5. Learners select (or are assigned) a patient with whom they will apply the nursing process by collecting baseline data and by correctly selecting a standard care protocol as well as identifying problem areas that are unusual.
6. Unusual problem areas are discussed with colleagues, and individualized expected outcomes and nursing orders are formulated only after further study and validation by the instructor.
7. Formulate care plans for several patients. Document progress according to expected outcomes, and make judgments as to the adequacy of the plan. Include an analysis of whether or not the plan, as implemented, was a substantial variable influencing the patient's progress. Hypothesize about what other variables may have been crucial.

Over the span of one or more early nursing courses, many learning processes can be designed to suit the instructor's style, the course content, or the teaching–learning philosophy. Several excellent teaching aids are available to assist in preparing nursing process-care planning classes. These teaching aids are listed and annotated at the end of this chapter.

Intermediate Courses

Suggested learner objectives for intermediate phases are:

1. Given descriptive patient data (written or videotaped), formulate a comprehensive, well-phrased nursing care plan for a patient experiencing a complex situation.
2. Utilizing reference and expert input, compose a standard care plan for patients of a specific clinical or nursing diagnostic category.
3. Criticize a standard care plan formualted by someone else. Write a complete analysis, including comprehensiveness of usual problems, validity of expected outcomes, and appropriateness of nursing orders.
4. Given a set of outcomes on several plans of care, evaluate and

document the associated patient's status. Make supportable judgments as to the appropriateness of the plan of care.

To accomplish these objectives:

1. For most or all clinically assigned patients, the student formulates a detailed plan of care including scientific principles and other supporting rationale. Include analysis of the patients' progress or lack of progress. Suggest revised plans of care based upon these judgments. Criticize these papers in small group sessions to add collegial input to each learner's planning and evaluating efforts.
2. In small groups, compose one or more standard care plans for groups of patients representative of the clinical problems under study in the intermediate courses.
3. Review and criticize the charting of patients' progress by learner, colleagues, or nursing staff. Verbally report on charting adequacy relative to outcome criteria. Make suggestions for improvements if needed and methods for achieving the improvements, ie, classes on care planning and outcome charting, flow sheets, POMR, and so forth.
4. Provide the students with an overview of retrospective and concurrent audit processes. Draw relationships from these audit methods to the standard care plans and charting that the learners have been formulating and analyzing.

Other variations of the suggested learning processes can be devised by faculty members. The incorporation of nursing audit principles can be enlarged upon in greater detail than has been suggested. Annotated references for teaching aids are provided at the end of this chapter.

Advanced Courses

Suggested learner objectives for advanced courses for the nursing process theme are:

1. Given examples of two or more standard care plans, correctly associate them with the theoretical frame of references from which they are derived.
2. Given descriptive patient data (written or videotaped), choose an appropriate theory for care and provide a supportable rationale for the choice.
3. Analyze a colleague's plan of care, assess the patient, and criticize the plan for relevant theory base, application of theory in plan, success of plan, variables affecting success (nursing or physician

interventions, patient's level of growth and development, patient's value system, patient's clinical status—past and present—and socioeconomic factors. Conclude the critique by summarizing and synthesizing the relevance, to this patient, of the variables that are most likely to have been crucial to the ultimate outcomes.

4. Demonstrate effectiveness in group leadership (colleagues and staff nurses) in conducting an analysis of a patient's plan of care and of making necessary adjustments as a result of group input, literature review, and consideration for the theoretical basis for care.

5. Conduct a retrospective audit on a sample of charts. Report findings to colleagues and staff nurses. Facilitate the formulation of a remedial action plan.

To accomplish these objectives:

1. Learners read about and discuss current nursing theories and formulate one or more plans of care (standard combined with unusual problems) for specifically assigned patients.

2. Implement a plan of care for one or more patients and analyze it for its theoretical validity and its relevance to the patients' situations and hypothesize what variables were the most crucial in achieving the actual outcomes.

3. Participate in an agency's nursing audit committee and the quality monitoring processes that are ongoing. Criticize these processes for their effectiveness. Suggest improvements if needed. Ascertain what importance the agency places upon quality assurance processes. Identify the administrative and staff levels and their support of quality enhancement efforts.

In advanced courses, the learners themselves will design learning processes of their own that can add immeasurably to the value of this sequence of advanced application of the nursing process. Annotated references for suggested teaching aids appear at the end of this chapter.

SUMMARY

The preceding pages have suggested certain values, objectives, and learning activities that can reinforce the nursing process as a theme throughout a series of courses in a nursing curriculum.

Early phases focus on simple concepts applied to relatively simple clincial data in order to establish an organized way of thinking and to learn the language of care planning. Intermediate phases reinforce comprehension, terminology, and systematic thinking and focus on discrimination and analysis. Advanced courses focus on the comprehensive application of the nursing process through analysis and the synthesis of theories and human and social variables. Included also are applications to the quality assurance methodologies that represent another level of the nursing process in action.

REFERENCES

1. Torres G, Yura H: Today's Conceptual Framework: Its Relationship to the Curriculum Development Process. New York, National League for Nursing, Department of Baccalaureate and Higher Degree Programs, 1974
2. Bloom B (ed): Taxonomy of Cognitive Domain. New York, David McKay Co, 1971, pp 35-46

BIBLIOGRAPHY

Hegyvary S. Chamings P: The hospital setting and patient care outcomes. J Nurs Admin 5:29, March-April 1975; 5:36, May 1975
Hegyvary S, Haussmann R: Monitoring nursing care quality. J Nurs Admin 5:17, June 1975
Little D, Carnevali D: Nursing Care Planning. Philadelphia, Lippincott, 1976
Mayers M, Norby R, Watson A: Quality Assurance for Patient Care: Nursing Perspectives. New York, Appleton-Century-Crofts, 1977
Riehl J, Roy C: Conceptual Models for Nursing Practice, New York, Appleton-Century-Crofts, 1974
Woolley F, Warnick F, Kane R, and Dyer E: Problem-Oriented Nursing. New York, Springer, 1974
Yura H, Walsh M: The Nursing Process, 2nd ed. New York, Meredith, 1973
A Plan for Implementation of the Standards of Nursing Practice. Kansas City, American Nurses Association, 1975
Patient Care Planning: A Syllabus. Chicago, Nursing Care Systems, Medicus Corporation, 1974
Quality Assurance: A Syllabus. Chicago, Nursing Care Systems, Medicus Corporation, 1974

ANNOTATED BIBILIOGRAPHY OF TEACHING AIDS

Early Phases

Mayers M, El Camino Hospital Staff: Standard Nursing Care Plans. Stockton Cal, KP Co Medical Systems, 1977, Vol 3, Maternal-Child Health.

This volume provides approximately 80 standard care plans for both simple and complex diagnostic categories. A section on growth and development is included. These care plans can be used as references to help the beginning learner.

Watson A, Mayers M: How to Write Nursing Care Plans. Stockton Cal, KP Co Medical Systems, 1976

This 95-page workbook explains, illustrates, and interacts with the learner through programmed learning sequences and tests the learner's progress each step of the way. The learner interacts with the authors by use of a special marker pen that uncovers the instructors' feedback to the learner's decisions. This book can be completed independently by the learner, thus substantially reducing the instructor's classroom time for teaching basic care planning.

Nursing Care Planning: A Slide-Sound Program. Mt View Cal, El Camino Hospital, 1977

The 1½ hour autotutorial or small group self-teaching program is a delightfully illustrated series of slides with definitions, illustrations, and pauses for learner participation through the use of an accompanying handbook. This slide-sound program is designed to stand alone or to be used in conjunction with the Watson-Mayers workbook, *How to Write Nursing Care Plans.*

Taking the Pain out of Care Planning. Chicago Medicus Corporation, 1977

This 60-page booklet takes the learner quickly and easily through the basic steps of care planning. Occasional programmed learning tests occur at the end of major cognitive steps. It is designed to be used as a self-learning booklet, thus reducing the need for didactic classroom time.

Intermediate and Advanced Phases

Mayers M, El Camino Hosptial Staff: Standard Nursing Care Plans. Stockton Cal, KP Co Medical Systems, 1975, Vol 1, Medical-Surgical Care; 1976, Vol 2, Intensive Care

These two volumes together provide over 150 standard care plans which can assist students as a reference when formulating their own standard plans.

Mayers M, Norby R, Watson A: Quality Assurance for Patient Care: Nursing Perspectives. New York, Appleton-Century-Crofts, 1977

The entire 400-page book provides an excellent reference for learning quality assurance processes. However, Chapter 8, "Patient Outcome Charting," describes and illustrates charting as it relates to care planning. It illustrates POMR, narrative outcome recording, and the design and use of flow sheets.

Chapter 11, "Teaching Quality Assurance in Health Care Agencies," provides suggested learner objectives and learning processes and includes 27 full-page illustrations to be used as guides for creating transparencies or slides to illustrate the teaching-learning content.

Chapter 12, "Teaching Quality Assurance in a Nursing Curriculum," outlines three learning modules, including objectives and detailed content and learning activities for each module.

Watson A, Mayers M: The Essentials of Quality Assurance: An Illustrated Teaching-Learning Program. Stockton Cal, KP Co Medical Systems, 1977

This self-contained teaching packet is designed for classroom use. It includes 30 colorful transparencies which illustrate retrospective audit and related quality assurance concepts. The instructor is provided a handbook that outlines each area of content and the associated learning activities. Several pertinent article reprints are included. This teaching-learning program can minimize teacher preparation time and can help to standardize how the subject is taught from one student group to another.

11

The Data Base: Foundation for Judgment and Evaluation

RATIONALE FOR DATA GATHERING

The terms *data base, nursing history, admission interview, assessment interview format*, and the like are becoming increasingly common in the vocabulary of nursing. All refer to a variety of organized sets of questions or topics which serve as a guide for obtaining the data believed necessary for planning a patient's care.

Weed's definition[1] serves to clarify the meaning of *data base*. It is a systematic compilation of patient information which is used to identify patient problems and serves as a foundation for later evaluation of the patient's condition.

Inherent in the data-gathering process is judgment. Judgment refers to discernment and understanding. It is a thinking process whereby one compares ideas, facts, and concepts and ascertains relationships among them. The judgment process is continuous in nursing practice. Early judgments (such as those made upon admission), however, are crucial in that decisions about what data to collect, which facts to pursue, and what meaning to glean from the information establish the foundation for subsequent judgments and evaluative decisions.

Like other disciplines, nursing has found that in order to meet its responsibility to patients it must not leave to chance the collection of information that is basic to good care. Historically, physicians have used a format for history taking and physical examinations. As medical specialties have matured, variations on the basic "history and physical" have been developed. A neurologist uses a specific format for history taking which has been carefully designed to guide him in obtaining the information he needs in order to rule out or to refine a neurologic diagnosis. Similarly, a gynecologist has a routine set of questions and a method of examination that has been thoughtfully organized to facilitate his data gathering for diagnosis and patient care. The same is true of each medical specialty.

Paramedical disciplines, such as physical therapy, also have routine, systematic ways for assessing muscle strength, coordination, joint rotation, and so forth. Dietitians interview patients and assess their dietary status by utilizing a guide for the content and sequence of their questions. Nursing also has found that an organized system of data gathering assists profoundly in subsequent planning and evaluation.

Nursing History as an Assessment Guide

The phrase "nursing history" is a term frequently used in nursing to refer to an organized interview or data-collection format. The content and format of a nursing history vary from agency to agency or from one specialized type of care unit to another. It consists of a specific selection and sequence of questions or topics that serve as a reminder or guide to the interviewer. Nurses who use nursing histories consistently find that they can rapidly memorize the general topics. Therefore, they do not constantly have to refer to the questionnaire format after the first few interviews. They also learn quickly to deviate from the guide by covering the questions in a different order if a changed order is more appropriate for a given situation.

Most agencies use nursing histories for data gathering at the time a patient is admitted to a nursing service. Because of this, most nursing histories include questions about the patient's health and socioeconomic situation, as a way of establishing a background frame of reference for him. Then, depending upon the type of agency or special care unit, the questions become more specific and more relevant to the anticipated problems and concerns of patients in that care setting. The nursing history is an integral part of nursing's methodology toward the goal of rational and systematic intervention, for maximizing maintenance, comfort, and higher level wellness. Since two of the major and unique concerns of nursing are the patient's maintenance and his comfort, interview formats almost always contain questions about a patient's preferences and requirements relating to personal maintenance. Also there are questions about the physical and psychologic environments that the patient perceives as comforting. Nursing's concern for better health has different implications in various settings and circumstances. Therefore, information about a patient's family or a group's health-illness pattern is basic to the planning of further care. A nursing history should elicit information about an individual's or a family's usual health practices, their illnesses, their experiences with and feelings about health care, and their perceptions of the meaning of wellness for themselves or their family. The information that is collected is referred to as the "data base."

EFFECTS OF DATA GATHERING

An admission interview of a patient by a nurse using a nursing history guide has several direct beneficial results. Obviously, the information obtained gives the responsible nurse the necessary data for making a nursing diagnosis. The nursing diagnosis is a list of the patient's problems, usual and unusual, which fall within the independent jurisdiction of nursing. Such problems would be, among others, those relating to personal health maintenance.

But what is frequently overlooked and what in some cases may be more important, the very process of history taking itself can accomplish much besides data collection alone.

It Begins the Nurse-Patient Relationship

A nurse-patient dialogue such as occurs when an admission nursing history is being taken establishes the beginning of an important therapeutic relationship. Because the nurse and patient have talked together and have shared concerns about the patient's problems and his hopes, they will have a basis for effectively working through the discomforts or crises associated with an illness and its treatment. As a result of an admission interview, the patient learns exactly who is responsible for his nursing care. His trust and confidence increase as he sees that the nurse is concerned about him personally. He knows upon whom to call for assistance if he has problems. He is secure in the knowledge that someone he has met and talked with—someone who knows him as a person—is in charge of his care.

It Begins Patient Involvement

Because the nursing history interview opens the door to a give and take of information and concerns, it becomes the medium for beginning a patient's involvement in his own care. When the nurse explains to the patient that the information is needed to plan his care in ways most effective for him and when she actively secures his involvement in setting goals and in planning methods for reaching them, the entire plan of care is much more likely to succeed. If patients know what their care plan objectives are and agree that the objectives are, in fact, desirable, those objectives will be more readily achieved. Carefully guarded care plans, whose very existence may be unknown to the patient, cannot help but lead toward a high failure rate. Patients must be involved in setting their own goals and must be consulted on the activities designed to meet those goals. Obviously, there may be circumstances that temporarily limit a patient's involvement in his own care planning, but such situations are rare in most nursing care settings. As a general rule, the nurse should make every effort to involve the patient. A nurse-patient dialogue established with the initial nursing history interview creates a viable milieu for ongoing patient care planning.

It Begins the Nurse's Commitment

A further benefit of an admission nursing history interview is the psychologic commitment to the patient that the interviewing nurse experiences. Because she has talked with the patient and shared common concerns with him, she knows him as a person, not as a diagnosis. She will feel a personal, human desire to see that his care is the very best possible.

It Saves Time and Energy

Nurses who consistently take admission nursing histories feel severely handicapped if for some reason they are deprived of the opportunity to talk with each newly admitted patient. They know that time spent on a nursing history interview is an investment that pays off not only in time savings but also in good care. When a patient's problems are identified or his potential problems are prevented, a significant amount of time can be saved. When a patient knows what to anticipate and knows that someone is truly in charge and cares, he will be less anxious and more relaxed. He will be less likely to demand staff time for small duties. Frequent requests for errands from a patient may, for instance, be his only way of assuring himself that someone cares and knows that he exists. If he is relaxed, trusting, and involved, his recovery will generally be faster and less complicated. This saves time and frustration for the patient as well as for the nurse. Clearly, a nurse–patient dialogue based upon a nursing history interview format is an important and viable tool for good nursing care.

It Establishes a Contract

The idea of "making a contract" with a patient is attracting attention from nurses, particularly from nurses involved in psychiatric and community health care. It has implications for all other aspects of nursing.

"Making a contract" means making an agreement between the nurse and her patient regarding the purposes of their association for a specified period of time. It implies that, early in the relationship, both nurse and patient will know what to expect of the other.

More specifically, a nurse will explain to the patient why she is there, what her responsibilities are, what she is able to do, and what she cannot do. She clarifies how she can be contacted and at what time she is available.

In response, the patient approves or accepts the nurse's statement of her purposes and intended activities and requests revision or clarification of any aspects that worry him. He also will agree to be available at certain times, to meet certain appointments, to make known any ongoing need for clarification or revision, and to contribute his expectations of the nature of their association.

A public health nurse first meeting a family makes a general statement about her reasons for visiting. After the history taking, as she begins to formulate a plan of care, she must clarify with the family the nature of her tentative goals and methods. When these have been reviewed and revised, taking into account the patient's suggestions, and then approved by the family, the basis for a nurse–patient contract has been established.

Similarly, in hospital settings, a nurse should explain to her patient who she is, what she will be doing, how she will be helping the patient, and what her plan of care for him is.

In some situations, when it is too difficult to obtain enough information early in the nurse–patient relationship for a specific contract to be appropriate, the nurse should, as part of a more general contract, make it known that as she and the patient understand his situation better they will refine an agreement between one another.

Making known their mutual expectations and pinpointing the purposes of their association is a vital element in establishing that all-important relationship of trust.

The nursing history interview is an opportune and useful medium for establishing the nurse–patient contract.

THE PROCESS OF DATA COLLECTION

Who Collects the Information?

Given that nursing histories are essential, there are varying points of view about who should take them and under what circumstances. If it is true that nursing has primary responsibility for many aspects of care and that nursing has certain legal responsibilities to patients, the answers to those questions are clear.

When a nurse is planning and implementing a patient's care, she will want to gather necessary patient care information. In the hospital setting, she may quite appropriately delegate to a well-trained nursing assistant the task of meeting the patient, checking his vital signs, taking care of his valuables, and orienting him to the physical environment, but she herself must follow up very soon with an admission interview or nursing history. Only a registered nurse has the background to answer effectively a patient's questions about treatments and about anticipated medical and nursing care. Only a registered nurse knows how to follow up on certain patient clues. For example, a patient may mention taking digitalis or other medications. This information has many implications that a nursing assistant is not trained to recognize, let alone evaluate. Appeals for simple basic information may be made by the patient during history taking and can be answered on the spot by a registered nurse. This could not be done by a nursing assistant. Finally, and perhaps most crucial of all, only a personal interview with the registered nurse will reassure the patient that the person responsible for his care does indeed know him and his problems.

Physical Settings for History Taking

The best time and place for nursing history taking probably are usually determined by the patient care setting. In community nursing, history taking most frequently occurs in the patient's home. The patient's natural environment is an ideal setting for gathering information that leads toward a home-based nursing care process. In other nursing specialties, such as office, industry, and clinic nursing, histories are completed in the office, at the factory, and in the clinic. Frequently, overcrowding in these settings forces the nurse to look for interview space that is private and nondistracting, where she and the patient can sit and talk with ease.

In the hospital the most likely physical setting for history taking is the patient's room. In multiple-bed rooms and wards, appropriate screening should be provided to maximize privacy, to minimize distraction, and to reinforce the nurse–patient trust relationship that is just beginning. The interviewing nurse should seat herself so that she can devote her full attention to the interview process. A nurse who remains standing while she interviews communicates a sense of haste. She may in fact be rushed, but she need not convey that fact to the new patient. A sense of hurry will obviously limit the patient's ability to share his concerns and to involve himself in the care-planning process. If a nurse sincerely wishes to convey her concern and interest, she will free herself to sit and talk face to face with her patient. Doing this will, with a minimum expenditure of the nurse's time and energy, appreciably add to the patient's feelings of worth—a major plus.

When a patient is ambulatory, as many medical-surgical and psychiatric patients are, the history-taking interview may best be accomplished in the privacy of a conference room or in the nurse's office.

The hard realities of many nursing care settings make it necessary for nurses to set priorities for the timing of history-taking interviews. Patients admitted as emergencies or experiencing acute physical stress obviously should not be interviewed until their condition is more stable, leaving them mentally able to participate. However, their attending family should not be ruled out as interim, and frequently invaluable, sources of relevant information upon which to begin care planning.

When multiple admissions to a service are made within a short period of time, it may well be impossible for the responsible nurse to interview all her new patients as soon as she would like. When that occurs, it will be necessary for the nurse to set responsible priorities. For example, a patient admitted to have major surgery the following morning may hold priority over a patient admitted to have a routine diagnostic work-up. Appropriate mechanisms for priority setting may be developed for varying situations.

The Interview

A feeling of caring should be transmitted in an interview. Caring means giving serious attention to someone, which communicates that the patient is respected and seen as a worthy person. Caring encourages a person to talk about his beliefs and concerns.

The interviewer who cares is genuine, warm, and understanding and avoids intruding his beliefs and values on the psychologic field of the patient. Essential to interviewing also is "to accomplish being with and not acting for another person." The what and how of interviewing are to learn how to get out of the patient's way.

It is not the purpose of this book to teach interviewing: interview relationships, determinants influencing interviews or interview goals, phases, and structure. It also is not within the scope of this book to discuss the expressive skills of communication. However, communication skills, sensitivity, warmth, and humanness are so crucial to nurse–patient data gathering, planning, and interaction that all of the topical guides and theoretical frameworks for questioning and observing remain only intellectual playthings in the absence of these more crucial skills and traits.

Schulman's book, *Intervention in Human Services*,[2] is one helpful resource for understanding and practicing the processes of observing, interviewing, and interacting. Little and Carnevali[3] summarize some of the major elements of data gathering and its contexts.

Documenting Data Base Information

A concern among nurses about history taking is whether actually to write on the history form as the interview unfolds. Some nurses believe that making notations during the interview may distract or worry the patient. However, nurses who have developed expertise in patient interviews are convinced that unwarranted patient worry can be prevented if they introduce themselves as the "nurse responsible for the patient's care" and if they explain fully their purpose for asking the questions. Expert nurses explain to the patient that, in order to make the nursing care most appropriate for him, they need certain information. They explain that they will be writing the information during the interview so they will not overlook it or forget it later. Patients respond to this approach with a sense of appreciation that their care is important.

Furthermore, leaving to a fallible memory the recall of important patient care data is unsafe. In other disciplines it is accepted, in fact *expected*, that the professional interviewer will record data as it unfolds. In nursing also, the history form should be completed during the interview.

EXAMPLES OF DATA BASE GUIDES

Following are samples of data base guides or nursing history forms that are applicable to various major patient care settings. Included in this chapter are guides for emergency room, operating room, acute medical-surgical, obstetrics, extended care, community health, home nursing, office nursing, and nursing education. None of the examples is intended to reflect a comprehensive treatment of the subject. They are designed to serve as guides for ideas and topics for data-collection forms.

These examples are not derived from an identifiable theoretical framework. Rather, they tend to represent (in question or topical form) those concerns that could be expected to arise as a result of physiologic illness, surgical procedures, or intrusions. A later section of this chapter illustrates how a standard care plan provides cues for initial data gathering. Another section of this chapter illustrates an assessment guide that is derived from a specific theoretical model. Whatever data base guide is used, the nurse's goal is to understand the patient's difficulties and concerns.

For Emergency Room

In emergency care settings, the nurse-patient interview must be timed and varied according to the patient's condition. But in order for a nurse intelligently to anticipate a patient's problems and to facilitate his maintenance, comfort, safety, and well-being, certain information must be obtained. If the patient is unable to respond, as much information as possible should be elicited from the family or from close friends, depending upon who is available at the time.

Emergency Room Example

Name: _____   Birthdate: _____
Address: _____   Occupation: _____
Phone: _____
Closest relative or friend: _____
Address: _____
Phone: _____

1. What happened that caused you to come here? _____

_____

2. What were you doing when this happened? _____

_____

3. Who helped you? What did they do? _____

4. How did you get here? _____

5. Who is with you? _____

6. Is there anyone you want very much to be with you now who isn't here?

_____

   How can they be located? _____

7. Is there anyone who needs to know you are here who doesn't now know?

_____

8. Has anything like this ever happened before? If so, what? _____

_____

9. How much pain or discomfort do you have now? _____

_____

10. How long have you been feeling this pain or discomfort? _____

_____

11. Do you want or need anything that will make you more comfortable?

_____

12. What do you know about what the doctor is planning for your continued
    care? _____

13. What problems are you likely to have following his advice? _____

_____

14. To what extent has this accident (or illness) disrupted your life? _____

_____

15. What problems do you expect to have getting your life back to normal again,
    and how do you plan to manage? _____

16. Have you any concerns about the cost of your emergency care? _____

_____

17. How do you plan to manage the cost problem? _____

_____

18. Do you have any questions or problems? _____

19. Is there anything more that you can think of that you would like us to do for
    you? _____

For Operating Room

Nursing history interviews by operating room personnel are usually completed the evening before surgery or at some appropriate earlier time if the patient is admitted more than a day in advance of surgery. The history interview is done by an operating room nurse who assumes responsibility for the immediate follow-up of any special concerns relevant to the surgical phase of hospitalization. She makes any other relevant care-planning information available to the surgical unit staff and, of course, to the operating room staff.

Operating Room Example

(Patient identification as needed)

1. What is your understanding of the surgery you are to have tomorrow? Do you know why it is being done? _____
2. What don't you understand or are not sure about? _____
_____
3. What do you expect will happen between now and the time you go to surgery? _____
4. How do you feel about having this particular surgery? Was it a difficult decision to make? _____
5. How does you husband (or wife, or family, or closest friend) feel about it?
_____
6. Will someone be with you tomorrow? Who? _____
7. Do you expect to see your doctor again before the surgery? Do you especially want to see him before the surgery for any reason?_____
_____
8. What do you know about the anesthetic you will be having? _____
_____
9. Have you ever had surgery before? What do you recall about it? _____
_____
10. Is there anything you are especially concerned about this time? If so, explain. _____
11. Is there anything you can think of that we can do or that you would like to have done that will make things better for you before or after surgery?
_____
12. Do you have any other questions or concerns? _____
_____

For Medical-Surgical

The rapid turnover of patients who are experiencing acute biologic crises creates a major challenge to medical-surgical nurses. It is obvious that there is a critical need to obtain care-planning information and to start a plan of care very early if nursing intends to contribute significantly to a patient's care before he is discharged.

Many factors should enter into the decision about the length and content of a medical-surgical nursing history—factors such as the usual types of physical problems, length of hospital stay, intensity of care, and staffing patterns.

The following four examples of nursing histories for medical-surgical care settings provide a variety of possible alternatives.

Example 1

Name: _____ Date of History: _____

Diagnosis: _____ Admission Date: _____

Age: _____ Sex: _____ Religion: _____ Ethnic Origin: _____

Marital Status: _____ Children living in home—ages: _____

Occupation: _____ Recreational Interests: _____

Previous Hospitalization:

    When: _____ Where: _____ Diagnosis: _____

Orientation: _____ Attention Span: _____

Ability to Understand Questions and Ideas: _____

Emotional Status (√ and explain)

    Anxiety: _____

    Aggression: _____

    Depression: _____

    Repression: _____

    Rationalization: _____

    Regression: _____

    Sublimation: _____

    Other: _____

    Effect of illness upon self-concept: _____

    Ability to relate: _____

Physical Problems (√ and explain)

    Hearing: _____

    Sight: _____

    Touch: _____

    Smell: _____

    Taste: _____

    Movement: _____

    Equilibrium: _____

    Swallowing: _____

Skin Problems (√ and explain)

    Dehydrated: _____

    Edema: _____ Where? _____

    Discoloration: _____ Where? _____

    Broken areas: _____ Where? _____

    Cleanliness: _____

    Localized temperature changes: _____ Where? _____

Oral Hygiene and Problems (√ and explain)

    Condition and appearance of oral cavity: _____

    _____

    Condition of teeth: _____

    Dentures: _____

    Oral hygiene (habits, time, preparation, etc): _____

    _____

Nutrition:
   General appearance (obese, thin, emaciated, normal, etc) _____
   _____

   Appetite: _____ How many meals: _____ Snacks: _____
   Food likes: _____
      dislikes: _____
   Food allergies: _____
   Use of alcoholic beverages: _____ What? _____
                                        Frequency: _____
Elimination:
   Bowel habits: _____
   Cathartics: _____ Kind used: _____ Frequency: _____
   Usual pattern of urinary elimination (√ and explain)
   Frequency: _____
   Amount: _____
   Pain: _____
   Retention: _____
   Color: _____
   Catheter: _____
   Other: _____
Menstrual History (as appropriate):
   Interval: _____
   Flow: _____
   Menopause: _____
Rest and Sleep:
   Normal sleep pattern: _____
      Easily disturbed? _____
      Device for getting to sleep? _____
   Naps or rest periods? _____
Comfort:
   Current pain: _____ Location: _____ Severity: _____
   Analgesic: _____ What type: _____ How often: _____
   History of pain: _____ Location: _____ Severity: _____
   Analgesic: _____ What type: _____ How often: _____
   Other pain-relieving devices found to be effective: _____
   _____

Significant observations made while taking history: _____
_____

Patient's degree of understanding of illness and purpose of contemplated
therapy: _____
Patient's plan for care after discharge: _____
Family involvement and understanding of problems: _____
_____

Analysis.   The above sample nursing history is arranged by topics
to serve as a reminder to the nurse. She phrases the questions approp-

riately to elicit the necessary information. The history includes topics regarding discharge planning and family involvement.

Example 2

How long have you known you were to be admitted to the hospital?
What kind of problems have you had and how long have you been feeling this way?
Have you been hospitalized before?   When and where?
What sort of things help you to be more comfortable when you are not feeling well?
Is there anything in particular you would like the nurses to do?
Do you have difficulties other than your present illness that restrict your activities?
Do you have any habits that will be affected by your hospitalization?
Were you on any special medications or diet before you came to the hospital?
Do you usually eat three meals a day?
Have you ever had any unfavorable reactions to foods or medications?
Do you have any difficulties with sleeping?
Does anything special help?
Do you have any difficulties with eliminations? Bowels: Urine:
Do you take laxatives regularly?
Do you have family nearby?   Will they be coming to visit?
Do you have any questions about the hospital?

Analysis. This is an example of a brief nursing history that many agencies believe is a way of meeting both the realities of time limitations and the need to gather patient-care information. It assumes that the nurse will go into more detail as needed.

Example 3

Patient's Name: _____ Date: _____
Time of arrival: _____ Room: _____ Admitted from: _____ How arrived: _____
Accompanied by: _____ Relationship: _____
Phone: _____ Height: _____ Weight: _____
T _____ P_____ BP _____
Allergy to medicines (list): _____
            Allergy to Food: _____
            Allergy to Other: _____
Asthma?   Yes: _____ No: _____ Diabetic?   Yes: _____ No: _____
Epilepsy?   Yes: _____ No: _____

Ever been on cortisone? Yes: _____ No: _____

If yes, when? _____

Previous hospital experience and date. _____

Any prosthesis? (√ and explain)

  Dentures: _____

  Artificial eye: _____

  Contact lens: _____

  Artificial limbs: _____

  Glasses: _____

  Hearing aid: _____

Fluid preferences: _____

Hobbies or Interests: _____

Dislikes: _____

Medications brought to hospital—disposition: _____

Medication taken just prior to admission (past 24 hours): _____

_____

Condition of Hair: _____ Nails: _____ Skin: _____

Nurse's observation and inspection of patient's general physical condition:

_____

Nurse's impression of patient's attitude and emotional status: _____

_____

Knowledge about present illness: _____

What does patient expect of this hospitalization? _____

_____

Patient plans for home care: _____

Outstanding experiences from previous hospitalizations: _____

_____

Typical day (activity pattern): _____

Patient's statement of how he reacts when he becomes upset: _____

_____

Comfort needs, preferences, and requirements: _____

Preference for visitor or family contact: _____

Preference for tub or shower bath and usual time for this: _____

_____

Usual teeth care routine: _____

Usual bowel habits. If irregularities, what ususally helps? _____

_____

Any bladder irregularities? _____

Social and family history: _____

Education: _____

Occupation: _____

Any other patient questions (record significant questions): _____

_____

Analysis.   This history is arranged by topic to remind the nurse to phrase the appropriate questions. It includes topics that refer to the patient's emotional as well as physical status. It is brief but quite comprehensive.

Example 4

A. Patient's Understanding of Illness and Hospitalization
   1. Why did it become necessary for you to come to the hospital or go to the doctor? _____
   2. What do you think caused you to get sick? _____
   3. What does your doctor say caused you to get sick? _____
   _____
   4. What have you been told about what to expect here? _____
   _____
   5. How do you feel about it? _____
   6. Have you been told how long you are likely to be here? How long?
   _____
   7. With whom do you live? _____
   8. Who is the most important person(s) to you? _____
   9. What effect has your coming here had on your family (or closest person)? _____
   10. Will they be able to visit? _____
   11. How do you expect to get along after you leave the hospital? _____
   _____

B. Comfort and Maintenance
   1. Comfort
      a. Pain/Discomfort
         1) Have you had any pain or discomfort recently? Yes___ No___
            If yes, explain: _____
         2) What did you do to relieve the pain/discomfort? _____
         _____
         3) Did it help? How much? _____
         4) If you have pain/discomfort while here what would you like nurse to do to relieve it? _____
      b. Rest/Sleep
         1) Do you usually have trouble getting to sleep or staying asleep? Yes_____ No _____
         2) What would you like us to do to help you get the rest and sleep you need while in the hospital? _____
      c. Hygiene
         1) Do you need help with your bath while here? Yes____ No____
            Hair? _____
            Tub or shower? _____
            How often do you usually like to bathe? _____
            What time of day? _____
         2) Do you need help with your teeth? Yes_____ No_____
            How? _____

      3) Do you use anything on your face or skin (lotions, astringents)? _____

2. Safety and Ambulation
  a. Ambulation
    1) Do you have any problems walking or moving about?
      Yes_____ No_____
      If yes, explain: _____
    2) How do you feel about staying in bed while here? _____
    3) Do you know how much the doctor wants you in or out of bed while you are here? _____
  b. Eyesight
    Do you have any difficulty with your eyesight? Yes____ No____
    If yes, explain: _____
  c. Hearing
    Do you have any trouble with your hearing? Yes_____ No_____
    If yes, explain: _____

3. Fluids
  a. How much liquid do you drink each day when you are well? ____
  b. What liquids do you like to drink?
    Water: _____   Coffee: _____
    Milk: _____   Tea: _____
    Fruit juice:_____   Soft drinks: _____
  c. What fluids do you dislike? _____
  d. Do you drink alcoholic beverages? Yes_____ No_____
    If yes, explain: _____

4. Oral Hygiene
  a. Teeth/Mouth
    1) What is condition of your teeth and gums? _____
    2) Do you wear dentures or partial plates? _____
    3) Do you have any trouble eating because of your teeth?
      Yes____ No____ If yes, explain: _____
    4) Do you have any soreness or swelling in your mouth?
      Yes____ No____ If yes, explain: _____
  b. Diet
    1) Has your illness made any difference in your eating?
      Yes____ No____ If yes, explain: _____
    2) What foods do you usually eat? _____
    3) Are there any foods you do not eat? Yes_____ No_____
      If yes, explain: _____
    4) Are you on a special diet? Yes_____ No_____
      If yes, what kind? _____
      Did you have any problems with your diet? Yes____ No____
      If yes, explain: _____
    5) Do you believe yourself to be overweight or underweight?
      Yes____ No____ If yes, explain (how much and why):
      _____

5. Elimination
   a. Bowels
      1) How often do your bowels usually move?_____
      2) What time of day? _____
      3) Do you take a laxative?_____   or an enema? _____
                          Regularly _____   Regularly _____
                          Frequently _____   Frequently _____
                          Occasionally _____   Occasionally _____
                          Never _____   Never _____
         What kind? _____
      4) Do you do anything else to help you have a bowel move-
         ment? Yes_____ No_____
         If yes, explain: _____
      5) Has being sick changed your bowel functions? Yes___ No___
         If yes, explain: _____
      6) Do you ever have any difficulty with your urine or passing
         your urine? Yes ___ No ___
         If yes, explain: _____
         What do you do about it? _____
6. Aeration
   a. Have you ever had any difficulty with your breathing? Yes___
      No___ If yes, explain:_____
   b. Has being sick caused any changes in your breathing? Yes___
      No___ If yes, explain:_____
7. Sex and close relationships (Ask according to marital status and
   appropriateness to the patient)
   a. (If married) Has being sick caused you any problems with your
      being a husband_____ wife_____ Yes ___ No___
      father_____ mother_____ Yes ___ No ___
      If yes, explain: _____
      (If single and appropriate) Has being sick made any difference in
      your relationships with other people, including close relationships
      with the opposite sex? Yes___ No___
      If yes, explain: _____
   b. (If appropriate) Has being sick caused any change in your sexual
      functioning (sex life)? Yes___ No___
      If yes, explain: _____
   c. Do you expect your sex life to be changed in any way after you leave
      the hospital? Yes___ No___ Don't know___
      If yes, explain: _____
   d. Do you expect your ability to function as a husband, wife, father,
      mother, or in a social relationship to be changed in any way after
      you leave the hospital? Yes___ No___ Don't know___
      If yes, explain: _____
C. Other
   1. Do you have any allergies? Yes___ No___

If yes, what kind? _____

How have you manged? _____

To what extent does the allergy handicap you? _____

2. How far did you go in school? _____

Can you read and write? (Ask only if indicated) Yes___ No___

3. Is there anything else you wish to tell me that would help with your nursing care? _____

Analysis. This is an example of a nursing history that elicits a large amount of detailed information about the patient. Nurses using a lengthy history such as this learn to phrase the questions appropriately and to move smoothly from item to item as the information unfolds. Frequently the answer to one question will answer other questions appearing later in the interview. In this case the question is not repeated. A note is made to refer to the previous question.

A comprehensive and detailed nursing history such as this one provides excellent data for effective and time-saving nursing care planning.

For Obstetrics

Obstetric nursing in the hospital often changes rapidly in short periods of time. To anticipate and to prevent problems, a nursing history is necessary upon admission to the labor area and later upon admission to the postpartum service. Upon admission to labor it is generally not advisable to interview regarding specific postpartum problems because of the patient's physical and psychologic preoccupation with the task at hand, that is, labor and delivery.

Labor and Delivery Example

(Patient Identification)

(Usual physiologic data, vital signs, vaginal discharge, contractions, EDC, gravida, and so forth)

1. What do you expect and know about labor and delivery? _____

2. Do you know what is happening in your body now? _____

3. If you have had previous experience with labor and delivery, what do you recall? _____

4. What do you believe the nurses did that was most helpful? _____

5. Have you prepared for labor in any special way, such as exercises, classes, and so forth? If so, explain: _____

6. Is there anyone you want to stay with you during labor? _____
   Will this be possible? _____
7. Is there anyone who needs to know you are here who does not know?
   How can they be reached? _____
8. Is everything taken care of at home so you don't have to worry? If not, what
   is it? _____
9. Have you had a chance to think carefully about how you wish to feed your
   baby—breast or bottle? Do you have any questions about that now? __

10. Are there any other question or concerns?_____
11. Is there anything special we can do for you that will make you more com-
    fortable or that will assist in making this a happy and satisfying event for
    you? _____

Analysis. This questionnaire is devoted to eliciting information about the patient's psychologic as well as her physical preparation for labor, which is crucial in supporting her throughout this experience. It includes a query regarding her wishes regarding breast or bottle-feeding so as to avoid leaving that question until the split-second after delivering the placenta, during the delivery phase, when she may or may not really know what she is saying.

Because of its content, this history begins a strong nurse-patient relationship that is so crucial during the subsequent, frequently long and arduous hours of labor.

Postpartum Example

1. Now that you have had your baby, how do you feel? _____
2. Have you had a chance to see and to hold your baby? If yes, when and for
   how long? _____
   If no, why not? _____
3. How does he (or she) look to you? _____
4. (If appropriate) Has your husband seen the baby? _____
   What did he say? _____
5. How do you feel about your labor and delivery experience? _____

6. Is there anything about it (labor and delivery) that you didn't (and still don't)
   understand?_____
7. Now that you have had your baby, do you know how long you will be in the
   hospital? What do you expect to happen while you are here? _____

8. (If infant is a boy) Have you (and your husband, if appropriate) had an
   opportunity to thoroughly discuss whether or not you wish your baby
   circumcised? _____

9. What questions do you have about circumcision? _____
_____

10. Have you thought about using a birth control method until such time as you want another baby? If yes, which method? _____
11. Have you discussed birth control with your doctor? If yes, what did he say?
_____

12. Do you foresee any difficulties with using a birth control method when you go home? _____
13. Have you any problems, questions, or concerns about how you will manage when you go home? _____
14. Have you any problems, questions, or concerns about your hospital stay? If so, what are they? _____
15. Is there anything special we can do that will make your stay here pleasant and comfortable? _____

Analysis. This interview format initiates the all-important subjects of the mother–child relationship, feelings about labor and delivery, specific care expectations, fertility regulation, and infant care. It establishes the psychologic environment for ongoing anticipatory guidance and mutual (patient and nurse) care planning.

For Psychiatric Nursing

The variable mental and emotional stresses that are experienced by most psychiatric patients at the time of their admission to a nursing unit make formal history taking a difficult and possibly unreliable process for obtaining helpful information.

It may well be that, in many cases, the family of a psychiatric patient may be a resource for certain information of the personal health maintenance and personal preferences variety. The psychiatric patient who already is unable to cope with the stresses of life must not be threatened further by an environment unnecessarily unacceptable to him. The family can offer excellent ideas for humanizing and personalizing the patient's care. They know his likes and dislikes, his personal idiosyncrasies, and his peculiar irritations, and they know what causes him to fell comfortable and secure. To overlook the family, however inadequate they may seem to be, is to overlook the only possible source of any relevant information about the personal care needs of the patient.

This is not to rule out the possibility that many psychiatric patients can effectively respond to queries about their personal care needs, their previous experiences with hospitalization, their previous health problems, the medications they may be taking, and so forth. Whenever a patient is willing and able to participate in nursing history taking, he certainly should be interviewed. All of the general principles that apply to history taking in other settings also apply to the patient being admitted to a psychiatric unit.

Gathering specific information for identifying a patient's psychologic problems, as a basis for planning therapeutic psychiatric strategies, usually occurs during a series of admission interviews held by members of the various disciplines. Their interview frameworks and methods vary from discipline to discipline and from professional to professional. Because this is such a highly specialized and sensitive area, a suggested format for a psychiatric nursing history is not included here.

For Extended Care

Nurses in extended care settings find that a nursing history designed to assess the patient's usual and unusual problems is an invaluable tool for facilitating care planning. The patient as well as his family should be interviewed in order to obtain useful information.

Extended Care Example

1. What is your current understanding of this health problem (cause, treatment, prognosis, time element)? _____

2. What is there about it that you don't understand or that you find confusing?
_____

3. How has this health problem changed you way of life? _____

4. How do you intend to cope with the changes? _____

5. What difficulties have you encountered in making or accepting the decision for extended care? _____

6. Have the difficulties been resolved? If not, how do you intend to cope with them? _____

7. What is your customary daily pattern of activities (time of eating, sleeping, and so forth)? _____

8. What things do you like to have around you to feel comfortable (Records, radio, books, people, pillows, comforters, and so forth)?
_____

9. Have you had previous experience in an extended care facility? If so, what do you recall about it? _____
If so, what did the doctors and nurses do that was not helpful?
_____
If so, what did they do that was helpful? _____

10. What can we do that will be most helpful to you while you are here?
_____

Analysis. Admission to an extended care facility, because of its long-term nature, is frequently a difficult reality for patients to accept. The importance of effective information to extended care planning cannot be emphasized too strongly.

This nursing history initiates topics that are highly relevant to the subsequent satisfactory adjustment of a patient to a convalescent care unit. It is a medium for understanding the patient's perceptions and feelings about his illness, his changes in life style, his coping abilities, his requirements for a sense of comfort, and his feelings about medical and nursing care. In addition to these questions, nurses in an extended care facility should select and modify certain other questions which are generally included as part of medical-surgical nursing histories.

For Community Health

Nurses in community health settings have become familiar with "opening a family to service," which involves an assessment of a family's health status. The interview follows a generally organized format that aids in obtaining the required socioeconomic and specific health problem information. This data provides a basis for specific care planning.

Because community health nurses are family-centered and because they see their role as one that helps the family attain a higher level of wellness, questions such as the ones presented in the nursing history format below would be helpful if added to the more traditional public health nursing history.

Community Health Example

What would you say is the general health status of your family?
    Very good:____ Good:____ Fair:____ Poor:____
Was your family's health better at some other time than it is now? If so, what do you believe is the reason for the change? _____
Is your family's health better now than it has been in the past? If yes, what do you believe is the reason for the change? _____
What are your hopes for yourself and your family? (What are the things that you and your family would like to do—jobs, finances, kind of housing, how much education for children, travel, social activities, and so forth?) _____
_____
What are you doing now that will help your hopes become a reality? _____
_____

What other things do you need to do to turn your hopes into a reality? ____
_____

What seem to be some real obstacles to making your hopes become a reality?
_____

What does you family like to do for fun? _____
Do you have a chance to have fun as often as you would like? _____
Do you know someone who will help you and your family in a crisis? Someone
you can count on? Do they live nearby? _____
How much contact have you had with doctors and nurses for medical care?
_____

What have doctors and nurses done that you believe has been the most helpful?
_____

What have the doctors and nurses done that seemed unhelpful? _____
_____

How could doctors and nurses be of help to you now? _____

Analysis. This community health nursing history format initiates topics for discussion that lead to a better understanding by both the nurse and the family of the basic dynamics and feelings basic to a family's progress or lack of progress. The format makes it possible to perceive overall trends in the family's illness and wellness and to identify the possible causative factors of both. It stimulates thinking about overall goals important to the family, not just to the nurse. It elicits feelings about medical and nursing care that could be crucial in an ongoing nurse–family relationship.

For Home Nursing

Visiting nurses, like community health nurses, have long used some form of assessment guide when they open a new case. Depending upon the reason for the physician's referral, visiting nurses conduct detailed interviews to appraise the patient's problems as well as the family's resources for caring for the patient. However, in addition to trying to manage the presenting problems, visiting nurses are also attempting to expand their role. They want to place greater emphasis on becoming a catalyst for progress and for change within the entire family. They see a need to establish a rationale for supporting the whole family as it copes with the multifaceted problems of long-term chronic illness. They must also develop greater skills for doing so.

Certain nursing history questions might well be added to the usual assessment guide to elicit the information and to create the environment necessary for the expanding role of the visiting nurse. A selection of these questions is included in the following format.

Home Nursing Example

1. What is your understanding of this health problem? What caused it? How long will it last? _____
2. What do you understand about the physician's plan for treatment and care? _____
3. How has this health problem changed your family's way of life? _____ _____
4. What do you see as some of the real problems of the family in dealing with the problem? _____
5. What are the things you are doing or the plans you have made to solve the problem? _____
6. What seem to be some real obstacles or insurmountable problems? _____
7. What are your family's strengths that will help? _____
8. Do you know someone who will help in a crisis or when you need a helping hand?_____
9. What changes has this health problem caused in your close family relationships (with husband, wife, parent, child)? _____
10. Has this health problem caused a change in your family's social life? If so, what kinds of changes? _____ How do you foresee coping with these changes?_____
11. In your previous contacts with nurses, what have they done that seemed to be the most helpful to you? _____
12. How do you think we can be the most helpful to you?_____ _____

Analysis. The preceding questions initiate a dialogue that can result in a real understanding of the family's perceptions of the meaning of the illness. It refers to the changes in a family's way of life, their weaknesses and strengths in coping with the problems, their discouragements, their outside resources, the changes in internal relationships, and so forth.

Unquestionably, the discussion and clarification of these topics cannot help but lead to deeper insights and a more growth-producing nurse–family relationship.

For Office Nursing

The office nurse has a special advantage in her unique position as a viable resource to her patient. Her long association, frequently of many years or a lifetime, with the patients who see a particular physician provides her a nurse-patient relationship that is, in many ways, similar to the physician-patient relationship. Her insight into patients' problems, together with her ready access to the physician, creates an environment for nursing intervention that is unparalleled.

A nursing history provides an excellent tool for gaining insight, assessing problems, and intervening successfully. Based upon the patient's presenting health problem, the nurse is able to develop specific plans for his care and treatment. In addition, however, certain more general questions may be very useful in assessing the patient's and his family's ability to cope successfully.

Office Nursing Example

1. What is your understanding of the health problem for which you are seeing the doctor (cause, treatment, prognosis)? _____
   _____

2. What medications are you taking? Which ones were prescribed by another doctor? _____

3. What is the reason for taking each of the medications? _____
   _____

4. What new instructions did the doctor give you today? _____
   _____

5. What is there about the instructions that you don't understand?
   _____

6. Are there any instructions that you will find difficult to follow or that you will be unable to follow? _____

7. Has this health problem interfered with your way of life? _____
   If so, what plans have you made to cope with it? _____
   _____

8. Has this health problem change any of your close family or friend relationships (with husband, wife, parent, child, friend)? If so, in what way?
   _____
   If so, have you thought of how to cope with these changes? _____
   _____

Analysis. These questions specifically elicit information that helps the nurse appraise a patient's understanding of his illness, its treatment, and his ability to follow through successfully. It also opens the subject of the illness and its influence upon the patient's way of life. A significant alteration in life style, with which a patient seems unable to cope satisfactorily, is certainly a problem a nurse needs to know about and to deal with effectively.

For Nursing Education

Students of nursing routinely interview patients during their usual preparation of nursing care plans as an educational tool. They follow a general interview format designed to help them understand the patient's health problems. To assist students in gathering more specific data for understanding illness-wellness and its influence upon a person's way of life, an educational interview format, or nursing history, can be developed. Depending upon the patient care setting, interview questions can be gleaned from the histories used by staff nurses. In addition, a student might ask certain other questions of her own devising.

Nursing Education Example

1. What is your understanding of your current health problem (cause, treatment, prognosis)? _____
2. Are there parts of the health problem that you don't understand or that seem confusing? If so, what specifically? _____
   _____
3. Over your lifetime, what are the health problems that stand out in your mind as being the most troublesome or difficult to manage? Why? _____
   _____
4. Have these health problems changed your life in any significant ways?
   _____
   How specifically? _____
5. Did the health problems change any of your close relationships with family, friends? _____
6. How did you finally manage the problems? _____
7. What would you do differently in relation to your health problem if you were to do it again? _____
8. What do you think about having frequent medical and dental checkups?
   _____
9. What has prevented you from having the recommended medical and dental checkups? _____
10. What have been some of the good experiences you have had with doctors and nurses and health care? _____
11. What have been some of the bad experiences you have had with doctors and nurses and health care? _____
12. How can doctors and nurses be most helpful to you now? _____
    _____
13. On the average, what percentage of your income goes for health care?
    _____

14. What are your hopes and dreams for yourself and your family (travel, housing, food, education, jobs)? _____

15. Do you foresee any health problems becoming obstacles to achieving the kind of life you want for yourself? If so, in what way? _____

16. How do you intend to manage the foreseeable health problems in order to achieve your desired way of life? _____

Analysis.   The questions listed in the preceding example are geared toward gathering information that will aid a student to gain an understanding of the larger dimensions of a specific health problem. The questions refer to a patient's understanding of his illness, his trends of illness and wellness over his lifetime, the alterations in his life style and his personal relationships, the economic implications of illness, and his hopes for the future. All of these dimensions influence the progress of a current health–illness situation, and as part of the learning process, a student must consistently find ways to seek out and evaluate its importance and meaning.

CONCEPTUAL MODELS AS FRAMEWORKS FOR DATA COLLECTION

Riehl and Roy[4] present several theoretical frameworks or conceptual models for nursing practice that illustrate the meaning and potential value of theories for practice. In the foreword to the Riehl and Roy book, de Tornyay says:

> The need to develop a conceptual framework for the systematic investigation of problems related to practice, and means for transmitting nursing knowledge remains a high priority for the profession of nursing. The development of conceptual models linked together facts and phenomena by means of an organized framework in order to assist the practitioner and the scholar of nursing in the study of outcomes of nursing actions and interventions with a minimum of error.[5]

One model is called, "A Total Person Approach to Viewing Patient Problems," formulated by Betty Neuman.[6] The model can be applied to individuals, groups, and communities. The following summary describes the model as it relates to an individual. The person is seen as an entity with many basic factors: normal temperature range, genetic structure, response pattern, ego structure, and so forth. This entity is surrounded by concentric circles of defenses and coping mechanisms which react and respond to stressors. Stressors can be one or several of many possibilities, such as pain, loss, or cultural change. Under certain circumstances, stressors may penetrate the lines of defense and disturb or incapacitate the person's equilibrium. When a stressor is suspected or identified, nursing interventions can take the form of primary prevention (reducing the probability of encountering the stressor), secondary prevention (treatment of the symptoms of stress and stabilizing the environment), or tertiary prevention (facilitating reconstitution or adaptation), which follows active treatment or secondary prevention. Figure 11-1 illustrates this model in graphic form.

An assessment tool derived from this model is a list of questions that assist the caregiver in identifying the patient's perceptions of his situation, thereby making possible the identification of stressors and their implications for the person's equilibrium or wholeness. The assessment/intervention tool suggested by Neuman follows:

Assessment/Intervention Tool Based on the Neuman Health Care Systems Model: A Total Approach to Patient Problems

A. Intake Summary
    1. Name _____
       Age _____
       Sex _____
       Marital _____
    2. Referral source and related information
B. Stressors
    Identified by and based on the patient's perception of his circumstances. (If patient is incapacitated, secure data from family or other resources).
    1. What do you consider your major problem, stress area, or areas of concern? (Identify problem areas)
    2. How do present circumstances differ from your usual pattern of living? (Identify life style patterns)
    3. Have you ever experienced a similar problem? If so, what was that problem and how did you handle it? Were you successful? (Identify past coping patterns)
    4. What do you anticipate for yourself in the future as a consequence of your present situation? (Identify perceptual factors, ie, reality versus distortions—expectations, present and possible future coping patterns)
    5. What are you doing and what can you do to help yourself? (Identify perceptual factors, ie, reality versus distortions—expectations, present and possible future coping patterns)

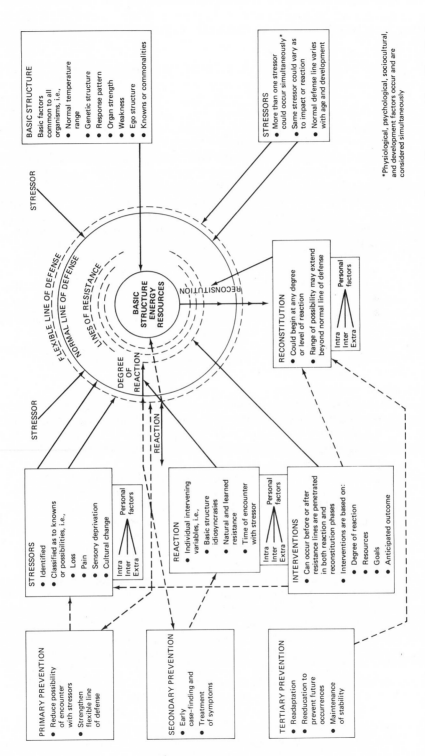

FIGURE 11-1. The Betty Neuman model: A Total Person Approach to Viewing Patient Problems. (From Neuman: *Nurs Res* 21:3, 1972, used by permission)

C. Stressors

Identified by and based on the caregiver's perception of the patient's circumstances.

1. What do you consider to be the major problem, stress area, or areas of concern? (Identify problem areas)
2. How do present circumstances seem to differ from the patient's usual pattern of living? (Identify life style patterns)
3. Has the patient ever experienced a similar situation? If so, how would you evaluate what the patient did? How successful do you think it was? (Identify past coping patterns)
4. What do you anticipate for the future as a consequence of the patient's present situation? (Identify perceptual factors, ie, reality versus distortions—expectations, present and possible future coping patterns)
5. What can the patient do to help himself? (Identify perceptual factors, ie, reality versus distortions—expectations, present and possible future coping patterns)
6. What do you think the patient expects from caregivers, family, friends, or other resources? (Identify perceptual factors, ie, reality versus distortions—expectations, present and possible future coping patterns)

Summary of Impressions: Note any discrepancies or distortions between the patient's perception and that of the caregiver related to the situation.

D. Intrapersonal Factors
1. Physical (examples: degree of mobility, range of body function)
2. Psychosociocultural (examples: attitudes, values, expectations, behavior patterns, and nature of coping patterns)
3. Developmental (examples: age, degree of normalcy, factors related to present situation)

E. Interpersonal Factors: Resources and relationship of family, friends, or caregivers which either influence or could influence area D.

F. Extrapersonal Factors: Resources and relationship of community facilities, finances, employment, or other areas which either influence or could influence areas D and E.

G. Formulation of the Problem: Identify and rank the priority of needs based on the total data obtained from the patient's perception, the caregiver's perception, and/or other resources, ie, laboratory reports, other caregivers, or agencies. With this format, reassessment is a continuous process and is related to the effectiveness of intervention based upon the stated goals. Effective reassessment would include the following as they relate to the total patient situation: (1) changes in nature of stressors and priority assignments, (2) changes in intrapersonal factors, (3) changes in interpersonal factors, and (4) changes in extrapersonal factors. In reassessment it is important to note the change of priority of goals in relation to the primary, secondary, and tertiary prevention categories. An assessment tool of this nature should offer a current, progressive, and comprehensive analysis of the patient's total circumstances or relationships of the four variables (physical, psychologic, sociocultural, and developmental).

STANDARD CARE PLANS AS FRAMEWORKS
FOR DATA COLLECTION*

How do you know that a patient has usual or unusual problems? Do you find out by chance or design? Certainly, by design would be preferable. Of course, much useful information does appear unexpectedly. However, for purposes of data gathering by design, you can use an organizer, such as a list of questions or topics that can be derived from some basic nursing goals.

The organizer comes from the standard care planning model. The sequential steps of data gathering generally are (1) obtaining evidence of *usual problems*, (2) obtaining evidence of *unusual problems*, and (3) considering special *daily living requirements*.

Obtaining Evidence of Usual Problems

Because on admission or shortly thereafter most patients have a physician's diagnosis, the standard care plan for that diagnosis can provide cues for questions and physical inspection. The problems and expected outcomes elements of the care plan are the specific cues to areas for investigation.

To illustrate, let us assume that a woman, age 32 and married, has been admitted with a diagnosis of ulcerative colitis. To effectively gather data for care planning, use the standard care plan for ulcerative colitis and refer to the problems and expected outcomes as cues for formulating questions and to perform specific physical assessments. Following are some questions and physical assessment suggestions that are derived from the standard care plan that is shown in Figure 11-2. Refer to the care plan as you read the assessment questions so that the relationships become clear.

Interview Questions and Physical Inspections—Ulcerative Colitis

Problem and Expected Outcomes 1
  How many bowel movements are you having now?
  How many do you have when you feel well?
  Are they liquid or formed?
Problem and Expected Outcomes 2
  Weigh patient
  What is your normal weight?

___

* This section is adapted from an unpublished paper, "Data Gathering for Problem Identification," by A. Watson and M. Mayers, 1976.

Date	Usual problems	Expected outcomes	Dead-lines	Nursing Orders
	1. Diarrhea and possible abdominal cramping	1. Decrease in number of stools to one daily Stools of normal consistency	Discharge q 8 hr	1. Chart color, consistency, and frequency of all stools
	2. Potential weight loss from anorexia nausea, and/or vomiting	2. Maintain at admission weight Taking most of all meals without nausea or vomiting Verbalizes understanding of diet	Discharge q 8 hr	**2A.** Weigh daily **B.** Encourage diet high in protein, calories, and vitamins and low in residue: have dietician discuss with patient the diet, likes, and dislikes **C.** Get order for antiemetic if needed and give as needed
	3. Dehydration	3. Intake at least 2,000 ml per day Moist mucous membranes Good skin turgor	Day 2 q 8 hr	**3A.** Record intake and output **B.** Have fluids at bedside (flow residue fluids) **C.** Force fluids to 2,000 ml per day
	4. Potential perianal discomfort, skin breakdown, or rectal bleeding	4. Healthy skin around anus No rectal bleeding	Discharge q 8 hr	**4A.** If needed, get order for: —Sitz bath —Vaseline around anus **B.** Instruct in good hygiene (for example, clean self after each bowel movement)

5. Weakness due to gastrointestinal malabsorption	**5.** Ambulates without assistance Doing own activities of daily living	Day 3 daily	**5A.** Encourage self-care **B.** Establish plan with patient for doing activities of daily living **C.** Monitor plan every shift and adjust as necessary **D.** Increase ambulation as tolerated
6. Frustration due to diarrhea and possible interference with life style	**6.** Verbalizes tolerance of situation Demonstrates relaxed manner Verbalizes realistic plans for activities after discharge	Discharge q day and PM shift	**6.** Delegate nurse to spend 15 minutes twice a day with patient in active listening and guidance regarding home management Nurse to provide relaxed, unhurried, peaceful environment
7. Potential development of complications: hemorrhage and/or perforation	**7.** Vital signs stable Temperature normal No severe pain or sudden increase in pain	Discharge q 8 hr	**7.** Check at least every 4 hours temperature, pulse, respirations, bowel sounds, level of comfort

DISCHARGE CRITERIA
1. Verbalize understanding of and willingness to follow MD's outpatient regimen.
2. Verbalize understanding of and willingness to follow diet at home and make correct selection from a food list.
3. Verbalize understanding of medication regimen.
4. Verbalize realistic plans for coping with stressful situations after discharge (for example, family, job, etc).

FIGURE 11-2. Standard care plan, ulcerative colitis. (Courtesy of Marlene Mayers and El Camino Hospital, used by permission)

How well have you been eating?

What type of diet are you on and why?

Problem and Expected Outcomes 3

How many glasses of liquid have you been drinking per day?

Check lips for dryness

Do pinch test on back of hand

Problem and Expected Outcomes 4

Have you any tenderness or sore skin?

In the rectal area?

What about bleeding?

(An affirmative answer requires physical inspection of the area)

Problem and Expected Outcomes 5

Are you keeping up with your regular activities at home and work?

Problem and Expected Outcomes 6

Observe body posture and facial expressions for signs of tension or relaxation

How has your colitis problem interfered with your daily routine or your life style?

How have you been coping with your symptoms and treatment?

Problem and Expected Outcomes 7

Check vital signs: temperature, pulse, respiration, and blood pressure

Have you ever had any large amounts of bleeding which has frightened or concerned you?

The Discharge Criteria provide reminders for asking

Are there certain foods that upset you or cause you to have diarrhea?

What medications are you taking now? Do you know what they are for?

What are the situations in your daily life which seem to upset you?

It is not necessary in actual practice to tediously handwrite all the interview questions that have been illustrated here for the purposes of demonstration. Of course, once a set of data-gathering questions or physical inspection topics have been defined, they could be typed, duplicated, and used as a nursing history guide for patients with colitis. Information obtained can be handwritten on the form which could become part of the chart. Another alternative would be to summarize the patient information in the nursing or progress notes as part of admission assessment data.

If your patient exhibits the typical, predictable problems, you could then implement the standard care plan.

Obtaining Evidence of Unusual Problems

To identify unusual problems that could otherwise remain obscure, further queries and observations are necessary.

Suggested observations or open-ended questions related to all or some of the following topics aid in learning about a patient's usual difficulties:

Other physiologic disorders or disabilities
Impaired ability to focus or understand
Emotional stresses and reactions
Financial concerns
Interaction or communication difficulties
Feelings derived from previous experiences with health care
Expectations of health care versus its reality
Extenuating problems in family
Inability to cope with usual problems

If your patient exhibits evidence of difficulties related to any of the topics listed above, you would enter them as unusual problems on your care plan.

Obtaining Evidence of Special Living Requirements

Virtually any therapeutic regimen interrupts or disrupts a person's normal, preferred life style. Therefore, to minimize this disruption, consider preferences. To identify potential areas of disruption, make observations or ask questions about the patient's preferences regarding:

Personal habits—eating, sleeping, bathing, elimination, and so forth
Daily schedule or routine
Comfort preferences
Personal interests and leisure activities
Occupation

The topics mentioned as evidence of unusual problems and as evidence of special living requirements can be condensed into one brief form which has headings for identifying unusual problems and special living requirements. This form can be used in conjunction with the standard care plan for data-gathering purposes (Fig. 11-2).

SUMMARY

The nursing history is an important tool for obtaining a broad spectrum of information about a patient and his health problems preliminary to problem identification and care planning. This information is referred to as the "data base." It is an organized selection of predetermined questions or topics that guide the nurse in data collection at the time of a patient's admission to a service. The content of a nursing history varies from agency to agency and from one specialized type of care unit to another.

Besides the nursing history's obvious benefit of eliciting information about a patient, it has other very important side benefits. The admission history interview creates a milieu for beginning the nurse-patient relationship. It makes possible the early involvement of the patient in his own plan of care, and it creates within the nurse a sense of commitment and personal involvement. Making a contract with a patient is also facilitated when it is done within the context of a nursing history.

History taking is done in many physical settings and under many conditions. But certain principles should underlie any selection of the time and place for taking a history. Attention must be given to privacy, to a sense of caring and commitment, and to timing the interview so it produces the most satisfactory results.

The selection of questions or topics suitable for nursing histories in various agencies and care settings is an important process and must receive high priorities of time and attention if nursing is to be a viable and positive force for the improvement of health care. Choice of topics and questions can be derived from a conceptual framework for nursing practice.

REFERENCES

1. Weed L: Medical Records, Medical Education, and Patient Care, Chicago Year Book, 1974.
2. Schulman E: Intervention in Human Services, St. Louis, Mosby, 1974, p 41
3. Little D, Carnevali D: Nursing Care Planning, Philadelphia, Lippincott, 1976, pp 32-146
4. Riehl J, Roy C: Conceptual Models for Nursing Practice, New York, Appleton-Century-Crofts, 1974
5. Ibid. p xi
6. Ibid. pp 99-114

BIBLIOGRAPHY

Cady J, Goldfogel L, Mayers M: Syllabus for Integrating Nursing Care Planning and Problem-oriented Medical Records. Chicago, Medicus Systems Corp, 1974

Doona M: The judgment process in nursing, Image 8:27, June 1976

Doona M: A Philosophical Study of Judgment for Use in Nursing. (Ed D dissertation, Boston University, 1975)

Froelich R, Bishop F: Medical Interviewing: A Programmed Manual, 2nd ed. Louis, Mosby, 1972

Kelly K: Clinical inference in nursing. Nurs Res p 23, Winter 1966

Klug CA: Judgment and creative thinking. Image 5:10, 1973

Mills E: Judgment in nursing practice. S Carolina Nurse p 120, 161, Summer 1971

Regan WA (ed): Standing orders and nursing judgment. Regan Rep Nurs Law 11:1, Nov 1970

Runyan J Jr: Primary Care Guide. New York, Harper, 1975

12

Implementation: Putting the Process Into Practice

Many factors must be taken into account when a new system of patient care planning is going to be implemented. The agency's philosophy, its usual kinds of patient problems, its staffing patterns, and its staff's degree of readiness must be known and understood. The ability and probable support of the in-service education and supervisory staff must be evaluated. The time and energy costs of implementing the new system must be identified and planned for in a way that will insure a successful transition.

PHILOSOPHY

Before it designs and implements a system of care, an agency must review its official philosophy of nursing. The agency must ascertain that its philosophy represents the current beliefs of the nursing staff about patients, staffing, and nursing as a profession. The broad philosophic beliefs of an agency set the basic framework for more specialized, more narrowly focused statements by subunits within the agency.

A well-defined philosophy is critical to a nursing agency. It determines the assumptions that underlie the basic principles of care and the relevance of the nursing methods that are employed.

The Significance of a Philosophy of Nursing Service

A philosophy of patient care is not a hastily conceived set of vague and ambiguous statements to be accepted uncritically and then forgotten or ignored in actual practice.

It should, instead, represent a thoughtful point of view regarding patient care policies and practices. It should provide the foundation for daily nursing practice within the agency. To achieve the best nursing care outcomes, the premises of an agency's philosophy should be carefully thought through and should be consistently and rationally applied by all staff under the agency's auspices who assume responsibility for patient care.

A well-developed philosophy of nursing will guide patient care by stimulating continual evaluation of the overall nursing service, administration, and staff-development policies and practices, providing a basis for organizing patient care services, and influencing the type of nursing actions and interventions as well as the methods for evaluating care.

The way statements of philosophy ultimately influence patient care can be demonstrated.

For example, suppose that an agency's stated policy is that patients achieve improved health more successfully when they are involved in self-appraisal of their own care. In that case, the nursing methods will be fashioned to employ nurse-patient dialogues for assessing the patient's illness-wellness status, to stimulate patient participation in decisions about the patient's own overall and interim objectives, and to maximize the patient's involvement in his own care regimen. To support its philosophy, the agency will develop relevant personnel policies, job specifications, staffing patterns, and staff development programs. Additionally, the agency will include representatives of consumer groups on as many as possible of its policy and care planning committees. In the absence of such a stated policy, nursing intervention methodology relative to a patient's involvement in his own pattern of illness and wellness would likely be internally inconsistent.

Or suppose that an agency openly declares its philosophy that nurses have a right to a sense of personal and professional satisfaction and that this is achieved through growth, learning, encouragement, and positive reinforcement of individual abilities. Then the personnel policies, administrative support, and job requirements ought to reflect this belief. Staff nurses would be involved in self-evaluation and would be encouraged to develop their individual skills. Punitive measures would be minimal. Staff nurses would be actively encouraged to acquire new knowledge and skills. Staffing patterns would be designed to maximize a nurse's potential for excellence and her personal satisfaction from providing good patient care. In the absence of a stated belief about nurses as persons and professionals, the administrative system would by default be inconsistent or, more probably, would negatively influence personal and professional growth.

An agency's philosophy provides the structure upon which its subunits can develop their statements of belief; these will be more specific and more relevant to the subunit's particular client system and nursing processes. For instance, a psychiatric unit will have a somewhat different statement of specific beliefs from that of an acute medical-surgical unit of the same agency.

From agency to agency, specific beliefs vary because of differences among their client populations and differences in their rationales for care. Home nursing agencies will have a commitment to the wellness of persons and families, with particular respect to long-term problems in the home. They will have beliefs about the nursing processes that are uniquely applicable to home settings. By way of contrast, an inpatient acute care agency will be guided by specific beliefs about the wellness of patients in an institutional setting. It will have committed its philosophy to the nursing processes in that environment.

Today, because of the rapidly changing social climate, agencies and their subunits must frequently reexamine their beliefs. They must assure themselves, their clients, and their staffs that basic assumptions for care upon which they function actually do reflect their current philosophy.

The contemporary social issue of unequal care among various socioeconomic groups is an issue most nursing services will want covered in their statements of belief. If an agency believes that persons of all races and socioeconomic groups are equal and are thus entitled to receive care which will reinforce their self-respect and dignity, the agency will develop services that guarantee this result. The agency's facilities and staffing for the poor will be the same as that for the more affluent. Or, better still, the agency's care will represent a sensitive awareness by the agency of the special problems relating to various minority groups and will vary appropriately. It is conceivable that staff ratios and care intensities will be greater for certain minority-group clients than for average middle-class clients, who may be assumed to have learned to cope well with social and health care systems. The unequal, greater intensity of care will result in an equal sense of dignity and self-worth among various races and groups to whom it is given.

An agency's proclamation that all races and groups have much to offer to nursing care and to nursing as a profession should logically be followed by an accelerated recruitment of, and provision of incentives for employment among, minority-group nurses and other staff.

In short, an agency's statement of beliefs—its philosophy—represents the agency's special commitments to its clients and staff and to the processes that occur within its jurisdiction.

SERVICES AND STAFFING VARIABLES

Diversity of Services

Before a system of patient care planning is implemented, an appraisal should be made of general and specialized nursing services, of staffing patterns, and of staff readiness.

An agency with a multitude of complex and differing nursing services should evaluate the problems that highly varied care units anticipate when they utilize the same care-planning format. A trial or pilot study of the proposed system will yield information about potential problems and their solutions. Each major service can, after a trial run, develop a variation of the basic system, a variation which will provide the best tool for it. It is entirely possible that standard care for a given problem may vary from one unit to another within a single agency. The differences in standard care from unit to unit are less important than whether or not the staff of each unit has thought through, developed, and written their own plan of care.

It is almost certain that the configurations of standard care protocols will vary from one major service to another. This is likely to be especially true in agencies which have segregated services; these are services that follow the pattern of the common medical specialties. Thoracic care, neurology, eye, ear, nose, and throat, or gynecology, for example, will all have significantly different listings of standard care protocols.

Nursing units whose patients consistently have a high rate of unusual problems may need to plan for, and devote more attention to, unusual problems. Units that are highly specialized and whose patients are consistently well prepared may have a longer listing of standard care plans. As a general rule, surgical or orthopedic units are the best candidates for trying out and developing a prototype care-planning system.

Staffing Patterns

Staffing patterns should also be analyzed. The ratio of registered nurses to auxiliary staff and the ratio of staff to patients will influence the success or failure of a care-planning system. When units are short-staffed and overworked, the addition of another task—care planning—may be difficult. When a staff is harried and pressured, it is not likely to want to spend the extra energy and time for learning the system. Even though in the long run the care-planning system will probably save the staff's time and energy, the overwhelming demands made on them by the current day-to-day system (or non-system) make the transition virtually impossible.

Many agencies have mistakenly overlooked the need to change staffing patterns when a system of patient care planning has been introduced. A nurse will be frustrated in her efforts if she is not provided the appropriate supporting staff. If she is still expected to carry a heavy medications and treatment regimen in addition to all her new responsibilities, obviously the pressure on her time will force her to relegate her nursing assessment and care-planning activities to the small fragments of time she may have left over.

Staff Readiness

A further element that must be given serious consideration before a care-planning system can be introduced is staff readiness. The staff's intellectual and psychologic capacities will determine the degree to which the staff accepts and involves itself with the new way of functioning.

A group of nurses accustomed by long practice and conditioning to the more traditional nursing processes will find it difficult to move toward greater independence. The nurses' unique needs and strengths must be, accounted for when the nurses are oriented to systematic care planning. Nurses traditionally have tended to understand, and to do well with, the concept of usual problems and standard care plans. Their long experiences with nursing care provide them a basis for recognizing typical signs and symptoms and associated standard care. Because of their generally good understanding of typical expected problems, nurses also quite readily recognize unusual problems. Their greatest difficulty tends to be stating unusual problems succinctly, systematically arriving at expected outcomes and deadlines, and writing nursing orders which are independent of medical orders.

Recent graduates of nursing programs tend to be skilled at stating problems and expected outcomes. They generally understand the independent functions of nursing, and they can develop nursing orders. However, because of their comparatively limited experience with patient problems, they tend to have trouble differentiating between usual and unusual problems and understanding the validity of standard care routines.

People's psychologic limitations must be recognized. Care must be taken not to introduce too many new ideas or projects at the same time. Members of a staff who are already deeply involved in a special project are unlikely to adapt well to another demand upon their psychologic reserves. One agency which wanted to implement a new system of care planning decided to postpone it because the staff was at the time significantly involved in a personnel standards and practices project. The project was taking a great deal of time and energy. The nurses were interested in it and well motivated. It was a wise administrative decision to postpone another major project until the current one had been completed.

Staff readiness is important and relevant to the success or failure of a new system. It must be seriously considered before a patient care-planning program is implemented.

IN-SERVICE EDUCATION AND ADMINISTRATIVE SUPPORT

The successful implementation of a system for care planning depends also upon the support of the administrative and in-service staffs. The system should be designed by responsible administrative persons in consultation with representative staff nurses, since it is designed to best meet their particular needs. Thus, the importance of staff's participation in helping the system to evolve cannot be overemphasized. When trial runs of the system are made, the staff's cooperation and suggestions will prove to be invaluable.

It is the job of the in-service education department, in cooperation with staff nurses and others, to plan an organized educational program whose aim is to aid the staff to discover how they can best put an effective care-planning system into operation.

LEARNING CARE-PLANNING SKILLS

Experience in teaching the system of nursing care planning described in this book has resulted in several models for teaching the system within an in-service educational structure. Variations of the models can be used by all nursing agencies and subunits.

The following general outline calls for a course of seven classes of two hours each. The course is to teach the nursing staff the principles of this method of nursing care planning. The general outline is followed by a detailed explanation of the content of each class session.

Course Outline

1. Overview of System
   a. Definitions
   b. Problem solving for care planning
   c. Example of how to start a plan of care
   d. Clinical assignment
2. Stating the Problems
   a. Usual and unusual
   b. Actual, potential, and possible
   c. Elements of a problem statement
   d. Clinical assignment
3. Stating the Expected Outcome (Objective)
   a. Elements of the statement of an objective
   b. Deadlines
   c. Clinical assignment
4. Nursing Orders
   a. Elements of nursing orders
   b. Specificity and brevity
   c. Clinical assignment
5. Evaluation and Nursing History
   a. Patient responses—how and when to document
   b. Clinical assignment
   c. Nursing history (assessment)
   d. Rationale for designing an assessment guide
   e. How to complete a nursing history
   f. Environment for history taking
   g. Clinical assignment
6. Standard Care Plans

    a. Usual problems
    b. How to develop standard care plans
    c. Clinical assignment
7. Review and Critique
    a. Review of problem solving and operational use of system
    b. Plans for implementing system

This guide for teaching nursing care planning requires that nurses be given outside clinical assignments. The teaching staff should devote extra time to reviewing and making notations on the written clinical assignments. Experience indicates that formal classes are best spaced at weekly intervals, with clinical assignments due each week.

Class 1. Class 1, "Overview of System," has the following learning objectives for nurse-students:

1. To demonstrate an understanding of the basic elements of problem solving by correctly writing each of the major steps, including a clarifying definition
2. To apply knowledge by correctly identifying problems portrayed in simulated clinical nurse-patient interview

Discussion. To accomplish these objectives, the teacher describes the basic system by using a sample care plan format. Each nurse-student has a copy of the format and makes notations on it for future reference. The basic system is most easily explained by the teacher's going over each portion of the sample care plan and describing the kind of data written in each section. Copies of the operational definitions for the system should be available to each student. Questions should be encouraged and specific answers should be given.

The overview should be followed by students role-playing a nurse–patient admission interview. The group would then start a sample care plan together. Groups of no fewer than three and no more than six persons seem to work most effectively with this assignment. Groups should have a resource person available to help them use the system. Many questions will arise during the first role-playing exercise. Misunderstandings should be clarified as they become evident. The teacher or resource person should be skilled at using the system in order to minimize confusion.

After approximately 20 minutes of group work, each subgroup reports on how it developed its care plan. The instructor clarifies any missteps, and the total group makes suggestions as each sub-group reports.

The session ends with a brief written examination that requires each major step (problem, expected outcome, nursing orders, and patient response) to be reiterated.

The group care plans are given to the instructor for her evaluation of the class members' ability to use the method successfully.

The clinical assignment for the week is for each nurse to select one of her patients, to identify *one* problem, to follow the problem through the major steps, and to write these on a sample care plan form.

Class 2.   Class 2, "Stating the Problems," has the following learning objectives for nurse-students:

1. To demonstrate an understanding of problem statements by correctly writing specific, concise problem statements based upon a model clinical example
2. To assign correctly the terms "usual," "unusual," "actual," "potential," and "possible" to a list of problem statements provided by the instructor

Discussion.   These objectives are met by starting the session with a review of the system as introduced in the previous class.

Following the review, the instructor refers to the definitions of usual, unusual, actual, potential, and possible problems and provides examples and explanations of each. Each example is used to show how specifically a problem statement should be written, including the cause of the problem.

The verbal presentation should be followed by group work. The groups listen to a description of a patient situation. They identify the patient's problems and write them as briefly and precisely as possible, applying all the criteria outlined in the lecture portion of the session. As in the first class, each work group reports on its selection of problem statements. The instructor and the entire group clarify and make suggestions.

A brief examination terminates this session. It consists of a list of problem statements with brief clarifying data. Each nurse assigns two terms to each one. She defines each as either usual or unusual. Secondly, she decides whether each problem is actual, potential, or possible.

For the clinical assignment, the nurses select one patient from their own caseloads and write brief, concise statements for each of the problems identified. They label the problems as usual or unusual and as actual, potential, or possible.

Class 3. Class 3, "Stating the Expected Outcome," is a lesson in writing care plan objectives. The goals or objectives for this class are:

1. To demonstrate an understanding of the process of developing objectives by correctly writing expected outcome statements based upon selected problem statements
2. To assign deadlines or checking intervals correctly to the expected outcome statements

Discussion. The instructor spends the first portion of class time describing the elements of an expected outcome statement. She utilizes examples of problem statements, writes them on the blackboard, and, with the assistance of the class, writes expected outcome statements along with deadlines or checking intervals.

When this is completed, each nurse is given a list of problem statements with brief clarifying data. She is asked to write expected outcomes and deadlines correctly. That is the examination for this session.

For the clincial assignment, the nurse takes last week's clinical assignment of problem statements and now writes the appropriate objectives or expected outcomes, including deadlines or checking intervals. In the process, she may need to revise or refine her problem statements.

Class 4. Class 4, "Nursing Orders," has the following objective:

1. To demonstrate ability to write nursing orders that are brief, clear, and itemized

Discussion. To meet this objective, the instructor utilizes one of the student's clinical assignments which has the problem and the expected outcome statements. The information is copied onto the blackboard. Together, she and the students write nursing orders for the case. They check each other for brevity, clarity, specificity, and for direct relevance to the problem.

Groups of from four to six nurses then devote the remainder of the time to writing nursing orders for the clincial assignment each has completed during the previous week. The separate groups go through the same process they went through jointly during the first half of the class with the instructor.

The clinical assignment to follow this class is for each nurse to select one patient from her own caseload, to identify one problem, and to follow it through with an expected outcome, deadline or checking interval, and nursing actions.

Class 5. Class 5, "Evaluation" and "Nursing History," follows. Its learning objectives for nurse-students are:

1. To demonstrate ability to write patient response evaluative statements on the patient's nursing notes, based upon a clinical example
2. To demonstrate a beginning skill in history taking by completing a nursing history and by starting a care plan

Discussion. For this class, the instructor reviews the rationale for observing the patient's response. She describes how expected outcome statements are the guides for subsequent evaluation at the required deadlines or checking intervals. Utilizing a clinical example, the instructor demonstrates how a nurse would make an appropriate notation of patient response on the nursing notes of the patient's record.

For the "Nursing History" portion of the class, the instructor reviews the principles of timing and environment for history taking. She then demonstrates how to take a nursing history by interviewing one of the nurses, who role-plays the part of a patient. The class then criticizes the role-playing situation, offering their observations and suggestions.

For the final portion of the session, the class divides into groups of two nurses each. Each nurse alternates with her partner at role-playing a nursing history interview. They share suggestions and ideas with one another. The instructor should have many copies of various nursing history formats for students to use in this activity.

The clinical assignment to follow this class is for each nurse to do a nursing history and to start a care plan for one of her patients.

Class 6. Class 6, "Standard Care Plans," has the following objectives:

1. To demonstrate ability to differentiate between usual and unusual problems
2. To demonstrate ability to utilize the problem-solving method for developing standard care plans

Discussion. To meet these objectives, the instructor reviews the rationale for standard care. She then uses the blackboard and develops a clinical example to show how the "problem, expected outcome, deadline, nursing orders" method is used to develop standard care plans.

The second portion of class activity is managed in groups of from three to six persons. Each group selects a problem area that is typical of a certain patient care setting and, utilizing the problem-solving method, develops a standard care routine. The groups usually need frequent assistance from the instructor or other resource person.

To end the session, a patient situation involving several problems is presented to the nurses. Their task is to assign the terms "usual" or "unusual" to all of the problems listed.

The clinical assignment to follow this class is for half the students to make a list of the problems or major diagnostic areas they believe may be the core of common problems for their nursing settings. The other half selects one problem or major diagnosis and uses it as a basis for designing a standard care plan.

Class 7. Class 7, "Review and Critique," is designed to meet the following objectives for nurse-students:

1. To refine and clarify an understanding of the operational use of the care-planning system. Demonstrate skill by responding appropriately to random questions regarding the system
2. To identify and discuss the implications of implementing care planning within one's own nursing setting. Discuss ways to resolve any predictable problems

Discussion. To meet these objectives, the nurses, again in groups, review and criticize the clinical assignments of their colleagues. In a general discussion that follows, they present any difficulties or concerns that are still apparent.

A final examination is comprised of patient situations, problem statements, and questions about definitions. The examination provides a final opportunity for the nurses to demonstrate their skill and understanding.

The last portion of time is used for discussing implications the system of care planning may have for various nursing settings in the agency. The group shares ideas for resolving problems and for establishing the care-planning system as a beneficial tool.

Other Teaching–Learning Models

Chapter 10 of this text reviews other teaching–learning guides that are applicable to the nursing service setting. An annotated bibliography at the end of Chapter 10 reviews several books, workbooks, and autotutorial learning tools that can be used to supplement an in-service program or that can be used as the in-service component for the care-planning process.

Follow-up Support

After a series of planned teaching sessions, the administrative and in-service staff should make themselves available to work with the staffs of the various units. Major subunits may proceed at different rates in varying ways, depending upon the many factors which influence each setting.

One of the first tasks of the agency and its subunits will be to establish standard care plans and to design its checklist of standard and frequently ordered care.

Another early task is to design a nursing history guide. This may be the same for every unit throughout an agency or may vary from one major area to another.

Once the standard care plans and the data base guides have been developed, the system can be put into operation.

COMMON IMPLEMENTATION PROBLEMS

Putting a system of care planning into operation, even with adequate preparation, frequently produces problems.

Role Confusion

One problem is role confusion. When done well, care planning results in some change of emphasis in patient care responsibilities. Nurses who were more desk oriented or more supervision oriented will become more patient oriented. More of their time will be spent assessing, evaluating, and teaching patients. More of their time will be spent assisting and supporting team members. As a result, the responsibilities of other nurses will shift. Medications and treatments may be delegated to another staff member. Communication of patient care data will be transmitted through different channels in different ways, which may take some time to learn. Clinical specialists and nurses with expertise from other areas will be called in to assist during care planning conferences.

All of these elements can, for a time, create some understandable role confusion. Leadership staff can be most helpful in anticipating these phenomena and in providing positive support and encouragement through the transitional phase.

Lack of Efficiency

Another common problem is lack of efficiency on the system's operational level. The work, the misunderstandings, and the frustrations of creating care plans for a large group of patients can result in discouragement. Persistence and patience gradually yield greater efficiency, greater skill, and greater energy savings. As experience grows, the method becomes easier—less energy is required and time is saved.

Once the system is efficiently operating and roles are stabilized, the resulting time saved and the satisfaction gained from better care are seen as rewards for all the effort expended throughout the transitional phase.

The Transition

Certain support strategies may be employed to minimize the problems of the transitional phase. Because of the increased time it takes to learn to use the system, a temporary period of heavier staffing may be most helpful. Another strategy is to implement the system gradually instead of all at once. For instance, a unit may start a care plan for each new patient until eventually all patients are covered. Or a unit may draw up care plans for only a small core of patients at the beginning. Various ways of easing the transition should be investigated.

Some agencies may find it wise to introduce a system of care planning one unit at a time. This would allow staff to be loaned to the selected unit and would insure adequate administrative and in-service staff support throughout the transitional phase. When an entire agency with many subunits goes into a new method of operation, it is better for maximum support and staff to be provided to each developing unit one at a time than for already short staffing and support to be spread over the entire agency.

When problems are anticipated and planned for, and when efficiency with the system is gained, patient care and nurses' satisfaction with their practice can be greatly enhanced.

CARE PLAN FORMS

Since a care plan is a written guideline for patient care, it can be organized in a variety of ways. Its format, the forms that are used, and its terminology are tools that should provide the most efficient and effective vehicles for nurses to actualize their care-planning skills.

In acute care settings the Kardex, Rand, or clipboard systems seem to be more readily accessible than charts. In psychiatry, community health, and other outpatient services, the chart may well be the best repository for the care plan. In service settings that have computerized information systems, the videoscreen at the terminal may be the most efficient place to assess displays of the plan of care.

Forms and Formats

The major purpose of a form and its format is to organize the important information in such a way that "anyone can visualize what care is needed and why." [1] Watson and Mayers indicate that forms should help to "organize your thoughts according to the patient's problems; what should be done about the problems; and how you will know when the problems are solved." These authors point out that the most facilitative forms have the following characteristics: [2]

Provide specific cues (headings) for the necessary content
Include spaces for writing the patient's problems, objectives, and
    nursing orders
Encourage brevity and discourage redundancy
Provide easy physical and visual access to information

Depending upon your service setting, how many persons require quick access, and how many patients' care is being managed simultaneously, and depending upon whether your service has a centralized (nursing station) or decentralized (patient's room) information system, your forms may need to be designed differently.

Unstructured Forms. Unstructured forms are those that provide few, if any, headings, cues, or columns. There may be only a heading

"Care Plan," with one or two topics to suggest entries, such as "History" and "Action Plan" or "Goals and Treatment Plan." The unstructured form provides great latitude for each professional to organize and phrase his or her thoughts. The advantages of an unstructured form are flexibility of organization and expression and freedom from biased or limited information which more structured forms might produce. Limitations are difficulty in understanding the logic of the writer's impressions, since the content is unlikely to follow a generally understood topical sequence. Thus, a second disadvantage of the unstructured form is that it is more time-consuming to find relevant information as it is needed. Figure 12-1 shows an example of an unstructured form.

Semistructured Forms. Semistructured forms ordinarily include four or five major headings: "Long-term Objectives," "Short-term Objectives," "Needs or Problems," and "Approaches." The semistructured form appears quite commonly in acute care settings and is generally patterned after a teacher's lesson plan. Figure 12-2 shows one example of a semistructured form.

The advantages of this partially structured form are freedom to phrase and place content in one or more areas of the plan and the fact that the simple headings communicate that the form demands only a few entries. The disadvantages are that the form encourages generalities rather than specifics and usually produces redundancy in content because of its lack of specificity.

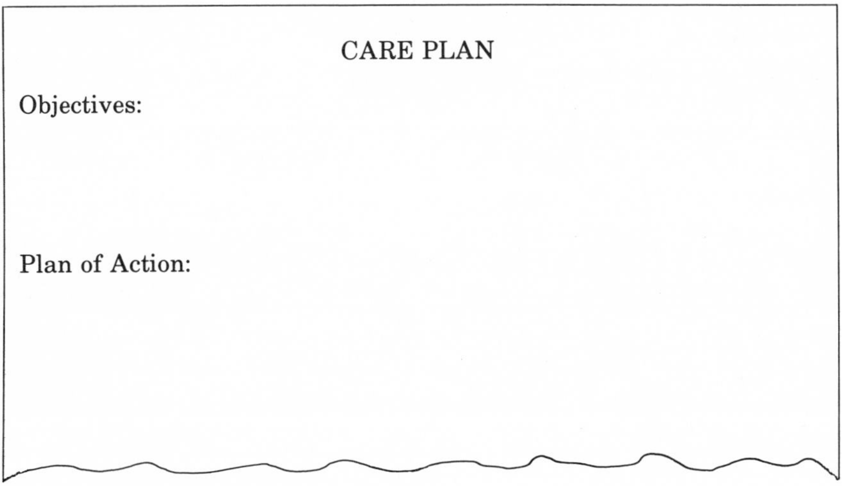

CARE PLAN

Objectives:

Plan of Action:

FIGURE 12-1. Unstructured care plan.

CARE PLAN

Long-term objectives:

Short-term objectives:

Needs or Problems   Approaches

FIGURE 12-2. Semistructured care plan.

PATIENT CARE PLAN

Physician's expectations regarding   Identifying Information: _____
treatment regimen or course of
convalescence: ( ) typical or routine   Diagnosis: _____
                ( ) atypical or
                    complicated
If atypical or complicated, in what way?
Criteria for discharge: _____

Home care coordination activities: _____

Date	Unusual Problems	Expected Outcomes	Dead-lines	Nursing Orders

FIGURE 12-3. Structured care plan.

The Structured Form.   A structured form is basically the one that has been utilized in this text. It has three major columns with one to three additional headings. Figure 12-3 shows an example of a structured form.

Advantages of a structured form are that headings and columns provide specific cues to the content that must be entered, and the reader of the care plan can quickly find exactly the information needed, since it will be entered in the predictable areas or columns. Disadvantages are that the form demands thought and attention to detail which may be time-consuming for the writer, especially in the early phases of learning how to formulate care plans. It also creates some wasted space (on an already crowded Kardex) because some columnar entries (nursing orders, for example) require more space than do other columns.

CARE-PLANNING TERMINOLOGY

The terms used by various authors and the topics provided on printed Kardex cards tend to vary substantially. Upon closer analysis, however, most of the varying terms are synonymous with the major problem-solving steps of the nursing process.

The following list summarizes the major steps of the nursing process and identifies the commonly used terms that are associated with each step.

Nursing Process and Associated Terminology

Data gathering	Nursing history
	Intake interview
	Admission interview
	Assessment
	Data Base
Problem identification	Needs
	Problems
	Problem list
	Nursing diagnosis
Goal setting	Objectives
	Short-term goals
	Long-term goals
	Expected outcomes
	Criteria
	Criteria for discharge

Intervention   Approaches
                          Methods
                          Solutions
                          Nursing orders
                          Plans of action
                          Nursing prescriptions
                          Treatment plan
                          Plan

Evaluation   Assessment
                          Patient response vs expected response
                          SOAP notes
                          Concurrent audit
                          Retrospective audit

Whichever terminology best reflects one's philosophy or preference is the terminology of choice. In this text the terms "data base" and "nursing history" are utilized because they are well understood and generally utilized in the health care field. The term "problems" is utilized because it focuses attention on the necessity to identify variances from satisfactory levels of health, creating an outline of priorities for professional attention. (Although the term "nursing diagnosis" is becoming popular, its real definition in terms of an official taxonomy of nursing practices remains unclear.)

In this text, the term "expected outcome" is used because it cues one to phrase objectives in terms of patients' behavior or clinical or situational manifestations. The phrases, "criteria for discharge" and "overall expected outcomes" are suggested because they again cue the care plan writer to formulate "behavioral (patient), clinical, or situational" statements that focus on observable or measurable phenomena. The "outcomes" terminology is also consistent with officially designed[3,4] patient care audit terminology. For the intervention element of nursing process, this text uses the term "nursing orders" to clearly communicate the required content of this prescriptive componenet of nursing.

For the evaluative element of the nursing process, this text puts into operation evaluation through the patient response/patient outcome charting guidelines. Chapter 13 describes the various levels of evaluation as they appear in quality assurance methodologies.

Computer-assisted Care Planning

As yet, few health care organizations have taken advantage of computerized information systems for nursing services. Yet nursing probably processes more diversified information per unit of time than does any other service. It is this author's opinion that computerized information systems are already a necessity and will become a reality in a majority of nursing and health care systems within the next decade.

A few developmental projects for computer-assisted care planning are available for review.

In rural Arizona a prototype for computerized care protocols is being developed.[5] The system is designed to assist nurses who function independently in isolated areas with the assistance and consultation of physicians via computer and video terminals, computerized medical care protocols, and nursing protocols.

In Texas a group has created an experimental prototype for the components of care planning that are uniquely related to rehabilitation.[6] Their care planning data are task oriented, which minimizes memory bank storage space. It also may limit their computerized applications for outcome assessments and auditing.

In North Carolina a hospital has designed components of care based on 200 or more initiators.[7] An initiator can be a symptom, a condition, a piece of equipment, a disability, a medication, or a treatment. This operational system makes it possible for a nurse to enter an initiator into the system, thereby producing from the computer a care plan which sets forth elements of care that are related to that initiator. This system has unique capabilities because of its initiator concept. Its limitations may relate to the fact that its care plans do not include expected outcomes and are not diagnosis related. Several other computer companies or organizations are involved in early developmental phases of nursing care-planning systems.[8-10] This is not an exhaustive review of computerized care-planning applications, since each year various organizations are adding to the knowledge base regarding nursing's unique needs for computer-assisted information systems.

A Computer-assisted, Outcomes-oriented Care-planning System

One example of a relatively well developed computer-assisted care-planning system is being evolved at a hospital in California. The following summary of this hospital's care-planning system* is taken from a report of a pilot study completed in 1976.[11]

For many years, the nursing profession itself, as well as the Joint

*This development is jointly sponsored by the hospital and by the vendor and is partially funded by grants from the US Dept of Health, Education, and Welfare.

Commission on Hospital Accreditation (JCHA), has required that each patient have a comprehensive and current plan of care, including statements of the patient's problems (nursing diagnoses), short- and long-term objectives (expected outcomes), and detailed statements of required nursing interventions (nursing orders). All but three or four nursing services in the United States handwrite the plans of care onto cards which are kept in a Rand or Kardex for easy access. Few nursing services are successful in keeping care plans updated, primarily due to the large amount of detailed, constantly changing information that should be written. This results in nurses giving token attention to the writing of care plans, relying primarily on word-of-mouth information transmission. Because in a typical hospital any one patient is likely to have 12 to 14 different nurses caring for him over a five-day average hospital stay, the word-of-mouth method is fraught with problems of faulty recall and fragmented information. The result is inadequate analytic and planning data available to a nurse as he or she cares for a patient.

The focus of this system is that of computerizing outcome oriented patient care planning so that the operational difficulties of manipulating large quantities of data can be made so efficient that care planning will actually be accomplished by nurses. Outcome-oriented care planning is also designed so that the computerized data can be used for both concurrent and retrospective audit purposes. This supports the goal of improving the quality of patient care and enhancing the effectiveness with which it is delivered. The system integrates (1) diagnosis-particular, outcomes-oriented standard nursing care plans, (2) outcomes-oriented systematic nursing care-planning processes, and (3) the computerized medical information system in use at this hospital. This integrated system* is designed to focus nursing care on patient outcomes rather than on nursing tasks and to compare actual patient outcomes against standards.

The Care-planning Scenario.   The nursing care-planning process begins when the patient arrives at the nursing unit. The first step is a

---

*This automated system is designed to reduce, avoid, and forestall the enormous costs of manual information processing. This real-time, comprehensive, integrated, medical information system operates from a large-scale computer located in the vendor's regional center, which is connected to video and printer terminals located throughout the hospital. Physicians, nurses, and other hospital professional and clerical personnel interact directly with the system by use of these terminals to enter, retrieve, and print clinical, financial, and administrative information. The system, either in whole or in part, takes over a great many of the patient-oriented information-processing tasks that are performed thousands of times daily in a hospital. Patient information is captured from admission through discharge. The system affects all nursing units and clinical ancillary departments as well as many administrative and support departments.

patient interview. Data from the interview, from other chart documents, e.g., the physician's history and physical, and from the standard care plans' data base (resident in the computer) are synthesized at the video terminal to produce this patient's nursing care plan, which reflects not only his diagnosis but also his unique problems.

The nursing care plan is formulated in terms of both real (actual) and potential problems, expected outcomes that reflect the predicted resolution of the problems, deadlines by which this resolution can be reached, and nursing orders representing necessary nursing actions to accomplish this resolution.

The nursing care plan is recorded at the video terminal by selecting the appropriate items from the standard care plan data base and by typing in any special problem(s) specific to this patient. Entering the nursing care plan via the terminal produces a printed version of this individualized care plan for use by the nurse caring for the patient. This printout includes all care-planning data as well as the expected date of discharge estimated by the nurse. It also includes the initials of the nurse responsible for the data and the plan. The printed version of the nursing care plan is produced once a day or on demand and serves as the nurse's work sheet as she cares for the patient. While caring for him, she determines, in conjunction with the patient, which expected outcomes have been or are being accomplished. She also determines whether deadlines are realistic and whether the nursing orders are effective.

The information gleaned from caring for the patient is documented via the computer in the nurse's notes and describes the patient's progress toward expected outcomes. At the same time, the nurse can (via the computer) update the nursing care plan. She completes those problems resolved and, if necessary, changes such other data as deadlines or nursing orders to reflect the patient's changing situation. The next printed care plan includes these changes. As the patient progresses toward health, this is reflected in the nursing care plan as expected outcomes are reached and no longer appear on the updated plan.

The video matrix features of the nursing care plan are as follows:

Standard care plans (diagnosis related) are stored in the computer memory bank

Standard care plans are easily adapted to each patient because unusual or nonstandard care plans are easily formulated

There are cross-reference indices between standard care plans and problems

Lists of real and potential problems are contained within each standard care plan

Problems that are common to several standard care plans are in-
dexed and listed separately
Abbreviations are incorporated to save time and space
Relative deadlines are readily translated into actual dates because
expected outcome time frames are provided

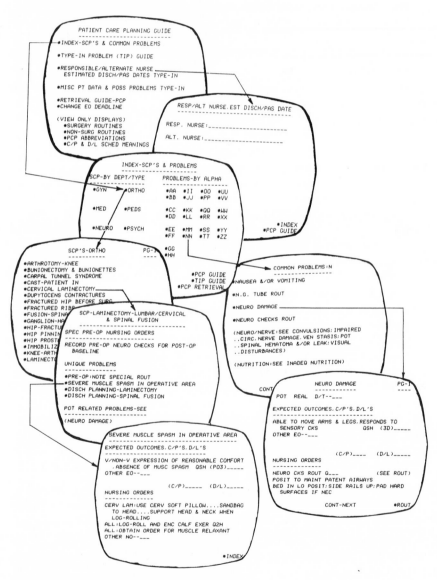

FIGURE 12-4. A typical matrix sequence.

Coordination between the responsible nurse and the utilization review nurse is facilitated

The nursing care plan includes the identity of the responsible and alternate nurse, the estimated discharge date, criteria for discharge, real and potential problems, expected outcomes, deadlines, and nursing orders. Also included are possible problems which require further data or watchfulness.

```
4WEST-8612-02        EL CAMINO HOSPITAL
  4/20/76  3:09 PM              PAGE 001              NURSING CARE PLAN
GAUDON JENNY                F 37      SERV, SURG
  301421      ADM, 04/05/76  WILLIAM CHILDS             7:00 AM  4/20/76
================================================================================

  RESP. NURSE:J. SCHUYLER                   ALT. NURSE:
DX: NON-UNION BACK FUSION...04-06-76:               **04/17  PAS:
    LAMINECTOMY L4, EXPLORE L5-S1,
    FORAMINOTOMY L4-5 BILATERALLY, FUSION L
    4-SACRUM....


REAL & POTENTIAL PROBLEMS:

   4/6   DISCH PLANNING-SPINAL FUSION                                  MCE
   EXPECTED OUTCOMES                              C/P:   D/L:
      4/6   DEMO PROPER TECHN                      QDE    4/15    MCE
   NURSING ORDERS
      4/6   INST RE PROPER BODY MECHANICS                             MCE
      4/6   INST RE APPLIC OF CORSET &/OR CHAIR-BACK
            BRACE                                                     MCE

   4/6   CONSTIPATION, D/T--IMMOBILITY                                MCE
   EXPECTED OUTCOMES                              C/P:   D/L:
      4/6   SOFT ABD.PASSING FLATUS,NORM STOOL,NORM
            BOWEL PATTERN FOR PT                   QDS    4/15    MCE
   NURSING ORDERS
      4/6   ENC FLDS,CK FOR BOWEL SOUNDS                             MCE
      4/6   GET APPROP ORD FOR R TUBE,HARRIS FLUSH,
            STOOL SOFTENER &/OR LAX,PRN                              MCE

   4/6   EMBOLUS FORMATION                                           MCE
   EXPECTED OUTCOMES                              C/P:   D/L:
      4/6   NEG HOMAN SGNS;NO SWELLING OR TENDERNESS
            OF EXTREM;NO SUDDEN RESP DISTRESS      QSH    4/15    MCE
   NURSING ORDERS
      4/6   GET ORD FOR A-E HOSE-REMOVE FOR BATH,HS
            CARE ONLY                                                MCE
      4/6   FOOT PEDAL,DB EXER Q2H-5X/SESSION, FROM 08
            :00PM                                                    MCE
      4/6   AVOID KNEE GATCH & PROLONGED HIP FLEXION                 MCE

MISC PT DATA & POSS. PROBLEMS:
   4/5   PRESENT ILLNESS--NON UNION BACK FUSION. CAST THORACIC
         AREA. CHIEF COMPLAINT ON ADMISSION 1. DIMINISHED MOBILITY
         DUE TOBACK PAIN 2. PAIN CONTINUOUS LUMBAR AREA.,
         ADDITIONAL DESCRIPTION--OTHERWISE HEALTHY AND ALERT,
         COOPERATIVE                                                 MCE
   4/5   MED-SURG-PSYCH HISTORY--HAS HAD PREVIOUS PULMONARY EMBOLI
         POST-OP                                                     MCE
   4/5   MED ALLERGY....MORPHINE                                     MCE
   4/5   RECORD PRE-OP NEURO CHECKS FOR POST-OP BASELINE             MCE

                          LAST PAGE
 -*-
```

FIGURE 12-5. A preoperative laminectomy care plan.

Figure 12-4 illustrates a typical matrix sequence, and Figure 12-5 shows a preoperative care plan for a laminectomy patient.

SUMMARY

Before any system of nursing care planning is implemented, many factors must be considered if the venture is to be successful.

The agency's philosophy—its basic beliefs about its patients, its nursing staff, and its nursing processes—must be appraised to ascertain that it accurately reflects the current beliefs and commitments of its staff. Because an agency's philosophy is the foundation for the daily practice of nursing within that agency, it significantly influences the type and quality of care planning that is performed.

That diversity of services and staffing patterns also has implications for the modifiction of a care-planning system to meet the unique needs of various kinds of nursing services. Probably there should be a somewhat different operational model for care planning in an intensive care unit from the model used in a convalescent care unit.

Staff readiness is critical to success or failure when a new system of care planning is to be introduced. The staff's previous experience with care planning, its educational and experience differences, and its preoccupation with other projects must be taken into consideration.

The successful implementation of a system for care planning also depends upon the ongoing support of administrative and in-service staffs. Many factors are crucial to the successful implementation of a new system. Noteworthy among these factors are the time required for learning how to do care planning, the feasibility of providing in-service education sessions, the ability of key staff to teach and to follow up, and the provision of additional interim staff support when the new system is phased in.

The design of a care-planning information system depends upon many variables. Forms, terminology, and definitions should reflect the philosophy and preference of the organization. Manual (paper and pen) systems should be designed for maximum efficiency to reduce time-consuming handwriting and to reduce errors of copying or of readability.

Computer-assisted prototypes under development in the early 1970s provide early breakthroughs for the ultimate incorporation of effective computer-assisted nursing information systems in the future. One computer-assisted care planning prototype is described in this chapter.

REFERENCES

1. Watson A, Mayers M: How to Write Nursing Care Plans. Stockton Cal, KP Co Medical Systems, 1976, p 9
2. Ibid, p 16
3. Joint Commission on Accreditation of Hospitals. Accreditation Manual for Hospitals. Chicago, CAA, 1975
4. A Plan for Implementation of the Standards of Nursing Practice. Kansas City, American Nurses Association, 1946
5. United States Indian Health Service, Tucson, Arizona
6. Demonstration of a Hospital Data Management System (Five-year summary program report, January 1967–June 1972). Houston, Texas Institute for Rehabilitation and Research
7. Somers J: Computerized Nursing Care System. Hospitals. p 93, April 1971
8. Spectra Information System. Chicago, Medicus Systems Corporation, 1977
9. National Data Communication: General Overview, Dallas, National Data Communication System, 1976
10. Technicon Medical Information Systems, Sunnyvale Cal, Technicon Corp, 1977
11. Cook M, Hushower G, Mayers M: Computerized Nursing and TMIS. Unpublished paper presented at the Technicon International Congress, New York, December 1976

BIBLIOGRAPHY

Hannah K: The computer and nursing practice. Nurs Outlook 24[9] 555, Sept 1976

US Public Health Service, National Center for Health Services Research and Development. Comprehensive Hospital Computer Assplications Program. National Technical Information Services, PB-211690. April 1972, Vol 2 pp 255-269

A Realistic Approach to the Teaching and Implementation of Care Planning. Chicago, Medicus/Nursing Care Systems, 1975

Taking the Pain out of Care Planning. Chicago, Medicus/Nursing Care Systems, 1975

13

Quality Assurance:
Evaluation and Accountability

EVALUATION OF PATIENT CARE

For centuries, the mystique associated with all of the healing arts intimidated patients and professionals alike, so that systematic evaluation of care has only recently been attempted. Valid and reliable methodologies are being developed and tested as part of a major ongoing effort among health care professionals.

An early pioneer in health care evaluation, Dr. Abraham Flexner published his famous report on the quality of medical schools in the United States in 1910. Thus began an evolution of projects and studies. The American College of Surgeons, in 1913, became an accrediting organization, formulating standards for physicians' practice and education. In 1952, the Joint Commission on Accreditation of Hospitals succeeded the American College of Surgeons and confronted the issue of developing audit methods that would define and measure quality.

In 1973, the American Nurses' Association set standards for nursing practice.[1] In 1976, the ANA published a model for quality assurance.[2] Concurrently, the National League for Nursing became the official accrediting body for nursing's educational processes.

All of these groups' efforts are directed toward establishing evaluation processes in the health care industry. Michnich et al refer to evaluation as

> the process of collecting data to produce information for decision-making . . .
> The purpose of quality evaluation is to point out those areas of acceptable performance and give credit to those involved in contributing to quality, and to locate those areas of unacceptable performance where improvement can be accomplished.[3]

Specific methodologies for evaluation have been set forth by many persons in the health care professions. Most methodologies can be classified as measures of structure, processes, or outcomes.

These three terms can be defined as follows:[4]

Structure: Referring to and formulating criteria for adequate physical facilities, good administrative processes, well-qualified staff, good communications, and staff development processes.

Process: Referring to and defining evaluative criteria according to desired or expected nursing tasks, functions, or activities.

Outcomes: Referring to those desired effects defined as specific clinical manifestations, mobility levels, patient knowledge, or self-care skills.

QUALITY ASSURANCE METHODS

There are several common methods for gathering measurement data for patient care evaluation: retrospective chart review, concurrent chart review, bedside audit, and patient questionnaires. Any of these methods requires that specific criteria be formulated to provide measurement yardsticks. "Criteria are descriptive statements of performance, behavior, circumstances, or clinical states that represent a satisfactory, positive, or excellent state of affairs. Criteria describe the assessable elements of care processes or patient outcomes that can be used to measure quality."[5]

This definition describes a direct link between patient care plans and evaluation criteria. To evaluate the care of an individual unusual patient, the nursing orders provide "process" criteria. The expected outcomes are "outcome" criteria. To evaluate large numbers of patients, standard care plans provide process and outcome criteria.

Although evaluation (audit) forms are designed in a different way than are care plans, the process and outcome criteria are basically the same. Figure 13-1 [6] shows several chart audit criteria for patients who are primiparas. The first column shows the criteria. The next columns ("P" and "O") denote which criteria measure nursing processes and which measure patient outcomes. The other columns show "Percent Desired Compliance," "Predictable Exceptions," and "Instructions to Auditor." Close inspection of the criteria reveals that these statements in a slightly different form would appear as nursing orders or expected outcomes on a standard care plan for primiparas. Conversely, if audit criteria have been formulated, it takes a few short steps to convert these into the basic content for a standard care plan. This linkage between operational care plans and audit criteria is crucial to a solid and mutually reinforcing quality assurance system.

The preceding paragraphs have described how criteria are the yardsticks for measuring the quality of care. Chart audits, bedside audits, and questionnaires are data-gathering methods which utilize these criteria. The percentages of charts or patients that are found in compliance with each criterion give indications of levels of quality. All of the preceding evaluative methods represent the assessment or measurement elements of evaluation. Assessment is not the same as quality assurance. According to Michnich,[7] most of the quality care efforts have been devoted to assessment. The quality assurance phases of evaluation require that something be done about any low compliance levels that are found. The assurance phases of evaluation include (1) identifying the source(s) of the problem, (2) formulating a remedial plan, (3) assigning responsibility for the plan, (4) implementing the plan, and (5) reassessing at periodic intervals, using the same criterion measures.[2,4]

This assurance process can be applied to the care of one patient, by identifying that the patient's status is at variance from the expected outcome. An analysis of the patient's situation, the care processes, and other relevant information leads to a hypothesis as to the source or reason for the variance. The plan of care is then changed so as to correct the cause. A nurse assumes responsibility for vigorous implementation of the plan of care, and, finally, the patient's status is evaluated at deadline or checkpoint intervals. This assurance process is exactly the same as the care-planning process that has been described throughout this text. This remedial action process represents how the process is continually repeated when expected outcomes are not reached as predicted. Mager's book, *Analyzing Performance Problems*,[8] provides an excellent model for identifying

Criteria	P	O	Percent Desired Compliance	Predictable Exceptions	Instructions to Auditor
Chart should show documentation of:					
Admission: (First 15 minutes)					
1. Height (fingers breadth) and firmness of fundus.	X		100	None	Admission notes or flow sheet
2. Amount and color of lochia. Lochia pad count per 8 hours and color (dark, bright) and clots—absence or presence.	X		100	None	Admission notes or flow sheet
3. Vital signs: Blood pressure, pulse, respirations.	X		100	None	Admission notes or flow sheet
4. Skin color and temperature.	X		100	None	Admission notes or flow sheet
5. Condition of episiotomy: intact and/or local bleeding.	X		100	None	Admission notes or flow sheet
Interim:					
(After first 15 minutes through postpartum day 2)					
6. Fundus firm when checked q 8 hours.		X	100	None	Nurses' notes or flow sheet
7. Normal voiding 6 to 8 hours postdelivery.		X	100	None	Nurses' notes or flow sheet
8. Normal bowel movement by 2 days postdelivery.		X	100	None	Nurses' notes or flow sheet
9. Patient verbalizes that she feels rested q day.		X	100	None	Nurses' notes or flow sheet
Discharge (Last day)					
10. Normal lochia: scant, brownish color, no foul odor.		X	100	None	Nurses' notes
11. Demonstrates bottle or breast-feeding technique.		X	100	Stillbirth	Nurses' notes
12. Demonstrates self-care: Breast and perineum.		X	100	None	Nurses' notes
13. Demonstrates correct baby bath technique.		X	100	Stillbirth	Nurses' notes
14. Verbalizes satisfaction with home care plans.		X	100	None	Nurses' notes
15. Verbalizes correct knowledge of potential pregnancy and choice of prevention.	X		100	None	Nurses' notes
16. Verbalizes knowledge of correct use of birth control methods or specific preference for no birth control.		X	100	None	Nurses' notes

FIGURE 13-1. Criteria for postpartum uncomplicated primipara. (From Mayers et al: *Quality Assurance for Patient Care: Nursing Perspective,* 1977.

reasons for variances and for following through with the most appropriate kinds of remedial action plans.

The American Nurses' Association provides a model[9] for implementing the quality assurance process in the care of a specific client. The model suggests a circular process, starting with values and then continuing to standards, criteria, measurement methods, judgments as to progress toward meeting criteria, and instituting action when problems are identified. The model also suggests sources, tools, references, and methods for each of the steps and elements in the circular process.

The ANA also provides a similar model and resources for implementing the quality assurance process for large numbers of clients on an institutional scale.[10]

For large numbers of patients, retrospective chart review is one evaluation method. Many charts of patients of a certain diagnosis or other classification are reviewed to check their compliance against outcome and process criteria, such as those illustrated in Figure 13-1. Statistical summaries show what percentage of the charts met each of the criteria. These data are then analyzed by an audit committee (or similar group).

Negative variances are identified, their sources or reasons are hypothesized, new compliance percentage goals are set, and an appropriate type of remedial action plan is implemented. Reaudits of charts, again using the low-compliance criteria as yardsticks, will show whether or not the reason or source was correctly identified and corrected.

Another method of retrospective review is that of patient questionnaires.[11] Large numbers of ex-patients receive mailed questionnaires which query them regarding many aspects of their care. Many of the questions are adapted from process and outcome criteria. Tallies of positive and negative responses to questions can be analyzed and related to standards or criteria. This information provides another important evaluative dimension.

Another evaluation method that can be applied to relatively large numbers of patients is referred to as "concurrent care review." Concurrent review is done while patients are still undergoing care, rather than after the fact as in retrospective review. Concurrent review can be accomplished through a number of measurement tools or scales. The ANA outlines these tools in their quality assurance model.[2]

The care-planning format outlined in this text not only provides guidelines for formulating patient care plans but also illustrates and implements the basic processes of quality assurance, thus aiding nursing professionals in meeting their responsibility for assuring high quality services to their patients and to the public at large.

DIMENSIONS OF ACCOUNTABILITY

Whose responsibility is it to assume leadership in the patient care-planning component of quality assurance? How the responsible person is chosen is important. The knowledge and skills required and the demands placed upon this person are manifold. Accountability must be clear.

Responsibility for Assessment

The skillful and perceptive assessment of a patient's health status demands that the nurse have a comprehensive understanding of specific health problems, their causes, usual signs and symptoms, diagnostic and treatment regimens, and their long-range implications. She needs to recognize, evaluate, and make judgments about the patient's socioeconomic and psychologic status and to predict, with reasonable accuracy, the effects these will have upon the success or failure of the medical and nursing interventions. She must be skilled in the techniques of interviewing and observation. Her interviewing skills must be based upon an intellectural rationale that accounts for a patient's readiness, his mental abilities, vocabulary differences, cultural variations, and psychologic influences. In interviewing, she must have a knowledge of and skill with the principles of logical progression, clarification, information giving, and active listening. All of this knowledge is acquired through a study of the theoretical rationales underlying each of the aforementioned principles and methods. Skill in applying them is acquired through well-directed experience.

Responsibility for Problem Solving

In order to continue the care-planning process beyond the assessment phase, the nurse must be a skillful problem solver. She must be able to analyze, to sort the data obtained, and to identify correctly the problems that exist. The effective statement of problems and expected outcomes and the sound planning of relevant nursing care require intellectual skill with the scientific process as well as thorough, up-to-date knowledge of the principles of therapeutic intervention.

Responsibility for Leadership

Another requirement for the nurse who assumes leadership in nursing care planning is that she have effective interpersonal and communication skills. When the plan of care has been developed the nurse must be able to implement it by directing the efforts of her staff. To do this, she must have their trust, confidence, and respect. She must be able to delegate, to assist, and to provide direct patient care herself. She must be able to demonstrate, to explain, and to clarify. She must be free to assist her staff as well as her patients if the care plan is to result in the expected outcomes for each patient.

This brief summary of the skills required of the nurse who assumes leadership in nursing care planning makes clear that that person must be well selected. In most patient care settings the registered nurse is responsible for planning care for her group of patients. It is she who should make patient assessments and write plans of care. Her job requirements should be designed to maximize her independent role. She must be available to assess and reassess patients' changing reponses. She must be free to write and update plans of care and be available to teach, to assist, and to problem solve with her staff.[1]

In order to free registered nurses for these critical leadership–patient care functions, many agencies are delegating medication-treatment routines to qualified licensed practical or vocational nurses. In most if not all states, licensed practical nurses are legally qualified to give medications and to perform the majority of treatment procedures, provided they are under the supervision of a registered nurse. If an agency believes in giving staff members opportunity to function to their maximum ability, delegation of specified nursing tasks to the licensed practical nurse reinforces this commendable approach. Relieving the nurse of certain traditional tasks frees her also to function at her maximum ability. Assessment, nursing diagnosis, care planning, staff development, teaching, and problem solving with patients and other staff represent those dimensions of the nursing role that cannot be delegated.

Legal and Professional Responsibility

The registered nurse who makes patient assessments and designs plans of care should be the person who actually writes or signs the nursing orders. Like the physician, the nurse must know first hand that the nursing care which is ordered via the care plan is, in fact, the care for which she is assuming responsibility. This responsibility cannot be delegated to other staff persons. Furthermore, when too many people independently care for the same patient, chaos results. Many agency administrators speak proudly of the fact that, in their hospital, everyone writes on the nursing care plan. It is their way of demonstrating that all levels of staff are involved in care planning and that everyone's ideas are welcome. Although their philosophy of total involvement is a good one, their method of demonstrating that philosophy is not. When everyone is welcome to write on the care plan, it no longer is a plan. It becomes a suggestion box. A suggestion box approach invites haphazard, nonrelated suggestions for care that a staff person may or may not be inclined to act upon. Nursing must function more responsibly. The only way that nursing as a profession can assume responsibility for patient care is for nurses to insist that care plans be designed by the delegated registered nurse.

Responsibility for Staffing

Staffing patterns are most frequently designed to "get the job done." This is certainly justifiable and appropriate. However, it is also well to consider staffing from the patient's point of view, and from the aspect of nursing process before final staffing decisions are made.

Hospital Staffing. In the hospital setting, where many patients are coping with acute biologic stress as well as with the emotional strain of new and unaccustomed dependency, there may be need for registered nurses to have more time for direct patient contact. Personnel with other levels of skills may be assigned to routine custodial and technical care and to ward administration activities. Too many nurses with excellent patient intervention skills are tied down to desks, records, and phones.

Clinical Specialists. Another possible innovation would be the freer interchange of expert nurses among units. Many medical-surgical patients with significant emotional problems could benefit from the attention of a nurse with psychiatric skills. Medical-surgical nurses might request a qualified nurse from the psychiatric unit to help construct a plan of care and to be a resource person as the plan is implemented. Conversely, psychiatric patients often have medical-surgical problems and the psychiatric staff might call upon a medical-surgical nurse for advice. In many hospitals, clinical specialists already fill this role. But even more multispeciality nursing involvement can be utilized for better care planning and implementation.

Clinical Coordinator. The traditional supervisory position is curently undergoing analysis in hospital nursing circles. Many supervisors find that their duties involve them with paperwork, making rounds to collect information, getting emergency supplies, reassigning staff, and many other nonnursing tasks. An emerging trend is for a clinical coordinator to replace the traditional supervisor. The clinical coordinator often assumes responsibility for the total 24-hour-a-day care of patients in her jurisdiction. She assesses patient and staff problems, plans individual and group care programs, works with staff development, and is a resource person for clinical care problems. She commits herself not in terms of time but in terms of responsibility for care. This means that her hours are planned to meet the needs of her patients and staff. She may not have an 8:00 AM TO 5:00 PM shift. To meet her responsibilities, she plans to be present on the nursing units at different times during all three shifts. She is "on call" similar to the way a physician is "on call." She can be reached at any time of the day or night through a telephone exchange. This type of nursing role has possibilities in all patient care settings and may prove to be a better way to use nursing skills than the traditional supervisor's role has been.

Coordinator of Patient Care Services. Yet another innovative administrative staffing pattern that some hospitals are now using is to appoint a nurse as coordinator of patient care services. This strategy is based upon the assumption that all personal care services, whether performed by dietitians, physical therapists, occupational therapists, or nurses, fall into the same broad category, and that the benefit of each is greater if all of them are coordinated by one administrative unit. The coordinator of personal care services assumes responsibility for overseeing all related paramedical patient care services. She works with a committee from all of the services, including nursing, and together they plan better coordination of the delivery of patient care.

Unit Patient Care Committee. In their quest for an improved multi-disciplinary team approach to care planning, a few hospitals have developed ward, or unit, patient care committees. The patient care committee is made up of representatives of each of the major services in a given hospital unit. On a typical medical-surgical unit, the representatives might be a nurse, a physician, a physical therapist, and a dietitian. The committee meets regularly at monthly intervals. They make it a point to meet somewhere within their specific patient care unit. By doing this, they reinforce their primary reason for being together—patient care on that unit.

Their general purpose is to improve patient care by analyzing critical incidents, analyzing patient care trends, reviewing current standard care protocols, trouble-shooting grievances between disciplines, and defining needs for staffing, scheduling, equipment, and physical facilities changes.

They make recommendations directly to administrative channels, as appropriate. Patient care committees have proven to be a workable mechanism for promoting the team approach to patient care. Fully implemented, each major hospital unit would have a patient care committee of this nature. The committees invite people in from other relevant disciplines when they need resource information or judgment outside their own competence. Committees sometimes invite patients to serve as sources for relevant information.

General Staffing Considerations. The acute health manpower shortage has resulted in every health care discipline reevaluating its traditional roles and responsibilities. Physicians are exploring ways to augment their services through the use of physician's assistants. Large medical practice groups are turning to automated mass screening systems. Physicians in many areas are employing electronic methods for instantaneous reading of electrocardiographs. Physicians are updating their knowledge by the systematic use of mailed or telephoned lecture and information tapes.

Similarly, nurses are revising staffing patterns to incorporate health aides, nurse specialists, and nurse coordinators. The traditional hierarchy of nursing organization is undergoing critical analysis and, in many places, is being replaced by a peer group, patient-oriented organizational structure. The traditional hierarchy of authority in nursing may be found to have too large an overhead of nonpatient-centered persons—a price perhaps too high to pay in these days of acute manpower shortage.

Contemporary attitudes among nurses also influence the reevaluation of traditional structures. Nurses' resistance to bureaucratic power structures, their growing sense of personal professional responsibility, their desire to be agents for change, and their positive attitude toward peer group responsibility are parts of this evolutionary change.

Staffs from all areas of nursing are seriously studying the part patients should play in their own care. The patient's involvement in his own care is not conceived as a method for saving the nurse's time but as a reflection of changing roles and responsibilities. The philosophy that patient involvement leads to more effective patient rehabilitation is the basis for this innovation. Some hospitals are setting up systems for patients to administer many of their own medications. When a patient is scheduled to go home on a certain medications regimen, it is particularly appropriate that he learn in the hospital how to manage that element of his care safely and correctly. Patient participation in setting up plans of care, an idea discussed in earlier chapters, is another aspect of this concept.

All of these philosophic, economic, and psychologic considerations are causing significant changes in staffing patterns for nursing care.

QUALITY IMPLICATIONS OF PRIMARY NURSING

Primary nursing is a care delivery modality that "assumes that the total care of an individual patient is the responsibility of one nurse—the primary nurse." Manthey describes primary nursing as "the delivery of comprehensive, continuous, coordinated and individualized patient care through the primary nurse who has autonomy, accountability and authority to act as the chief nurse for her patients." [12]

In reality there appear to be variations from hospital to hospital in how primary nursing is actually implemented. In its intended form, one nurse assumes the responsibility for the 24-hour plan of care for three to five patients. She is the caregiver for these patients when she is on duty and collaborates closely with her associate nurses who are the caregivers on other shifts or on her days off. Any one nurse may be the primary nurse for some patients and an associate for others. This concept assures that one nurse comprehends the patient's situation and has the authority to plan, implement, direct, and evaluate his care. Her authority lies in that her responsibility covers a patient's care 24 hours a day. She makes decisions and is accountable for them. She is autonomous in her nursing role, not subordinate. She is a colleague in her participation with others, such as therapists, nutritionists, physicians, and her associate nurses.

A study by Marram et al[13] reveals that primary nurses' care plans are substantially more complete and individualized than are those of team nurses.

Primary nurses are more likely to:[14]

1. Include the patient's perception in the descriptive reason for admission
2. Give a statement of general appearance which established an individualized picture of the patient
3. List more nursing needs or diagnoses of a wider variety on the assessment and to transfer these in the form of a care plan on the Kardex
4. Identify physical care needs significantly more often than team nurses
5. Provide an individualized patient profile on the Kardex
6. Supply a care plan on the Kardex, one which focuses on needs identified
7. Identify fewer psychosocial and anticipatory guidance needs

This last finding is puzzling in that it would seem that the more comprehensive assessments would lead to the identification of a higher proportion of psychosocial and learning needs.

Primary nursing is being studied and implemented in increasingly greater numbers so that some of these early questions ultimately will be answered. Early evidence does indicate, however, that primary nurses, because of their continuous involvement and their clear authority and accountability, are likely to provide higher quality plans of care and follow-through.

QUALITY IMPLICATIONS OF CASE METHOD NURSING

There is little or nothing in the literature as yet that discusses the case method approach and its contribution to the planning of nursing care. The case method modality can be described as the complete responsibility for one or more patients, providing all or part of the nursing care when on duty, delegating some aspects of care to colleagues or assistants, and updating the patient's care plan as part of the eight-hour responsibility. Authority and accountability are shared with colleagues on other shifts. The case method allows for the same nurses to care for the same patients from day to day or for changes in case loads and responsibility from day to day.

An enhancement of the case method approach in some hospitals has resulted in the term "responsible nurse." This variation provides for one nurse to be responsible for the care of one or more patients. She is responsible for initiating and updating the care plans for her patients and collaborates with her alternates, who manage the care on the other shifts. She may delegate all or some direct care to colleagues or assistants who are working with her. She, however, is accountable for her decisions that affect the patient's care, whether or not she is physically present. This variation of the case method approach does not allow the changing of case assignments from day to day among either the responsible or alternate nurses, thus enhancing continuity for the patients and nurses.

In many respects, this variation is similar to primary nursing. Its differences lie in the fact that the responsible or alternate nurse may delegate all or part of a patient's care to assistants who are assigned to help her with her case load. The professional responsibility for assessing, planning, implementing, and evaluating care is, however, not a function that can be delegated to another by the responsible nurse.

ACCOUNTABILITY FOR CLEAR COMMUNICATION

The care plan is a vehicle for effective communication. It provides an effective medium for transmitting planned care information. It must be designed so that the staff persons utilizing it can quickly and accurately perceive and implement the intended care.

Devices for Filing Care Plans

Perhaps the most commonly used device for filing care plans is a Kardex or Rand which is kept within easy access to all staff. The disadvantages of a Kardex are related to the fact that it contains data for 15 or more patients. When a staff person uses it to secure data regarding just one patient, she limits availability of the data concerning the 14 other patients. The person who is transferring orders and receiving and transmitting patient care information at the main desk frequently needs the Kardex for relatively long periods or needs to use it at a moment's notice for clarifying or checking orders. This again limits its accessibility to other staff members. On busy care units, there often are a number of staff persons waiting to see the Kardex. Knowing that it is in demand, a staff nurse will, upon gaining access to it, tend to use it hurriedly. Obviously this greatly increases the potential for error. In situations where there is a large number of staff and where time pressures are great, the potential exists for unsafe care and wasted time and energy.

The practice of filing care plans individually and separately is gaining favor as an alternative to the Kardex. A revolving metal file with slots designed to hold clipboards is one innovation. The care plan for each patient is attached to the clipboard and placed in its identified slot. The revolving file is mounted on a desk or deck, to be within easy reach of everyone. The ward clerk or head nurse can pull care plans as needed, leaving the rest free for use at the same time by other staff.

Sometimes certain parts of care plans are kept in notebooks or card files, while other parts, such as medication and treatment orders, are kept in the usual Kardex. This way of dividing up patient care data is generally contraindicated. It fragments what should be a total understanding and management of the patient. If Xeroxing or duplicating methods are easily available, care plans can be duplicated so that each nurse can clip her copies of care plans to a clipboard. These plans are used by her wherever she is. She can make notations for update on these copies as her judgment dictates.

Whatever filing or data-retrieval system is used, whether a notebook, Kardex, or multiple clipboards, it is essential that patient care information be organized in such a way that it can be easily read and understood. In Chapters 8 and 9, examples of the elements of a total care plan were given. A total care plan consists of all the relevant data needed for patient care. These include medications, treatments, diagnostic tests, standard and frequently ordered care, and unusual problems. It includes spaces for patient preferences and miscellaneous data, for the physician's expectations of the course of convalescence, and for nursing's criteria for discharge. The recommended method is to have all of these elements on the patient care plan. When all necessary patient care information is abstracted onto one accessible Kardex or onto a page or two attached to a clipboard, it saves time and energy. It also provides a comprehensive picture of the patient, his problems, and his care.

Care-planning Conferences

An integral part of the system of transmitting nursing care information is the patient care conference. Sharing ideas, clarifying standard and specialized care, and analyzing data for problem identification are vital functions that can be facilitated in team conferences. Conferences can and should be of varying types to meet the multifaceted needs of staff and patients.

The One-to-One Conference. The individual or one-to-one conference is undoubtedly the type of conference most frequently used in nursing. One-to-one conferences occur continuously and are usually brief and unplanned.

A one-to-one conference can take place by the water cooler, in the cafeteria, or in hospital corridors. These conferences are frequently just as productive as more formally structured meetings. A one-to-one conference can also be a deliberately arranged meeting, effectively utilized by team leaders, head nurses, or clinical specialists. A team leader can brief a staff nurse on the current plan of care, teach an unfamiliar procedure, and clarify misunderstandings on a one-to-one basis. An excellent purpose for the individual conference is to share feelings of satisfaction over care well done. Positive reinforcement techniques should be consciously employed in nursing. The individual conference is an excellent medium in which they can be used.

The Team Conference. The "team conference" is perhaps the most commonly used term and the least used method for transmitting information in nursing. The time pressures of patient care force the average nursing staff to abandon hope of ever being able to follow consistently a schedule of team conferences. There are, however, seldom-considered variations of the team conference that might tend to minimize the limitations imposed by the pressures of time and staff shortages. One variation is the partial team conference. That is, half of the team carries the patient care load while the other half has a conference. Subsequently, the two halves exchange roles. Thus, at periodic intervals everyone on the team has an opportunity to become involved in the care-planning process. Nursing units with two or more teams can quite easily set up a rotation schedule for conferences so that one team covers for the other during the conference period.

However, for effective team functioning there should be a meeting of the entire team at periodic intervals.

Team conferences have many purposes. They are most effectively used for:

1. Exchanging data about patients who present unusual or challenging problems. Information-sharing is geared to the task of reaching more precise identifications of problems.

2. Reviewing the specialized nursing actions for a particular patient. When the specialized nursing actions are complex, the team leader can utilize the team conference for orienting everyone to the designated patient care.
3. Reviewing and clarifying misconceptions of the staff regarding standard care plans. In order to maximize staff efficiency and good standard nursing care, the team members need periodic reinforcement of their knowledge of, and responsibility to follow, the standard care plans.
4. Reviewing the team's entire caseload, in order to update information relating to progress and problems.
5. Analyzing critical incidents that have occurred recently. It is essential to safe care that the entire team periodically review critical incidents that have occurred. Together, the team identifies causes and plans strategies that will prevent the incidents from recurring.
6. Reviewing the recent instances of excellent care. When the team evaluates its experiences with good care, the team members can identify the factors that contributed to it. They can then incorporate those factors into their regular care plans. This results in positive group planning, and it motivates members to provide excellent care.
7. Expressing feelings about interpersonal relationships among the team. Prevention or resolution of major interpersonal problems can be accomplished by this kind of conference.
8. Expressing and discussing team education needs.

Many of these purposes can best be accomplished if conferences occur on a regularly scheduled basis. Between scheduled conferences, impromptu conferences can be called to meet critical patient and staff needs as they arise.

Walking Rounds.   Another variation of the team conference is what some staffs call "walking rounds." At the beginning of each shift, the team makes rounds with the team leader. Each patient is visited and briefly interviewed, and the day's care is outlined and discussed with the patient. This method incorporates the patient into the care planning and minimizes confusion among both patients and staff. Most nurses who use walking rounds find that the time spent on rounds is minimal compared with the resulting time that is saved and the patient and staff satisfaction that is gained.

Trouble-shooting Conferences.   A further variation of the team conference is referred to as "trouble shooting." For this, a team meets briefly for 10 or 15 minutes some time during the shift. They quickly review every patient and talk about only the concerns that each staff member may have about patients. The team members do not attempt to resolve their concerns; they merely express them. The team leader then follows up the clues and rules them important or unimportant after evaluating the patient. This method has proven very effective for the prevention, early identification, and resolution of patients' problems.

These variations may not be applicable to every nursing care setting. However, every patient care unit can utilize a variety of conference methods that best meet its patient and staff needs. Flexibility of scheduling and timing, combined with good leadership and a sense of purpose, can result in significantly improved patient care.

Multidisciplinary Team Conferences. Care planning among multidisciplinary groups is another kind of conferencing that is critical to a coherent and coordinated plan of patient care. Frequently nurses, physicians, dietitians, physical therapists, and patients share and exchange information of care planning on all levels. The nursing care plan is an invaluable aid to the nurse who wishes to contribute specific, relevant information to a multidisciplinary conference. New information obtained out of these team conferences can be used to revise and update the nursing care plan.

The Conference Phone Call. A variation of the multidisciplinary team approach to care planning is the conference phone call. Nurses in community health settings, who frequently need to exchange information with several persons about a patient or family, can utilize the conference call much more extensively than they generally do at present. It is very costly to bring together professionals from many locations to discuss a patient. A conference call can accomplish the same purpose at a fraction of the cost. Nursing should assume more initiative in the use of telephone conferences.

Communicating Care-planning Data to Other Agencies and Services

Intraagency and Interagency Referrals. A referral is a verbal or written statement of a patient's problems and relevant background data which transfers all or a portion of the responsibility for that patient's care. The information is transmitted to an appropriate service or agency.

A referral is an integral part of the daily activities of community health nurses. They recognize its value and use it constantly. Nurses in other settings also find that referrals are a useful tool for transmitting care-planning information.

When patients are transferred from one place to another, or when additional health professional services are required, a summary of problems and reasons for referral is needed to facilitate the continuum of care.

A patient care plan can serve as the source of relevant information for referrals. In many cases an abstract of the unusual problems section of the patient care plan can provide the new service or agency with a clear perception of the patient's status and progress.

Communicating with Physicians. Discussing patient problems and care planning data with physicians is an activity of critical importance to the ultimate well-being of patients. Nurses and physicians, as colleagues, participate in an ongoing exchange of ideas and concerns. Nurses who deal with patients minute by minute, day after day, have important observations and data to offer. Physicians, with their clinical expertise and understanding of patients over a different time span and at a different professional-interpersonal level, have much to share with nursing.

Nursing's need to communicate effectively with physicians implies a responsibility for them to consider the matter thoughtfully. Frequently, the pressures of a care setting militate against effective dialogue. Nurses and physicians who exchange ideas in an environment of distraction are unlikely to reach any real understanding of each other's concerns. When a nurse needs well-considered assistance from the physician, she should provide the setting for an effective conference. In a hospital she can invite the physician to an office or conference room to discuss a particular subject relating to his patient. It is important that she abstract and summarize her main points in order most effectively to transmit her perceptions to the physician and to do so in an environment free from distraction. Thus the time and effort of both professionals is more likely to be well spent. A nurse's well-intentioned concern for the physician's time, however, need not result in poor communication.

Nurses in convalescent, home care, and community health settings most frequently communicate with physicians by telephone. Their skill in abstracting and summarizing information or questions can facilitate telephone conversations immeasurably. The mental process of problem identification outlined in this book offers nurses a method for concisely stating a patient's problems. Before picking up the phone, the nurse can briefly outline on paper the problems and observations she wishes to relate. This will help her transmit the message effectively to the physician and will maximize his willingness to respond thoughtfully.

Thoughtful, aggressive, dynamic efforts by nurses to create an environment for effective dialogue with physicians can ultimately result in more effective patient care.

Communicating with Paramedical and Administrative Services. As a professional group, nurses recognize the need to participate actively in patient care planning on a policy-making and administrative level. In every health care agency there are many disciplines associated with overall policy planning for patient care. Each discipline has its own expertise and data to contribute to the total effort. Nurses must convincingly express their unique concerns and recommendations when they help plan overall patient care strategies. When they are involved in group planning, whether with medical and paramedical personnel within an agency, with representatives of various agencies, or more comprehensively with groups on the community, county, or state level, nurses need basic specific data to justify their ideas and recommendations.

The information that is documented on patient care plans can be abstracted, summarized, and analyzed through concurrent and retrospective audit processes. It then can be used as a source of concrete data to support the recommendations of nursing. When problems, expected outcomes, deadlines, nursing orders, and patients' responses are well documented via the problem-solving approach, successes, failures, and needs can be identified and clearly articulated to other disciplines and to higher levels of nursing administration. It is no longer necessary to resort to generalities and ambiguous statements about patients' problems and needs. Nurses on every level can present audit data as justification for recommending staff changes, personnel and care policy changes, job description changes, and organizational changes.

As they plan budgets for patient care, nursing directors are increasingly faced with the task of explaining patients' nursing needs to administrators and budget experts. Budget analysts are particularly oriented toward specific objectives and the methodologies for meeting them. When a nursing director has quality audit data at her disposal, she can more effectively communicate the rationale for her recommendations in language that is readily understood by administrators and budget analysts. As a result, more constructive and realistic budget allocations will be made for patient care services.

SUMMARY

To actually achieve high levels of quality, formal monitoring and evaluation systems are necessary. Concurrent and retrospective review methods are being developed and refined. A model for quality assurance has been set forth by the American Nurses' Association. It outlines the evaluation cycle and recommends how to implement and measure the structure, process, and outcome elements of nursing services.

Requisite to actualizing the benefits of quality assurance methods is the concept of accountability. There must be clear definition and delegation of accountability for all levels and processes of care. Accountability means responsibility and answerability for one's actions and personal responsibility for the outcomes of one's actions.

REFERENCES

1. ANA: Standards of Nursing Practice. Kansas City, American Nurses' Association, Commission on Nursing Services, 1973
2. ANA: A Plan for Implementation of the Standards of Nursing Practice. Kansas City, American Nurses' Association, 1976
3. Michnich M, Harris M, Willis L, Williams J: Ambulatory Care Evaluation. The ACE Project, School of Public Health, University of California. Los Angeles, Regents of the University of California, 1976, p 11
4. Mayers M, Norby L, Watson A: Quality Assurance for Patient Care: Nursing Perspectives. New York, Appleton-Century-Crofts, 1977
5. Ibid. p 17
6. Ibid. p 256
7. Michnich. Op cit. p 8
8. Mager R: Analyzing Performance Problems. Belmont Cal, Fearon Publishers, 1972
9. ANA: Op cit. 1976, p 21
10. Ibid. p 20
11. Mayers et al: Op cit. pp 14, 15
12. Manthey M: Primary nursing is alive and well in the hospital. Am J Nurs 73 [No 1]:83, 1973
13. Marram G, Flynn, K, Abaravich W, and Carey S: Cost Effectiveness of Primary and Team Nursing. Wakefield Mass, Contemporary Publishing, 1976
14. Ibid. pp 75, 76

BIBLIOGRAPHY

Accreditation Manual for Hospitals. Chicago, Joint Commission on Accreditation of Hospitals 1975

ANA: Standard of Nursing Practice. Kansas City, American Nurses' Association, Commission on Nursing Services, 1973

ANA: A Plan for Implementation of the Standards of Nursing Practice. Kansas City, American Nurses' Association, 1976

Aydelotte M: Identifying critical points in the process of care and nursing activities at these points. In Proceedings of Joint Institute, ANA, AHA: Quality Assurance for Nursing Care. Kansas City, 1973

Daeffler RJ: Patients' perceptions of care under team and primary nursing. J Nurs Admin 5[No 3]:20, 1975

Donabedian A: Evaluating the quality of medical care. Milbank Mem Fund Q 44:166 [Part 2], 1966

Douglass L: Review of Team Nursing. St. Louis, Mosby, 1973, p 2

Dyer E: Nurse Performance Description: Criteria, Predictors and Correlates. Salt Lake City, Univ Utah Press, 1967

Guidelines for Review of Nursing Care at the Local Level. US Dept of Health, Education, and Welfare, Bureau of Quality Assurance, 1974

Hemphill D: The relationship between research and evaluation studies. In Tyler RW (ed): Educational Evaluation: New Roles, New Means. Chicago, Univ Chicago Press, 1969, Part 2

Iowa Lutheran Medical Center: Quality assurance bedside audit. Des Moines Iowa

Maas M: Nursing autonomy and accountability in organized nursing services. Nurs Forum 12 [No 3]:237, 1973

Medicus/Nursing Care Systems: Nursing Audit/Quality Assurance Syllabus (notebook). Chicago, Medicus Systems, 1974

Methodology for Monitoring Quality of Nursing Care. Bethesda Md, US Dept of Health, Education, and Welfare, 1974

Ohio Nurses Association: The Patient's Rights to Nursing Care. Am J Nurs 75 [No 7]:1112, 1975

Payne D (ed): Curriculum Evaluation. Lexington Mass, Heath, 1974

Phaneuf MC: The Nursing Audit—Profile for Excellence. New York, Appleton-Century-Crofts, 1976

Procedure for Retrospective Patient Care Audit in Hospitals. Nursing Edition. Chicago, Joint Commission on Accreditation of Hospitals, 1973

Quest for Quality: A Self Evaluation Guide to Patient Care. New York, National League for Nursing, 1966

Riehl J, Roy C: Conceptual Modes for Nursing Practice. New York, Appleton-Century-Crofts, 1974

SCALE: A Quality Control Plan for Nursing Service. Ann Arbor, Univ Michigan, 1965

Scriven M: The methodology of evaluation. Perspectives of Curriculum Evaluation. AERA Monograph Series on Curriculum Evaluation No 1. Chicago, Rand McNally, 1967

Suchman E: Evaluation Research Principles and Practice in Public Service and Social Action Programs. New York, Russell Sage Foundation, 1967

Tate B: Test of a Nursing Performance Evaluation Instrument. New York, National League for Nursing, undated

Veterans' Administration: Nursing Care Quality Evaluation. VA Form 10-204663, 1969

Wandelt M, Stewart D: The Slater Nursing Competencies Rating Scale. New York, Appleton-Century-Crofts, 1975

Wandelt M, Ager J: Quality Patient Care Scales. New York, Appleton-Century-Crofts, 1974

Weiss CH: Evaluation Research. Englewood Cliffs NJ, Prentice-Hall, 1972

Index